Rochester Symposium on
Developmental Psychopathology

Volume 4

DEVELOPMENTAL PERSPECTIVES
ON DEPRESSION

Rochester Symposium on Developmental Psychopathology

Volume 4

DEVELOPMENTAL PERSPECTIVES ON DEPRESSION

EDITED BY

DANTE CICCHETTI & SHEREE L. TOTH

Mt. Hope Family Center
University of Rochester

UNIVERSITY OF ROCHESTER PRESS

First published 1992

University of Rochester Press
200 Administration Building, University of Rochester
Rochester, New York 14627, USA
and at PO Box 9, Woodbridge, Suffolk IP12 3DF, UK

ISBN 1 878822 16 0

Library of Congress Catalog Card Number: 92–18117

British Library Cataloguing-in-Publication Data
Developmental Perspectives on Depression.
– (Rochester Symposium on Developmental
Psychopathology Series, v.4, ISSN
1056–6511)
    I. Cicchetti, Dante II. Toth, Sheree L.
III. Series
616.85
ISBN 1–878822–16–0

Rochester Symposium on
Developmental Psychopathology
ISSN 1056–6511

This publication is printed on acid-free paper

Printed in the United States of America

Table of Contents

List of Contributors

LYN Y. ABRAMSON, Ph.D.
Department of Psychology, University of Wisconsin
Madison, WI 53706
JULES R. BEMPORAD, M.D.
Cornell University Medical Center, New York Hospital
White Plains, NY 10605
JULIE BOERGERS
Department of Psychology, University of Denver
Denver, CO 80208
SUSAN B. CAMPBELL, Ph.D.
Clinical Psychology Center, University of Pittsburgh
Pittsburgh, PA 15260
DANTE CICCHETTI, Ph.D.
Mt. Hope Family Center, University of Rochester
Rochester, NY 14608
JEFFREY F. COHN, Ph.D.
Clinical Psychology Center, University of Pittsburgh
Pittsburgh, PA 15260
PAMELA M. COLE, Ph.D.
Laboratory of Developmental Psychology
National Institute of Mental Health
Bethesda, MD 20892
PAUL F. COLLINS
Department of Psychology, University of Minnesota
Minneapolis, MN 55455
JAMES C. COYNE, Ph.D.
Institute for Social Research
University of Michigan
Ann Arbor, MI 48106
E. MARK CUMMINGS, Ph.D.
Department of Psychology, West Virginia University
Morgantown, WV 26506–6040
PATRICK T. DAVIES
Department of Psychology, West Virginia University
Morgantown, WV 26506–6040

RICHARD A. DEPUE, Ph.D.
    Department of Psychology, University of Minnesota
    Minneapolis, MN 55455
GERALDINE DOWNEY, Ph.D.
    Department of Psychology, Columbia University
    New York, NY 10025
CONSTANCE HAMMEN, Ph.D.
    Department of Psychology
    University of California at Los Angeles
    Los Angeles, CA 90024
KARLEN LYONS-RUTH, Ph.D.
    Department of Psychiatry
    The Cambridge Hospital at Harvard Medical School
    Cambridge, MA 02139
BARRY NURCOMBE, M.D.
    Division of Child and Adolescent Psychiatry,
    Vanderbilt University
    Nashville, TN 37203
STEVEN J. ROMANO, M.D.
    Cornell University Medical Center
    New York Hospital
    White Plains, NY 10605
DONNA T. ROSE, Ph.D.
    Department of Psychology, University of Wisconsin
    Madison, WI 53706
SHEREE L. TOTH. Ph.D.
    Mt. Hope Family Center, University of Rochester
    Rochester, NY 14608
CAROLYN ZAHN-WAXLER, Ph.D.
    Laboratory of Developmental Psychology
    National Institute of Mental Health
    Bethesda, MD 20892

ACKNOWLEDGEMENTS

We wish to acknowledge
the Prevention Research Branch of the
National Institute of Mental Health
(R01 MH45027–01A1),
the W.T. Grant Foundation,
the Smith-Richardson Foundation, Inc.,
and the Spunk Fund, Inc.

DEDICATION

This volume is dedicated to the memory of
Joaquim Puig-Antich.
Kim's pioneering theoretical
and research contributions greatly advanced
our understanding of
development and depression.
His loss to the field is great,
but his work lives on.

Preface

The contributors to this volume present theory and research relevant to a developmental psychopathology approach to depression. The application of this perspective to depression necessitates a consideration of those components that are inherent in this new field of study. In the lead chapter to *The Emergence of a Discipline*, Cicchetti (1989) describes the central tenets of developmental psychopathology. Specifically, the importance of recognizing the links between normal and abnormal developmental processes, an attention to the underlying mechanisms and processes that contribute to adaptive or maladaptive outcomes, and an understanding of developmental continuities and discontinuities all are integral to a developmental psychopathology approach (Cicchetti, 1984; Cicchetti & Toth, 1991a; Rutter, 1986a; Sroufe & Rutter, 1984). Additionally, the focus of inquiry for developmental psychopathology is by no means limited to children, but rather requires an understanding of ontogenesis across the lifespan (Cicchetti, 1990a; Rutter, 1986a; Zigler & Glick, 1986). Inquiries into developmental continuities and discontinuities and the emphasis on the interplay between normal and abnormal functioning expand the populations of interest for developmental psychopathology to include subjects drawn from normal, atypical, and high risk samples. Finally a developmental psychopathology perspective strives to bridge the historical separation between scientific research and clinical intervention.

In efforts to impart a developmental perspective to the area of childhood depression, an important volume, entitled *Depression in Young People: Developmental and Clinical Perspectives*, was published by Rutter, Izard, and Read (1986). In that volume, the developmental psychopathology of depression is addressed and issues are raised that continue to be relevant to our growing understanding of the etiology, course, and sequelae of depression across the lifespan (Cicchetti & Schneider-Rosen, 1986; Rutter, 1986b).

A developmental approach to depression requires that attention be directed to the general course of normal biological and psychological development as it relates to depression (Cicchetti, 1990b). In this regard, issues such as the processes by which emotion expression and experience unfold and the developmental transformations underlying children's understanding of emotions such as sadness, anger, guilt, and hopelessness must be examined (see, for example, Cicchetti & Schneider-Rosen, 1986; Harris, 1989; Zahn-Waxler & Kochanska, 1990). Developmental considerations have been especially relevant to the study of childhood depression because early controversy existed regarding the capacity of children to experience an actual depressive disorder prior to the attainment of a requisite level of developmental maturity (Lefkowitz & Burton, 1978; Nurcombe, this volume; Rie, 1966). In many ways, the questions emanating from discussions related to childhood depression caused psychopathologists to examine the appropriateness of relying on downward extensions of adult criteria to the assessment of disorders of childhood and forced theoreticians, researchers, and clinicians to become increasingly aware of developmentally-specific manifestations of disorder.

The historical reliance of developmentalists on normative ontogenetic progressions also has implications for a developmental psychopathology of depression. Although group normative data are important, it is equally necessary to examine departures from the group mean. With respect to depression, questions regarding, for example, infant attachment classification and future psychopathology become important (see Cicchetti & Greenberg, 1991). Although many insecurely attached infants evidence psychopathology in later life, not all do (Cummings & Cicchetti, 1990). It is the individual differences question that becomes relevant for developmental psychopathology. What internal and/or situational factors may come into play that modify the course of individual development away from the expected group norm?

In addressing the importance of a lifespan approach to psychopathology, Rutter (1981) discusses the role that early experience plays in the etiology of future disorder. According to this formulation, early experience may result in a vulnerability to a depressive disorder through either direct or indirect mechanisms and the disorder may ultimately be precipitated by the individual's response to stress. Similar approaches have been articulated by Cicchetti and his colleagues, who have discussed potentiating and compensatory factors for the development of depression (Cicchetti & Aber, 1986; Cicchetti & Schneider-Rosen, 1986). Conceptualizations such as these underscore the complexities involved in understanding the course of development in relation to psychopathology.

In an article discussing developmental continuity, Sroufe and Jacobvitz (1989) examine four issues that must be resolved if the nature of coherence in individual development is to be understood adequately. These include: (1) developmental transformation; (2) branching developmental pathways; (3) increasing complexity of behavioral organization; and (4) multiple etiologies. Currently, little is known about the mechanisms through which genetic and environmental factors converge to delimit pathways to adaptation and maladaptation. The more simple and linear "main effect" models positing a direct pathway from biologic or environmental insult to psychopathology have been largely discarded. In their place, more sophisticated multi-factor causal models that seek to define varied pathways to health or psychopathology have been posited. However, due to their complexity, inclusion of multiple variables, the need for longitudinal follow-up, and the importance of recruiting appropriately large samples, the findings substantiating or challenging the utility of these models have been slow to emerge. Despite the difficulties inherent in conducting research in this area, a developmental psychopathology approach to depression must seek to incorporate these elements.

With these general aspects and goals of a developmental psychopathology focus in mind, more specific ways in which this perspective can enhance our understanding of depression can be undertaken. In fact, since the publication of *Depression in Young People* (Rutter, Izard, & Read, 1986), an increased recognition of the importance of including aspects of a developmental psychopathology approach into theories and research on depression has occurred. Questions related to the comorbidity of depression and aggression and the implications of this for examining multiple pathways to depression (Garber, Quiggle, Panak, & Dodge, 1991), the continuity of depressive symptomatology and disorders over development (Kovacs, Feinberg, Crouse-Novak, Paulauskas, & Finkelstein, 1984; Kovacs, Feinberg, Crouse-Novak, Paulauskas, Pollack, & Finkelstein, 1984), the developmental epidemiology of depression (Angold & Rutter, 1992), and the developmental neuropsychology of affective disorders (Davidson, 1991), are but a few of the areas that have been addressed by scholars who are applying principles of developmental psychopathology to depression.

Research such as this has laid the groundwork for the current volume, which is one of the few works on depression that has brought together research and theory pertinent to a developmental psychopathology perspective on depression across the lifespan. In accord with this approach, an evaluation of multiple intra- and extra-organismic factors (e.g., biological, individual, familial, societal), the role that they exert on the continuity of adaptation and maladaptation, their effect on the emergence of individual differences, and their influence on the complex pathways through which the same developmental outcome may be achieved must be undertaken. We believe that the contributors to the current volume demonstrate that such an approach is indeed possible, and that, when implemented, holds great promise for advancing our understanding of the mechanisms underlying depression.

The volume begins with a chapter by Barry Nurcombe, who addresses issues related to the developmental capacity of children to experience depressive disorders. The questions raised by Nurcombe hearken back to the early controversy over the validity of childhood depression and the appropriateness of viewing depression as a disorder of childhood. Although Nurcombe stresses that children suffer from emotional problems in which depressive mood is a prominent feature, he questions whether a categorical depressive disorder with a predictable genetic background, psychobiology, and natural history, and that is associated with a specific etiology and treatment response, exists in childhood. Nurcombe's chapter reminds us that premature closure on issues related to developmental considerations in childhood depression may be counter-productive in the absence of sufficient evidence.

In a chapter that integrates a developmental perspective on neurobiology and attachment across the lifespan, Paul F. Collins and Richard A. Depue discuss the behavioral facilitation system as forming the basis of a major component of human personality structure. After presenting data that support this hypothesized link, Collins and Depue discuss the implications of the system for conceptualizing affective disorders. This chapter epitomizes one of the goals of developmental psychopathology, namely the integration of multiple domains of functioning within an ontogenetic framework. Additionally, the articulation of the manner in which principles derived from normal psychobiology can inform and contribute to formulations regarding functioning in disordered populations provides a critical perspective that can facilitate the conduct of future work in this rich field of inquiry.

The importance of examining the course of development in populations considered to be at risk for psychopathology becomes clear in the chapter written by Jeffrey F. Cohn and Susan B. Campbell. In accord with the approach of Collins and Depue that builds upon a research base developed with nondisordered samples, Cohn and Campbell draw upon the seminal work that has been conducted with simulated depression in normal populations in their approach to exploring the effects of maternal depression on infants in clinical samples. After reviewing studies on the effects of maternal depressed affect on infants, these authors present their findings on the effects of maternal depression on infants. The approach that they employ with respect to sample selection begins to elucidate the varying perspectives that researchers use in their work with populations at risk for future psychopathology.

In their sample selection of depressed mothers, Cohn and Campbell sought to minimize the presence of risk factors other than depression so as to more clearly isolate the effects of depression per se on child development. In utilizing this approach, they conclude that the impact of maternal depression on children is reduced when related risk factors (i.e., poverty) are not present. The implications of these findings are significant with respect to both methodological and practical considerations and raise questions regarding how best to assess the effects of disorder on young children when related risk factors are typically present. Throughout the current volume, various approaches to this dilemma are presented and all possess merit for the conduct of investigations with depressed mothers. In order to begin to separate out the effects of single versus multiple risk factors, the utilization of similar developmental outcome measures in investigations that vary in sample composition with respect to the number of risk factors present will prove to be invaluable in answering questions regarding the effects of maternal depression on developmental outcome in offspring.

In a similar area of inquiry, yet with a very different sample, Karlen Lyons-Ruth reports her findings on a prospective longitudinal study of infants at risk due to the combined effects of poverty and maternal depressive symptoms. In contrast to the approach to minimize risk factors employed by the authors of the prior chapter, Lyons-Ruth explores the adaptation of children whose course of development is affected by maternal depression in conjunction with associated challengers. In accord with a developmental psychopathology focus, Lyons-Ruth's approach was spawned by prior research in normal development. In this chapter, she presents compelling findings on the interrelations among maternal depressive symptoms, disorganized attachment relationships in infancy, and future child adjustment. Consistent with emerging evidence on the continuity of adaptation or maladaptation, Lyons-Ruth found that assessments of maternal and child social-emotional functioning in infancy were predictive of later disordered behavior. In exploring the effects of risk factors, additive effects were found when both disorganized attachment relations and maternal psychosocial difficulties were present in infancy. In fact, in those cases the rate of aggressive child behavior evident during preschool doubled over that present when only maternal difficulties or child attachment insecurity was present. Lyons-Ruth also presents her findings on the positive effect of responsive relationship models provided through a program of intervention and discusses how new models of relationships were seen in parent-child relational patterns and, subsequently, in children's relationships with new social partners. In her use of a framework derived from normal developmental theory, her attention to continuity of adaptation and maladaptation, and her assessment of the effects of a program of intervention, Lyons-Ruth's work embodies many of the goals of a developmental psychopathology approach to a population at risk for developmental difficulties.

Pamela M. Cole and Carolyn Zahn-Waxler present a unique perspective on the relation between affective disorders and disruptive behavior during childhood. Like their colleagues in developmental psychopathology, Cole and Zahn-Waxler draw upon research and theory gleaned from normal populations and apply it to the area of affective disorders. In their chapter, Cole and Zahn-Waxler examine the underpinnings of disruptive behavior, explore the distinctness as well as overlap with traditional affective disorders, and identify developmental pathways that originate in early childhood and that lead to patterns of emotional dysregulation and stable disruptive behavior. The relation of disruptive behavior to affective disorders is especially interesting in view of the work being done on the comorbidity of aggression and depression during childhood and it relates to questions being asked regarding the possibility of various pathways leading to disorder that are frequently raised by developmental psychopathologists. These authors also strive to integrate an understanding of psychology and biology in their work, a goal very much in accord with developmental psychopathology's focus on multiple domains of development and the incorporation of an inter-disciplinary focus.

In moving from an exploration of parent-child functioning to a family systems perspective, James C. Coyne, Geraldine Downey, and Julie Boergers review the literature and present a model that articulates aspects of the relationship between depression and the family environment. These authors stress that depression affects the whole family system, as well as the broader ecology, and emphasize that it is the degree to which factors other than depression support or undermine the individual that determines the effects of depression. This perspective is consistent with that employed by other investigators in developmental psychopathology (Belsky, 1984; Cicchetti & Rizley, 1981) and underscores the importance of studying more than the depressed person and his or her child in order to fully understand the impact of depression on the developmental process. Methodological questions related to sample selection are again raised, as Coyne and his colleagues argue that having a depressed parent may be a marker for the presence of a family system that is characterized by adversity. These authors question whether the methodological quest for the minimization of risk factors may not alter the very nature of the disorder being investigated and advocate for "theory informed but phenomenon driven" research. According to Coyne and his colleagues, before any premature conclusions about the effects of depression on family members are drawn, the adequacy of the design being utilized must be determined.

In her own words, the author of the next chapter reflects someone who has "achieved" as well as had a developmental psychopathology perspective "thrust upon" her. Constance Hammen's roots emanate from the area of adult psychopathology, but her efforts to understand the effects of maternal psychopathology on children led her to incorporate a developmental focus into her work. In the course of this journey, Hammen's prior research on self-schemata and cognition has been integrated with attachment theory and the emergence of representational models (cf. Cummings & Cicchetti, 1990). Hammen concurs with the authors of the previous chapter in emphasizing the importance of understanding depression in the context of environmental, developmental, and historical processes and the need to view it as a dynamic process that alters people and their environments. In her description of research begun in the 1980s with depressed mothers, Hammen also grapples with the reality of multiple risk factors and presents models for isolating risk factors, as well as for exploring outcome when multiple risk factors are combined. In her study of depressed women and their children, Hammen found that some of the most fascinating findings emerged in relation to the interplay that occurred among multiple variables. The work of Hammen, as well as that of Collins and Depue and of Rose and Abramson, all represent the richness that can be brought to understanding developmental processes when traditionally non-developmental theorists incorporate aspects of a developmental psychopathology perspective into their thinking.

In their chapter on parental depression, family functioning, and child adjustment, E. Mark Cummings and Patrick T. Davies examine interactional and interpersonal mechanisms associated with the development of psychopathology in families having a depressed parent. They present a process-oriented framework for the investigation of the relations among parental depression, marital discord, and child adjustment problems. Like the authors of the prior two chapters, the importance of considering aspects of the broader family environment is emphasized. Additionally, Cummings and Davies draw upon a solid base of research with non-disordered populations and demonstrate the mutually enriching interplay that can occur between theories of development regarding normal and abnormal populations.

Similar to Hammen, the authors of the next chapter draw upon a rich body of work in the area of adult psychopathology in their application of helplessness and hopelessness theory to the emergence of depression. Donna T. Rose and Lyn Y. Abramson present a compelling discussion of developmental predictors of cognitive style in adult depressives. In their chapter, Rose and Abramson provide a theoretical background, review research regarding the heterogeneity of cognitive styles among depressives, and note links among aversive developmental events, cognitive style, and depression. Research that supports the proposed model for the development of negative cognitive styles in adults who have suffered trauma during childhood also is presented. After suggesting links among traumatic developmental events, cognitive style in adulthood, and adult depression, these authors discuss treatment implications of their findings.

The volume concludes with a chapter by Jules R. Bemporad and Steven J. Romano that comprehensively reviews the literature on childhood experience and vulnerability for depression. Specifically, Bemporad and Romano discuss studies that implicate the role of child maltreatment in the emergence of adult depression. These findings are interpreted as reflecting the creation of self-schema as the developmental link between child maltreatment and later depression. According to these authors, representational models of attachment figures and the self play a role in the development of depression.

This hypothesized link is supported in a cross-sectional study conducted by Toth, Todd Manly, and Cicchetti (1992), who provide evidence based on knowledge derived from the developmental sequelae of maltreatment that suggests that physically abused children are depressed due to the presence of poor representational models of attachment figures and of the self in relation to others. The fact that this link was not found to be present in neglected children suggests that different pathways to maladaptation may be present in children who have experienced different subtypes of maltreatment and emphasizes the importance of conducting prospective longitudinal studies that follow maltreated children who develop depression as well as those who manifest other types of psychopathology or who evidence adaptive outcomes. The review of Bemporad and Romano raises interesting questions regarding multiple pathways to adaptation and maladaptation that await the conduct of future prospective studies couched within a developmental psychopathology perspective.

In its entirety, *Developmental Perspectives on Depression* serves as a state of the art volume on the developmental psychopathology of depression. The authors address significant aspects inherent in a developmental psychopathology approach, including issues related to continuity of functioning, the exploration of multiple pathways to disorder and adaptive outcome, the reciprocity that can so richly occur between work conducted with normal and abnormal populations, and the importance of assessing multiple domains of functioning within an inter-disciplinary perspective. In accord with the recommendations of Cicchetti and Toth (1991b), an exciting aspect of this volume relates to the incorporation of a developmental psychopathology approach into the work of some scholars who have not traditionally explored the implications of their research from a developmental perspective. Commensurate with the goals of developmental psychopathology, an integration of theoretical, empirical, and clinical considerations can be found throughout this volume. The contributors provide thought provoking data as well as lucid discussions of theoretical and methodological issues that will enhance our understanding of the mechanisms involved in depression and that will certainly further important work in the area of development and depression.

Dante Cicchetti
Sheree L. Toth

REFERENCES

Angold, A., & Rutter, M. (1992). Effects of age and pubertal status on depression in a large clinical sample. *Development and Psychopathology, 4,* 5–28.

Belsky, J. (1984). The determinants of parenting: A process model. *Child Development, 55,* 83–96.

Cicchetti, D. (1989). Developmental Psychopathology: Past, Present, and Future. In D. Cicchetti (ed.), *Rochester Symposium on Developmental Psychopathology, Vol.1: The emergence of a discipline* (pp. 1–12). Hillsdale, NJ: Erlbaum Associates.

Cicchetti, D. (1990a). A Historical Perspective on the Discipline of Developmental Psychopathology. In J. Rolf, A. Masten, D. Cicchetti, K. Nuechterlein, and S. Weintraub (eds.), *Risk and Protective Factors in the Development of Psychopathology* (pp. 2–28) New York: Cambridge University Press.

Cicchetti, D. (1990b). Developmental psychopathology and the prevention of serious mental disorders: Overdue detente and illustrations through the affective disorders. In P. Muehrer (ed.), *Conceptual Research Models for Prevention of Mental Disorders* (pp. 215–254). Rockville, MD: NIMH.

Cicchetti, D., & Aber, J.L. (1986). Early precursors to later depression: An organizational perspective. In L. Lipsitt & C. Rovee-Collier (eds.), *Advances in Infancy* (Vol. 4, pp. 87–137). Norwood, NJ: Ablex.

Cicchetti, D., & Greenberg, M. (eds.) (1991). Attachment and Developmental Psychopathology. *Development and Psychopathology, 3* (4).

Cicchetti, D., & Rizley, R. (1981). Developmental Perspectives on the Etiology, Intergenerational Transmission and Sequelae of Child Maltreatment. *New Directions for Child Development, 11,* 32–59.

Cicchetti, D., & Schneider-Rosen, K. (1986). An Organizational Approach to Childhood Depression. In M. Rutter, C. Izard, and P. Read (eds.), *Depression in Young People: Developmental and Clinical Perspectives* (pp. 77–134). New York: Guilford.

Cicchetti, D., & Toth, S.L., (eds.) (1991a). *Rochester Symposium on Developmental Psychopathology, Vol. 2: Internalizing and Externalizing Expressions of Dysfunction.* Hillsdale, NJ: Erlbaum Associates.

Cicchetti, D., & Toth S.L., (1991b). The making of a Developmental Psychopathologist. In J. Cantor, C. Spiker, and L. Lipsitt (eds.), *Child Behavior and Development: Training for Diversity* (pp. 34–72). Norwood, NJ: Ablex.

Cummings, E.M., & Cicchetti, D. (1990). Attachment, Depression, and the Transmission of Depression. In M.T. Greenberg, D. Cicchetti, and E.M. Cummings (eds.), *Attachment in the Preschool Years* (pp. 339–372). Chicago: University of Chicago Press.

Davidson, R.J. (1991). Cerebral asymmetry and affective disorders: A developmental perspective. In D. Cicchetti and S.L. Toth (eds.), *Rochester Symposium on Developmental Psychopathology: Internalizing and Externalizing expressions of dysfunction* (pp. 123–154). Hillsdale, NJ: Erlbaum Associates.

Garber, J., Quiggle, N.L., Panak, W., & Dodge, D.A. (1991). Aggression and depression in children: Comorbidity, specificity, and social cognitive processing. In D. Cicchetti and S.L. Toth (eds.) *Rochester Symposium on Developmental Psychopathology: Internalizing and Externalizing expression of dysfunction* (pp. 225–264). Hillsdale, NJ: Erlbaum Associates.

Harris, P.L., (1989). *Children and Emotion: The Development of Psychological Understanding.* New York: Basil Blackwell.

Kovacs, M., Feinberg, T.L., Crouse-Novak, M.A., Paulauskas, S.L., & Finkelstein, R. (1984). Depressive disorders in childhood. I. A longitudinal prospective study of characteristics and recovery. *Archives of General Psychiatry, 41,* 229–237.

Kovacs, M., Feinberg, T.L., Crouse-Novak, M.A., Paulauskas, S.L., Pollack, M., & Finkelstein, R. (1984). II. A longitudinal study of the risk for a subsequent major depression. *Archives of General Psychiatry, 41,* 643–649.

Lefkowitz, M.M., & Burton, N. (1978). Childhood depression: A critique of the concept. *Psychological Bulletin, 85,* 716–726.

Rie, H.E. (1966). Depression in childhood: A survey of some pertinent contributions. *Journal of the American Academy of Child Psychiatry, 5,* 653–685.

Rutter, M. (1981). Stress, coping, and development: Some issues and some questions. *Journal of Child Psychology and Child Psychiatry, 22,* 324–356.

Rutter, M. (1986a). Child psychiatry: The interface between clinical and developmental research. *Psychological Medicine, 16,* 151–160.

Rutter, M. (1986b). The developmental psychopathology of depression: Issues and perspectives. In M. Rutter, C.E. Izard, & P.B. Read (eds.). *Depression in young people: Developmental and Clinical Perspectives* (pp. 3–30). New York: Guilford Press.

Rutter, M., Izard, C.E., & Read, P.B. (eds.) (1986). *Depression in young people: Developmental and Clinical Perspectives.* New York: Guilford Press.

Sroufe, L.A., & Jacobvitz, D. (1989). Diverging pathways, developmental transformation, multiple etiologies and the problem of continuity in development. *Human Development, 32,* 196–203.

Sroufe, L.A., & Rutter, M. (1984). The domain of developmental psychopathology. *Child Development, 55,* 17–29.

Toth, S.L., Manly J., & Cicchetti, D. (1992). Child maltreatment and vulnerability to depression. *Development and Psychopathology, 4,* 97–112.

Zahn-Waxler, C., & Kochanska, G. (1990). The origins of guilt. In R. Thompson (ed.), *Nebraska Symposium on Motivation, Vol.36: Socioemotional development* (pp. 183–258). Lincoln: University of Nebraska Press.

Zigler, E., & Glick, M. (1986). *A developmental approach to adult psychopathology.* New York: Wiley.

I The Evolution and Validity of the Diagnosis of Major Depression in Childhood and Adolescence

BARRY NURCOMBE

Il n'y a pas de maladie, il n'y a que des malades.
Rousseau

Historical Introduction

Can melancholia be distinguished from misery in children and adolescents? This paper will discuss the evolution of the concept of depression in British and American psychiatry, and the recent application of nosological and biological ideas from adult psychiatry to children. A method of validating the diagnostic concept of depression will be described, and the evidence that the taxon of major depression is true will be weighed for adults and for children and adolescents.

Much of the paper concerns attempts to establish empirically that major depressive disorder is qualitatively distinct from other forms of depression. Of what concern is that? Is it no more than a matter of taste whether one thinks of psychopathology in dimensional or categorical terms? This paper contends that dimensionality reflects genetic and phenotypic heterogeneity, whereas categoricality is a manifestation of phenotypic homogeneity. Categoricality implies pathochemistry, pathophysiology or abnormal structure; qualitative distinctness, therefore, represents a prima facie case in favor of a biological substrate for the condition in question. We will return to this point later.

ACKNOWLEDGEMENTS. The author would like to express his appreciation to Drs Thomas Ban, Judy Garber, Peter Loosen, Bahr Weiss, Robert Begtrup, Lawrence Gaines, and Dante Cicchetti for their help in the preparation of this paper.

Psychoanalytic Theory

Parents and clinicians have been long aware that children can be sad. However, psychoanalysis fostered the idea that some infants and children exhibit a true depressive syndrome. Working on the basis of speculative elaborations derived from play therapy, Melanie Klein (1948, 1949) proposed that, during the second half of the first year, the normal infant fuses previously split good and bad part objects. Consequently, the infant's ambivalence toward the caregiver leads to a depressive position in which the child fears his rage will destroy the whole maternal object. From a different psychoanalytic perspective, Anna Freud and Dorothy Burlingham (1944) observed the emotional disturbance of children separated from their parents and evacuated to the country during the London Blitz. Noting that multiple fostering was especially unfavorable, Freud and Burlingham remarked that some aspects of the children's emotional disturbance resembled adult melancholia.

The shift of focus in psychoanalysis from the oedipus complex to pre-oedipal development, which was initiated by Klein, foreshadowed the contemporary interest in object relations, strongly influenced the research of Spitz and Wolf (1946) on anaclitic depression, and flowered into the work of Bowlby (1952, 1969, 1973, 1980) on attachment, separation and loss.

Thus, it became attractive to speculate that early bereavement or separation trauma might predispose children to adult depression. Brown and Harris (1978), for example, postulated that early loss creates a vulnerability to depression through the medium of a pessimistic, self-derogating mental set. Tennant & Bebbington (1978) and Richards and Dyson (1982) have disputed Brown and Harris's conclusions, provoking a continuing debate.

Descriptive Psychiatry

By the middle of the nineteenth century, psychiatry was a hotbed of controversy (Lehmann, 1971; Ban, 1990). Should psychiatric disorders be classified by symptoms or by cause? Was mental illness caused by brain disease or by psychological stress? Was psychosis unitary (Griesinger, 1861), or should it be divided into types (e.g., Esquirol, 1838)? At the turn of the century, "exogenous" psychoses (mental illnesses caused by physical disease) had been identified (Bonhoeffer, 1909). The remaining "structurally determined" psychoses were divided into "reactive" (i.e., arising from conflictual experience or life stress) and "endogenous" (i.e., arising from inner, "autochthonous" causes). Endogenous psychoses were linked to innate biological defects (Morel, 1857) and to constitutionally determined predispositions (Moebius, 1893).

In 1896, Kraepelin cleaved structural psychosis into manic-depressive insanity and dementia praecox. He did so on the basis of course and outcome as well as symptomatology. Within manic-depressive insanity, Kraepelin grouped several forms of mania, several forms of depression, and mixed states of agitation and depression. Consequently, influenced by European descriptive psychiatry, British psychiatrists postulated a condition known as "endogenous" depression in contrast to "reactive" or "neurotic" depression (Gillespie, 1929). Endogenous depression was thought to arise internally, and reactive depression to be precipitated by life stress. Furthermore, the two conditions were thought to differ in terms of symptomatology (e.g., endogenous depression was associated with greater depth of depressive affect, diurnal variation, psychomotor retardation, vegetative signs, and mood-congruent delusions). Following the mid-1930s, as will be described, a lively debate arose between those who thought that endogenous depression was qualitatively distinct from reactive depression, and those who believed that the two conditions merged, differing only in degree.

Although in Europe the concept of childhood depression had long been utilized (e.g., Kuhn, 1963), the psychoanalytic view was that, prior to adolescence, children's superego development was too immature to allow the pathological guilt regarded as the central characteristic of adult melancholia (Rochlin, 1959; Finch, 1960; Rie, 1966). If pathological guilt were indeed the cardinal feature of melancholia, as in the psychoanalytic view of that time, this observation was correct; depressed children do not exhibit the self-torturing guilt typical of severe depressives. It was not until the 1960's that the issue was reopened when Toolan (1962), Glaser (1967), and Malmquist (1971) described "depressive equivalents" and "masked depression". Masked depression was thought to be the expression of an underlying dysphoria in the form of symptomatic equivalents such as somatic complaints, anxiety, hyperactivity, or conduct problems; pathological guilt was, thus, displaced as the cardinal feature of depression. Subsequently, Cytryn & McKnew (1972) asserted the existence of mood disorder in children, and divided childhood depression into three impressionistic types: masked, acute, and chronic. Soon afterward, McConville, Boag and Purohit (1973) proposed three different types: helpless, guilty, and self-deprecatory.

Biological Psychiatry

During the 1970s, excited by biological advances in adult psychiatry, several researchers examined disturbed children in order to determine whether any of them exhibited clinical features similar to those of adult melancholia. Ling et al. (1970), Weinberg et al. (1973), Cytryn and McKnew (1972), Poznanski and Zrull (1970), and Kovacs (1985) were pioneers in the adaptation of adult diagnostic criteria to child rating scales, while Puig-Antich & Chambers (1978), Herjanic and Campbell (1977), Hodges et al. (1982), Kovacs (1982), and Costello et al. (1982) introduced structured interviews designed to elicit children's psychopathology in a standard manner.

In a landmark study involving the use of a structured interview based on adult RDC criteria, Carlson and Cantwell (1980) found that children and adolescents could be identified as suffering from major depression. In other words, they demonstrated that depressive mood and vegetative signs could be unmasked by systematic interviewing. Since that time, DSM–III–R (1987) has recommended the use of adult criteria to diagnose both major depression and dysthymia in childhood and adolescence. As a result, many contemporary child psychiatrists think the matter is closed, and that the clinical features of major depression are prevalent among psychiatrically disturbed children and adolescents.

During the last decade, research into childhood depression has burgeoned, particularly with regard to its epidemiology (e.g., Kashani & Simonds, 1979; Kashani et al., 1983) and biochemistry (Puig-Antich, 1986). Child psychiatrists frequently diagnose depressive conditions, confidently distinguish major depression from dysthymia, and freely prescribe antidepressant drugs. This paper concerns the appropriateness of their doing so — the validity of distinguishing melancholia from misery in adults, in adolescents, and in children. Before doing so, however, it would be helpful to clarify several terms whose meaning has transmuted during the past one hundred years.

The Clinical Features of Depression

During the first half of this century, psychiatrists delineated melancholia, an especially severe form of endogenous depression characterized by a sadness blacker than mere misery, together with suicidality, impairment of appetitive functions, disturbed sleep, diurnal variation, and mood-congruent hallucinations and delusions. Melancholic patients were described as "agitated" or "retarded" in accordance with their psychomotor activity. The term "psychotic depression" was applied, rather loosely, to melancholia associated with hallucinations, delusions or suicidality. Because melancholia seemed to arise spontaneously, as described before, it was often termed "endogenous", in contrast to those depressions which appeared to be reactive to environmental stress. By the middle of this century, the association between suicidal depression, vegetative signs, and diurnal variation strongly suggested a biological etiology to many researchers. However, recent work has demonstrated that endogenous depression is often preceded by stress (Finlay-Jones, & Brown, 1981); consequently, the term "endogenous" has been largely discarded.

During the 1960s, both the discovery of lithium and family pedigree research allowed bipolar manic-depressive disorder to be separated from other affective disorders. The concept of polarity was taken, not altogether faithfully, from Leonhard's (1957) classificatory scheme. The term "unipolar depression" is currently used to contrast with "bipolar depression" which occurs in a cyclical bipolar disorder. According to DSM–III–R, a bipolar depressive episode is symptomatically indistinguishable from unipolar depression and can be diagnosed only if it is associated with mania in subsequent or preceding episodes. Dunner, Gershon and Goodwin (1976) have distinguished two forms of bipolar disorder. Bipolar I disorder is characterized by manic and depressive episodes, and bipolar II disorder by hypomanic and depressive episodes.

In DSM–III–R, endogenous depression has transmuted into the category of major depression. Major depression is defined by at least two weeks of depressed mood, anhedonia, weight change, sleep disturbance, psychomotor agitation or retardation, anergia, feelings of worthlessness, impaired concentration, and suicidality. The melancholic type of major depression is characterized by an even greater depth of depression, together with severe anhedonia, retardation or agitation, weight loss, and diurnal variation. Reactive, non-endogenous, neurotic depression has been re-designated "dysthymia". This term was taken from Kahlbaum (1863) who used it to describe a low mood of insidious onset, protracted duration, and non-episodic course. In DSM–III–R, dysthymia is defined by long-standing depressed mood, disturbance of appetite and sleep, impairment of energy and concentration, self-depreciation and feelings of helplessness. The only concession DSM–III–R makes to children is to substitute irritability for depression in both major depression and dysthymia, and, in the case of dysthymia, to reduce the time requirement from two years to one.

Are the symptoms of adult depression modified in childhood, or can most of them be identified? Cytryn, McKnew and Bunney (1980) concluded that the form and content of childhood depression are substantially similar to the form and content of adult depression. Carlson and Kashani (1988) found that, although age modified symptom frequency, it did not affect basic phenomenology: depressed mood, impaired concentration, insomnia, and suicidal ideation occurred with similar frequency at all ages, whereas anhedonia, diurnal variation, hopelessness, psychomotor retardation, delusions, depressed appearance, low self esteem, and somatic complaints were less common in childhood. Ryan et al. (1987) found no significant difference between children and adolescents in most symptoms; prepubertal children exhibited more somatic complaints, agitation, anxiety, phobias, and hallucinations, whereas adolescents evinced more anhedonia, hopelessness, hypersomnia, weight change, and drug usage. The acuity of suicidality was similar at the two levels. Developmental changes were thought to have little effect.

The common association of childhood depression with conduct disorder and separation anxiety disorder (Puig-Antich, 1982) is less apparent in adulthood. Rutter, Tizard and Whitmore (1970) demonstrated that, in the general population, the prevalence of depressive feelings increases markedly from childhood to adolescence. In clinic populations, depressed prepubertal boys outnumber girls two to one; whereas after puberty girls outnumber boys to the same degree (Pearce, 1978). In the general adult population, unipolar major depression can occur at any age but does not usually emerge until middle age. These age-related epidemiological changes are not explicable on the basis of a simple continuity between childhood and adult major depression.

Studies which apply adult depression criteria to children via structured interview or rating scale run the risk of several pitfalls. Many unhappy children are polysymptomatic; a restricted interview or scale may be identifying a spurious syndrome from a much larger set of signs and symptoms, particularly when the instrument is structured according to a particular condition such as depression. Clinicians affected by confirmatory bias may unwittingly suggest symptoms to patients, or endorse symptoms and signs which are dubious or marginal; and the halo effect can cause a clinician to detect other features of a favored syndrome once a cardinal feature has been elicited. Thus there is a danger that square pegs will be jammed into round pigeon holes. Moreover, Kovacs (1986) has described several metacognitive and semantic problems which plague the use of structured interviews with prepubertal children. For example, younger children do not tend to see themselves as patients: they may not appreciate that the clinician-patient relationship has a diagnostic purpose, or that the clinician is a helper. Younger children lack the introspective, relational, self-monitoring competence required to report affective symptoms reliably, and do not understand the concept that internal emotion can be expressed in behavior. Though able to label emotions correctly, younger children may be unable to separate them from external events; while temporal order and correct timing are not attained until preadolescence. All these problems are magnified when a miserable, angry, mistrustful, distracted, confused child is dislocated from home, taken to an unfamiliar office or hospital, and confronted by an inquisitive stranger who launches into an interminable, apparently irrelevant, interrogation. It is not surprising that the test-retest reliability of some structured interviews has been wrecked when, on retesting, subjects discover that they can deny trigger symptoms and spare themselves a tedious inquisition.

What does it matter whether depression is regarded as a symptom, a syndrome, or a disorder? The question is more than mere pedantic quibbling. A categorically distinct disorder is more likely to have a homogenous pathochemistry or pathophysiology. On the other hand, a continuously distributed dimensional syndrome is probably either heterogeneous or the outcome of variable mix of polygenic inheritance, temperamental vulnerability, stress reactions, and coping styles. Dimensional syndromes imply heterogeneity of etiology or expression. Categorical disorders may have more than one etiology, but they imply a medical model of disease expressed through the final common pathway of a specifiable biological dysfunction, a biological dysfunction which is the end result of pathochemistry, pathophysiology or structural abnormality, and which is constituted by distinctive clinical patterns arising from derangements of particular biological systems.

According to Kendell (1976), categorical distinctiveness indicates a natural boundary, point of rarity, or discontinuity between the disorder in question and other syndromes or disorders. If there were a boundary between major depression and dysthymia, for example, then patients with features of both conditions should be fewer than those with either. In other words, the blacks and whites should outnumber the grays. We shall return to this matter at several points during the forthcoming discussion.

Definitions

The term "depression" has been used in several different ways:

1. To refer to an *affect* or *mood*, a momentary or more enduring feeling state.
2. To refer to a *symptom* or *sign*, a subjective or objective mood recognized as abnormal in severity or quality.
3. To refer to a *dynamic*, a complex of conscious or unconscious ideas and feelings in response to actual or symbolic loss.
4. To refer to a *syndrome*, a constellation of symptoms and signs dominated by pervasively depressed mood.
5. To refer to a *disorder*, a depressive syndrome which defines a qualitatively distinct group of patients.
6. To refer to a *disease*, a depressive disorder that has been linked to a specific genetic, biochemical, physiological or structural abnormality.

Note particularly the difference between *syndrome*, *disorder*, and *disease*. Admittedly, the above definitions are, to some extent, idiosyncratic; many clinicians use these terms interchangeably. However, in view of the theoretical importance of differentiating the three concepts, they will be kept apart in the rest of this paper.

The abiding question has been whether major depression is qualitatively distinct from other depressive conditions or whether it merges continuously with them. As discussed before, the definition of a true categorical disorder provides a prima facie case for a biomedical disease model. This paper will first summarize the evidence for a categorical major depressive disorder in adulthood, and then consider in detail the validity of that diagnosis in children and adolescents.

Validating a Diagnostic Disorder

Taken together, the following ideal criteria support the validity of categorizing a syndrome as a disorder:

1. *Natural history.* Patients exhibiting the syndrome should have a characteristic clinical course, with a predictable onset, symptomatic configuration and outcome.
2. *Psychobiological markers.* The syndrome should be associated with paraclinical markers of pathochemistry, pathophysiology, or structural abnormality.

A *state marker* is an indication of active disorder; a *trait marker* indicates a predisposition to, or a residuum of, the putative disorder.

3. *Genetic studies.* If the syndrome has a genetic basis, it should be associated with a characteristic family pedigree, MZ-DZ twin divergence, and adoption pattern. Ultimately, it should be traceable to a defective chromosome or chromosomes.

4. *Construct validity.* The clinical syndrome upon which the disorder is based should be empirically isolable by multivariate analysis of the symptom patterns of diverse patients. The syndrome thus isolated should then be shown to characterize a qualitatively distinct group of people who exhibit the characteristic natural history, psychobiological markers, and genetic pattern described above.

5. *Response to treatment.* Patients with the disorder should respond predictably to specific treatment aimed at etiological factors.

Validating Major Depression in Adulthood

Natural History

Unipolar major depression has the following natural history:

1. It most often begins in middle life (Perris, 1966).
2. The average patient has three to five episodes (Perris, 1966).
3. The frequency of episodes increases as a function of previous episodes (Zis, Grof, & Goodwin, 1979; Zis & Goodwin, 1979; Grof, Angst, & Haimes, 1974; Cutler & Post, 1982).
4. Psychosocial stressors become less apparent with subsequent episodes (Zis & Goodwin, 1979).
5. Episodes in later life are more precipitous and severe (Cutler & Post, 1982).
6. Untreated episodes last seven to fourteen months, although 20% last longer than two years (Perris, 1966).
7. Before electroconvulsive therapy or drug treatment, the suicide rate in major depression was 15–30% (Tsuang, 1978).

No clear natural history has been defined for dysthymia; for, as we shall see, it is almost certainly heterogeneous.

Response to Treatment

Somatic therapies are required to relieve melancholia; psychosocial therapies are ineffective unless the depressive mood can be cleared. Akiskal (1986) summarizes numerous controlled studies as follows: electroconvulsive treatment aborts 90% of melancholic episodes; heterocyclic antidepressant drugs are effective in about 70%. If despite adequate blood level the patient does not respond to medication, antidepressant drugs may be augmented with lithium carbonate, thyroid hormone or psychostimulants. Dysthymic patients were thought to respond to antidepressants in a less predictable manner; however, recent studies have cast doubt upon this belief (Beukert, 1990).

Psychobiological Markers

Neurochemistry. Gold, Goodwin and Chrousos (1988) have reviewed the substantial amount of research into the biological markers of depression. The most consistent finding in major depression, and particularly in melancholia, is a hypersecretion of cortisol. The high blood levels of cortisol do not exhibit the diurnal rhythm normally observed, and are not suppressed, as in normal subjects, by the injection of the synthetic corticosteroid dexamethasone. Other biochemical findings have been less strongly corroborated; for example, diminished somatostatin and arginine vasopressin, a blunted response of growth hormone to clonidine or to insulin-induced hypoglycemia, and an attenuated response of thyroid-stimulating hormone (TSH) to thyrotropin-releasing hormone (TRH).

The hypercortisolism of major depression results from hypersecretion of corticotropin-releasing hormone (CRH). CRH secretion potentiates and is potentiated by the secretion of norepinephrine from the locus ceruleus. Gold, Goodwin and Chrousos hypothesize that stressors normally cause the release of CRH and norepinephrine, with consequent effect on both behavioral adaptation (via the hypothalamus, limbic system and neocortex) and peripheral adaptation (via the internal secretion of glucocorticoids and catecholamines). The animal is thus prepared for fight or flight. Circulating glucocorticoids feed back to restrain CRH and norepinephrine secretion, possibly via hippocampal receptor neurones. It is postulated that melancholia is a chronic, generalized stress response that has escaped counter-regulation by glucocorticoids.

Circadian Rhythms. Major depression is associated with an alteration of circadian rhythms. The abnormal sleep of melancholic patients is demonstrated by polysomnographic studies which reveal shortened REM latency, redistribution of REM sleep to the first half of the night, prolonged sleep latency, increased wakefulness, decreased arousal threshold, and early morning waking. It has been suggested that major depression is associated with an advance of the "strong" circadian oscillator in relation to the "weak" circadian oscillator, an advance that alters the timing of REM sleep (Wehr & Goodwin, 1981).

In short, major depression is associated with a profound dysregulation of central neuroendocrine and circadian functioning.

Genetic Studies

Affective illness congregates in the family trees of depressed patients. Although the rate of bipolar illness is highest in the relatives of bipolar depressives, it is still higher in the relatives of unipolar depressives than it is in the relatives of normals. In general, unipolar depression is five to ten times more common than bipolar illness in the relatives of unipolar depressives (see review by Rice & McGuffin, 1986). However, unipolar and bipolar depressive disorder may not be genetically distinct. Gershon et al. (1976) and Bertelsen, Hawald and Hauge (1977) found that 54% of MZ twins are concordant for unipolar depression, compared to 24% of DZ twins. Up to this point, all studies of twins reared apart concerned mixed bipolar-unipolar probands. No convincing evidence has been gathered of a genetic difference between major depression and dysthymia.

Attempts to associate depressive disorder with a particular gene locus have concentrated primarily on bipolar disorder. Bipolar disorder has been associated theoretically with an autosomal dominant gene on the X-chromosome (Slater, 1936), a red-green color blindness gene on the long arm of the X chromosome (Winokur & Tanna, 1969), the blood group "X" on the short arm of the X chromosome (Mendlewicz, Fleiss, & Fieve, 1972), a dominant gene on the short arm of chromosome 2 (Egeland et al., 1987), and a gene linked to the HLA–haplotype on chromosome 6 (Mathysse & Kidd, 1981). The true situation remains unclear.

Construct Validity

Despite the natural preference of clinicians for categorical systems such as DSM–III, empirical evidence for the categorically distinct nature of major depression has accrued only during the last thirty years. The following statistical techniques have been employed to investigate this matter (Trull, Widiger and Guthrie, 1990):

1. Principal component analysis
2. Cluster analysis
3. Bimodality analysis
4. Admixture analysis
5. Maximum covariance analysis

Principal component analysis (PCA) can validate a factorial syndrome, but it is not helpful in determining whether the syndrome is categorically distinctive, since all subjects score on all the factors derived. PCA serves best to isolate factors which can then be used as the basis for cluster or bimodality analysis.

Cluster analysis sorts out homogeneous, categorical subgroups on the basis of a measure of similarity such as a factor score. However, it is uncertain which of the numerous techniques of cluster analysis should be employed; nor is it clear how to determine the correct number of clusters. Grove and Andreason (1986) and Meehl (1979) suggest that cluster analysis should be used for hypothesis-testing rather than exploratory purposes.

Bimodality analysis (e.g. Wainer, 1978; Lord, 1958; Hasselblad, 1966) tests for a gap or gaps in the distribution of scores on a factor. However, bimodality emerges only if there is little overlap between two distributions; furthermore, Grayson (1987) asserts that, in some circumstances, bimodality can be exhibited by dimensional variables. Admixture analysis examines the distribution of canonical coefficient scores derived from discriminant function analysis in order to determine whether a distribution is best explained by one or more components. However, discriminant function analysis requires a prior diagnostic categorization, thus potentially introducing a circular logic. Maximum covariance analysis (MAXCOV) (Meehl, 1973), a form of latent class analysis, utilizes the concept that the covariance between two signs of a latent class variable will be minimized in homogeneous groups and maximized in mixed groups. Up to this point, principle components analysis, bimodality analysis, and cluster analysis have been the predominant techniques used in the search for a taxon of major depression.

Following World War II, the debate between the London and Newcastle schools of British psychiatry became more intense. At the Maudsley Hospital, Lewis (1934) and Curran (1937), had contended that neurotic and endogenous depression were merely arbitrary divisions of a continuous dimension, a view cautiously supported on empirical grounds by Kendell & Gourlay (1970). On the other hand, in a series of factor analytic studies of depressed patients at Newcastle-on-Tyne and Sydney, Kiloh and Garside (1963) and Kiloh et al. (1972) repeatedly extracted a bipolar factor contrasting "endogenous" with "neurotic" depression. When the distribution of patients along the bipolar factor was plotted, it tended to be bimodal. Subsequent cluster analyses of mixed samples (e.g., Pilowsky et al., 1969; Everitt et al., 1971; Paykel, 1971; Matussek et al., 1982; Grove et al., 1987) have repeatedly identified an "endogenous" subgroup which is distinct from other depressives. On the other hand, "neurotic depression" has repeatedly decomposed into different subtypes that collectively form a continuous distribution. Kiloh and Garside (1977) have suggested that the diagnosis of neurotic depression (i.e., dysthymia) is a by-product of clinicians' obsession with major depression, and that dysthymia represents a ragbag of spurious singularity. Others (e.g., Mullaney, 1984; Parker et al., 1990) have suggested that the so-called "neurotic depression" pole of the bipolar factor is composed of anxiety symptoms and coping style rather than depression per se.

In brief, multivariate analysis has repeatedly identified in adults a major depressive syndrome and category from mixed depressive samples; however, a pure category of neurotic depression or dysthymia has not been validated, and is almost certainly an artefact.

Validating Major Depression in Children and Adolescents

Natural History

Three studies have addressed the outcome of depression in childhood and adolescence. Zeitlin (1972, 1985) compared people who had been treated at the Maudsley Hospital both as children and as adults, with a sample who had attended only as children, and a sample treated only as adults. Of those depressed adults who had been treated as children, only a few had depressive conditions when younger. Of those children regarded as depressed, only a few were subsequently diagnosed as depressed in adulthood. However, among the small number of subjects who were depressed on both occasions, there was a clear continuity in the clinical picture (even though many of these children had not been originally labelled as depressed). Rutter (1986) noted that it is impossible to determine from this study whether depressive disorder should be diagnosed regardless of its associated symptomatology, or whether depression is best considered a response to stress rather than an illness. To complicate matters, one might add that either explanation could be valid, depending upon the child in question.

Kovacs et al. (1984 a, b) conducted a five-year followup of children diagnosed as having the three conditions: major depression, dysthymia, and adjustment disorder with depressed mood. Children with major depression and adjustment disorder recovered more quickly than those with dysthymia. Subsequent major depression was virtually restricted to those who had had major depression or dysthymia when younger, and occurred in about 70% of those who had. As Rutter (1986) points out, however, this study is flawed by a failure to ensure blind evaluation at followup. Garber et al. (1988) found that 100% of a sample of depressed adolescent inpatients had a subsequent depression over the next eight years. Kovacs et al. (1984b) found that 70% of child and adolescent major depressives had had a further major depression within five years.

Harrington et al. (1990) employed an operational definition of depression when they located from existing psychiatric records eighty child and adolescent depressives and eighty matched controls. Subjects were located an average of eighteen years after initial contact, using evaluators blind to the original diagnosis. There was a 58% incidence at followup of adult depression of any type, and a 35% incidence of major depression. Compared to the controls, the depressed group were five times more likely to exhibit any form of depression over twenty-one years of age, and seven times more likely as adults to suffer from major depression. It should be noted that the majority of the youthful depressives who exhibited major depression in adulthood were adolescent at the time of initial diagnosis.

Response to Treatment

Despite the enthusiasm with which antidepressant drugs are prescribed today, there have been only four controlled studies of their efficacy in children and adolescents. Puig-Antich et al. (1987) and Geller et al. (1989) found that imipramine and nortriptyline failed to surpass placebo in the treatment of prepubertal major depression; while Kramer and Feiguine (1981) and Geller (1989) found amitriptyline and nortriptyline to be no better than placebo in the treatment of adolescent depression. Thus far, no controlled study of antidepressant medication has demonstrated a significant experimental effect; indeed, placebo effects have been very impressive, an observation that indicates the need for skepticism about the results of uncontrolled drug trials. Nevertheless, despite these negative studies, no definite conclusion can be drawn. Further research is required.

Psychobiological Markers

Puig-Antich et al. (1981, 1984) found that, compared to dysthymic and nondepressed controls, a small group of prepubertal children with major depression secreted less growth hormone in response to insulin-induced hypoglycemia, and more growth hormone while asleep. In prepubertal major depressives, no evidence has been found for a blunting of the response of thyroid-stimulating hormone to thyrotropic-releasing hormone (Wagner et al., 1991). Cavallo et al. (1987) found lower nocturnal plasma levels of melatonin in a small sample of major depressive children compared to short-statured controls. After promising earlier studies (Puig-Antich et al., 1979; Puig-Antich, 1983), Puig-Antich et al. (1989) and Doherty et al. (1986) found no evidence of hypercortisolism when children with major depression were compared with non-affective psychiatric controls. However, Weller et al. (1985) has found evidence for hypercortisolism in a sample of hospitalized prepubertal major depressives.

Studies of dexamethasone suppression in childhood depression have been reviewed by Casat et al. (1989). The results have been contradictory; the specificity of the test has been questioned, and the sensitivity has varied between 40% and 60%.

Puig-Antich et al. (1982) and Young et al. (1982) found that the polysomnographic records of prepubertal major depressives did not reveal the decreased REM latency, decreased slow wave sleep, increased REM density, decreased sleep efficiency, or abnormal REM distribution that characterize adult depressives, and that the sleep architecture of depressed children did not differ from that of normal children. A recent study by Elmslie et al. (1990), however, has detected longer sleep latency, shorter REM latency, more individual short REM latency intervals, and a greater amount of REM sleep, in prepubertal major depressives compared to normal controls. Lahmeyer et al. (1983) and Goetz et al. (1987) found changes in the sleep patterns of depressed adolescents, but their results were not consistent.

In summary, psychobiological research into childhood and adolescent depression has yielded inconsistent findings. However, since too little is known concerning the effect of normal developmental neuroendocrine changes on the functions in question, these studies should be regarded as preliminary.

Genetic Studies

Puig-Antich et al. (1989) conducted a controlled study of the family history of prepubertal major depressives, non-affective psychiatric controls, and normals. Compared with major depression in later life, the diagnosis of major depression before twenty years of age was associated with an increased rate of major depression in first-degree relatives. Depressive children had significantly higher rates of major depression, alcoholism, and other diagnoses in first-degree and second-degree relatives. Puig-Antich has suggested that familial alcoholism potentiates prepubertal depression in genetically vulnerable children, that the search for a "pure" major depression in childhood might be futile, and that major depression allied to conduct disorder might be a non-genetic phenocopy of major depression. No twin or adoption studies have been undertaken with prepubertal or adolescent depressives.

Construct Validity

Multivariate Analysis. The results of multivariate analyses of child and adolescent symptomatology have been discussed by Achenbach and Edelbrock (1978), Dreger (1982), and Quay (1986). Quay reviewed 61 factor analyses of behavior ratings, case history studies, peer ratings, and self-reports in samples of both sexes from 3 to 18 years of age, derived from school, special classes, delinquency institutions, clinics and hospitals. The commonest factors isolated corresponded to *undersocialized aggression, socialized conduct problems, attention-deficit, mixed dysphoria, schizoid withdrawal* and *social ineptness*. The typical elements of the mixed dysphoria factor were, as follows: anxious, shy, depressed, sensitive, feeling worthless, self conscious, lacking in confidence, confused, weepy, aloof, and worrying. This factor appears to be an amalgam of anxiety, emotionality, sadness, and shyness. Of all the factors isolated, it is the closest to depression; but it is muddy at best.

Working from a large outpatient sample, Achenbach and Edelbrock (1983) isolated only a mixed *depressed-withdrawal-delinquent* factor for adolescent girls, and no depressive factor for adolescent boys; however, the following "depressive" factor was isolated from prepubertal boys: feeling worthless, guilty, needing to be perfect, feeling unloved, worrying, depressed, fearing own impulses, suicidal talk, and lonely. This factor is similar to the mixed dysphoria factor already described.

Lessing et al. (1981) isolated a depressive syndrome by cluster analyzing parents', teachers', and clinicians' ratings of a predominantly outpatient sample. Ryan et al. (1987) factor-analyzed K–SADS data elicited from prepubertal and adolescent patients attending an affective disorders clinic. The following factors were isolated: *depressed-anhedonia*; *negative cognition-suicide*; *anxious-insomniac-somatizing*; *appetite-weight*; and *irritable-agitated-antisocial*. The first factor was composed of the following items: anhedonia, fatigue, psychomotor retardation, withdrawal, depressed mood, hypersomnia, anorexia, decreased weight, and diurnal mood change.

In two related studies, Nurcombe et al. (1989) and Seifer et al. (1989) employed multivariate analysis to search for a depressive factor among adolescent and child outpatient and inpatient samples. In order to do so, they adapted the following ground rules from Ni Bhrolchain (1979):

1. Multivariate analysis should be used deductively, not to generate hypotheses.
2. Having stated a hypothesis every attempt should be made to maximize the chance of finding the reverse.
3. The data should be elicited by or from people with no preconception about the hypothesis. Omnibus instruments should be used in order to avoid the kind of circular logic that many structured interviews entail.
4. Principal components analysis is best used to identify syndromes. Cluster analysis lends itself to the isolation of categorical subgroups.
5. Syndromal factors and categorical clusters should be isolated from current symptomatology and mental status. Clusters can then be validated by associating them with other features such as family history, outcome, psychobiological characteristics, and response to treatment.
6. The results of one cluster analysis should be checked with a second clustering technique.

Data for the Nurcombe-Seifer analyses were derived from parental Child Behavior Checklists on 126 adolescent outpatients, 216 adolescent inpatients, 193 child outpatients, and 91 child inpatients. Principal components analysis of adolescent outpatients did not identify a convincing depressive factor. However, the analysis of adolescent inpatients yielded three factors: *conduct problems*, *depression*, and *social ineptness*. The depression factor was not bimodal in distribution. Table 1 lists the items that loaded most heavily on the depression factor.

Two separate hierarchical cluster analyses were then performed on Z-scaled factor scores. Both analyses isolated a depression cluster containing 11–15% of the sample. The cluster was validated against MMPI and CDI scores, but not against clinical diagnosis, suggesting a trend toward an overdiagnosis of depressive disorder by hospital clinicians. A similar multivariate analysis of 284 six- to twelve-year-old inpatients and outpatients extracted only a weak depressive component (see Table 2). Two separate cluster analyses failed to isolate a depressive category. There was no evidence of bimodality in the prepubertal depressive factor.

In summary, there have been many factor analytic studies of child and adolescent psychopathology but few have identified a convincing depressive

Table 1. Depression Factor Items and Factor Loadings Derived from Adolescent Inpatients (Nurcombe et al., 1989)

	Item	Loading
1.	Threatens suicide	(0.58)
2.	Depressed	(0.57)
3.	Worrying	(0.57)
4.	Anxious	(0.54)
5.	Feels worthless	(0.54)
6.	Trouble sleeping	(0.53)
7.	Shy	(0.52)
8.	Overtired	(0.52)
9.	Nightmares	(0.51)
10.	Fears doing bad	(0.51)
11.	Underactive	(0.51)

Table 2. Depression Factor Items and Factor Loadings Derived from Child Inpatients and Outpatients (Seifer et al., 1990)

	Item	Loading
1.	Worrying	(0.61)
2.	Must be perfect	(0.57)
3.	Feels worthless	(0.57)
4.	Too guilty	(0.57)
5.	Depressed	(0.54)
6.	Fears doing bad	(0.51)
7.	Nightmares	(0.50)
8.	Suicidal Ideation	(0.46)
9.	Anxious	(0.46)
10.	Self-conscious	(0.40)

factor. In most instances, depressive phenomena are commingled with anxiety, emotionality and social ineptitude. However, since most of these studies were of outpatients, pure depression may have been too uncommon to be detected. Two recent studies — one of adolescents in a mood disorders clinic and one of hospitalized adolescents — have identified cleaner depressive factors. Only the study of hospitalized adolescents has identified a categorically distinct depression cluster; however, it should be acknowledged that very few cluster analyses have been attempted in children and adolescents.

Discussion

The concept of major depression in adulthood, especially major depression with melancholia, is strongly supported by studies of its natural history and, to a lesser extent, by its response to specific treatments. It is reliably associated with specific changes in neuroendocrine function and with disruption of the circadian rhythm. The diagnosis is further supported by family aggregation and twin studies. Multivariate analyses of mixed data sets have repeatedly identified a bipolar factor which separates endogenous depression from neurotic symptoms, and isolated a subgroup of patients consistent with a categorical major depression; however, the essential components of this disorder have not yet been firmly established. On the other hand, dysthymia is apparently a diagnostic artefact that decomposes, on examination, into a mixture of temporary reactions to life crises, grief reactions, chronic personality traits, coping style, and the residua of major depression.

Contemporary enthusiasm for the diagnosis of major depression in childhood has come almost entirely from the application of adult criteria and techniques. However, this reasonable exercise in boot-strapping entails potential pitfalls. It is unlikely that the phenomenology of childhood depression will be completely isomorphic with that in adults. Furthermore, children — especially emotionally disturbed children — lack the metacognitive, introspective, motivational, attentional, discriminatory, relational, and temporal competencies required if they are to be reliable reporters of their own psychopathology. Therefore, it is essential to seek validation of apparently categorical disorders identified by techniques which do not presuppose the issue in question.

Three studies have demonstrated a continuity of depressive syndromes between childhood, adolescence, and adulthood; it appears that some depressive children grow up to become major depressives in adolescence or adulthood. These three studies represent the most impressive support for the validity of the diagnosis of major depression in childhood. However, there are numerous problems. The suicide rate is markedly higher in adolescents than in children, and has increased in the last twenty years. Among children, male depressives are twice as prevalent as female, the reverse of the sex ratio in adolescence. Furthermore, in children and adolescents, major depression and dysthymia are frequently entangled with aggressivity, antisocial behavior, anxiety, and substance abuse. The interaction between these problems is complicated — too complicated to be dismissed as "comorbidity".

The diagnosis of depression in childhood and adolescence has not been supported by antidepressant therapy and the psychobiological evidence in favor of this diagnosis is slim. However, it is fair to say that all the evidence is not yet to hand. The failure to find strong psychobiological support for the validity of the diagnosis could be explained by one or more of the following reasons:

1. *Type II error.* Sample sizes may have been too small to find significant differences.
2. *Insensitivity.* In contrast to adults, depressed children may not be responsive to the particular drug under investigation, or may not exhibit the particular psychobiological markers which have been tested for.
3. *Dosage variation.* Compared to adults, children may require a different relative dosage of the drugs or psychobiological probes in question.
4. *Faulty case detection.* Existing methods of case identification may be fraught with error, particularly if true cases are obscured by a large number of false diagnoses.
5. *Rarity.* The condition may be so rare that true cases are seldom detected.
6. *Invalidity.* The condition may not occur in children.

Many researchers (e.g., Puig-Antich, 1989) have failed to contemplate the last explanation.

One family pedigree study has found an aggregation of major depression, alcoholism, and other psychiatric disorders among the relatives of depressed children. As with the comorbidity question, the relationship between childhood depression and parental alcoholism, depression, and mental illness is probably complex. It is unlikely to be solely hereditary in nature.

Construct validity analyses have generally not supported the existence of a depressive syndrome. In most studies, depression emerges as part of an impure dysphoria factor, along with anxiety and social ineptitude or withdrawal. However, recent research has isolated an acceptable depressive syndrome from hospitalized or mood-disordered patients, possibly because these samples contained more severe or developed cases. In one study, a categorical depressive cluster was found in adolescent inpatients, but not in either adolescent outpatients or a mixed sample of prepubertal children. Among adolescents, the empirical evidence is consistent with the existence of a small group of patients who have a categorical depression and a larger group whose depression is dimensional and non-specific in nature. No evidence has yet emerged from multivariate analysis supporting a categorical depressive disorder in prepubertal children.

A Speculative Conclusion

The recent interest in childhood depression has trickled down from adult psychiatry. There is nothing wrong in that; even if the initial hypotheses were quite false — which is unlikely — something will come from the activity they have generated. Nevertheless, the proper scientific stance is one of constructive skepticism. There can no longer be any question that many children and adolescents suffer from emotional problems in which depressive mood is a prominent feature. The question remains, however, whether a true categorical depressive disorder can be isolated, linked to a predictable genetic background, psychobiology, and natural history, and eventually associated with a specific etiology and treatment. To pursue these ends, we require high-risk longitudinal studies (e.g., of the progeny of adult depressives) utilizing a variety of methods for gathering phenomenological data, and combining descriptive psychiatry with studies of the attitudes of high-risk children to themselves, their social environments, and their futures. At the same time, the search for family aggregations, psychobiological markers, and effective treatments should continue. How can development psychology provide a conceptual framework for research of this kind?

The panoramic developmental theories of Freud, Piaget, and Skinner are in decline. Contemporary developmental researchers move to and fro between their data and parsimonious constructs derived from information processing, social learning, and ethological theories. The scions of psychoanalysis, for example, examine abnormality in parent-child attachment as a predictor of later emotional disorder. They have little in common with descriptive psychiatrists and biological researchers who hunt for melancholic needles in the haystack of dysthymia. How can the two groups communicate?

Sroufe and Rutter (1984) Santosetfano (1978), and Cicchetti and Schneider-Rosen (1986) have proposed several guiding principles for a developmental psychopathology. Firstly, the meaning of behavior can be determined only within the total psychosocial and developmental context; for example, depressive mood following bereavement has a different significance from depressive mood following influenza. Secondly, later experience does not have a random effect upon individuals; it is perceived and reacted to in accordance with temperament, previous experience, and learned coping techniques. Thirdly, development is not linear; it results from the incorporation, reorganization, and subordination of old and new elements. Finally, development proceeds from global, inflexible, fragmentary origins towards increasingly specific, flexible and hierarchically organized ends. There is no need to postulate fixation or regression as the basis of psychopathology. The developmentally inappropriate quality of disturbed behavior results from a failure to reorganize and subordinate anachronistic elements which continue to operate in an inflexible or fragmented manner.

The attachment system represents a particularly promising field of research. It emerges early in life and may provide an anlage for other biosocial survival systems. Attachment is activated by the threat of danger and entails behavior that can be reincorporated and subordinated to later emerging systems such as mating and parenting. The link between early attachment experience and later behavior is conceivably via internal representations or "working models" of the self-in-relation-to-significant-others (Bowlby, 1969; Bretherton, 1985). Theoretically, then, disruption in early attachment could be linked to later

depressive psychopathology via global, inflexible, poorly organized, uninte-
grated, and dysfunctional self-other representations.

A number of questions spring to mind.

1. What is the influence of heredity in predisposing individuals to later depressive conditions? Does it operate by making some individuals more
   vulnerable to attachment disruption or to subsequent risk factors? Does it
   limit or define the coping techniques available? Does it render some individuals more likely to tip over from misery into melancholia?

2. If attachment disruption is a significant antecedent stress, does it act in an
   undifferentiated manner, or do such perturbations as parental depression,
   separation, bereavement, abandonment, rejection or abuse have differential effects?

3. If the effects of different types of attachment disruption are differentiated,
   can they be related to definable types of pathology in self-other representations? Does such inner pathology drive abnormal transactions with
   others, leading to self-fulfilling prophecies of failure, disappointment, rejection and self-hatred?

4. Can a depressive precursor condition be identified? Is it homotypic or
   heterotypic with later depression? Does it evolve into depression through
   invariant stages, with definable turning points?

5. If a precursor — outcome evolution can be delineated, what are the environmental, psychological, and biological factors which propel individuals
   toward a depressive outcome, or which protect them from moving in that
   direction.

6. Can protracted dysthymia tip over into a neuroendocrinologically decom-
   pensated melancholia? If so, what are the hereditary, biological or psychosocial factors which push individuals over the melancholic edge. At what
   age is such a decompensation possible?

7. How does helplessness relate to hopelessness? Why do some individuals
   give up hope, and how does that affect the neuroendocrine system?

The questions are numerous. The model suggests a linkage between genetic
predisposition, attachment disruption, representational pathology, dysfunctional social interaction, precursor state, risk/protective factors, depressive
outcome, and neuroendocrine decompensation. Naive perhaps. Nevertheless,
it provides a scaffolding upon which step-by-step studies can be erected, in
order to revise the model as the data emerge.

Let us finish with a metaphor. Picture a general hospital. Within it many
patients have fever: a syndrome involving high temperature, flushing, sweats,
and reduced output of urine. Although it is an index of ill-health and a
monitor of patient progress, many years have passed since physicians identified fever as a disease in its own right (? major fever disorder); instead, its
causes break down into a host of infections, inflammations, immunological
disorders and the like. However, within the diagnostic panorama of febrile
conditions, there is one disease — malignant hyperthermia — which is associated with characteristic dysregulation of temperature, a known etiology, and

specific treatment. If this metaphor is apt, the solution to the questions raised in this paper will not come easily. Meanwhile, as we hunt needles in a haystack, we are forgetting the hay. Many conditions congregate under the tatterdemalion cloak of "dysthymia". What predisposes a child to later dysthymia? What are the genetic, traumatic, and transactional forces which lead to the development of a pessimistic, self-depreciating personality? Can chronic demoralization evolve into melancholia? If so, what biochemical and physiological changes are involved, and how does puberty affect them? When the haydust settles, these may prove to be the questions of enduring importance.

REFERENCES

Achenbach, T.M., & Edelbrock, C.S. (1978). The classification of childhood psychopathology: A review and analysis of empirical efforts. *Psychological Bulletin*, 85:1275–1301.

Achenbach, T.M., & Edelbrock, C.S. (1983). *Manual for the child behavioral checklist and revised child behavioral profile*. Burlington, Vermont: Queen City Printers.

Akiskal, H.S. (1986). The clinical management of affective disorders. In J.E. Helzer & S.B. Guze (eds.), *Psychiatry: Volume II. Psychoses, affective disorders and dementia*. (pp. 119–146). New York: Basic Books.

Ban, T. (1991). *Psychiatric nosology Part I: Consensus — based classifications*. Nashville, Tennessee: Department of Psychiatry, Vanderbilt University.

Bertelsen, A., Harvald, B., & Haluge, M.A. (1977). A Danish twin study of manic-depressive disorders. *British Journal of Psychiatry*, 130:330–351.

Beukert, O. (1990). Functional classification and response to psychotropic drugs. In O.Beukert, W. Maier, & K. Rickels (eds.), *Methodology of the evaluation of psychotropic drugs*. Berlin: Springer.

Bouhoeffer, K. (1910). *Die symptomatischen Psychosen*. Leipzig: Deuticke.

Bowlby, J. (1952). *Maternal care and mental health*. Geneva: World Health Organization.

Bowlby, J. (1969). *Attachment and loss: Volume I. Attachment*. New York: Basic Books.

Bowlby, J. (1973). *Attachment and loss: Volume II. Separation, anxiety and anger*. New York: Basic Books.

Bowlby, J. (1980). *Attachment and loss: Volume III. Loss, sadness, and depression*. New York: Basic Books.

Bretherton, I. (1985). Attachment theory: Retrospect and Prospect. (pp. 3–38). I. Bretherton & E. Waters (eds.), *Growing points of attachment theory and research*. Monograph of the Society for Research in Child Development, Volume 50, Whole Number 1–2.

Brown, G.W., & Harris, T. (1978). *Social origins of depression*. London: Tavistock.

Carlson, G.A., & Kashani, J.H. (1988). Phenomenology of major depression from childhood through adulthood: Analysis of three studies. *American Journal of Psychiatry*, 1245:1222–1225.

Carlson, G.A., & Cantwell, D.P. (1980). Unmasking masked depression in children and adolescents. *American Journal of Psychiatry*, 137:445–449.

Casat, C.D., Arana, G.W., & Powell, K. (1989). The DST in children and adolescents with major depressive disorder. *American Journal of Psychiatry*, 146:503–507.

Cavallo, A., Hejazi, M.S., Richard, G.E., & Meyer, W.J. (1987). *Journal of the American Academy of Child and Adolescent Psychiatry.* 26:395–399.

Cicchetti, D., & Schneider-Rosen, K. (1986). An organizational approach to childhood depression. In M. Rutter, C.E. Izard, & P.B. Read (eds.), *Depression in young people: Clinical and developmental perspectives.* (pp. 71–134). New York: Guilford.

Costello, A.J., Edelbrock, C., Kalas, R., Kessler, M.D., & Klaric, S.H. (1982). *The NIMH Diagnostic Interview Schedule for Children (DISC).* Unpublished interview schedule. Pittsburgh: Department of Psychiatry, University of Pittsburgh.

Curran, D. (1937). *Psychological medicine.* Edinburgh: Livingstone.

Cummings, E.M. & Cicchetti, D. (1990) Toward a transactional model of relations between attachment and depression. In M. Greenberg, D. Cicchetti, & E.M. Cummings (eds.), *Attachment in the preschool years.* (pp. 339–372). Chicago: University of Chicago Press.

Cutler, N.R., & Post, R.M. (1982). Life course of illness in untreated manic-depressive illness. *Comprehensive Psychiatry,* 23:101–115.

Cytryn, L., & McKnew, D.H., (1972). Proposed classification of childhood depression. *American Journal of Psychiatry,* 129:149–155.

Cytryn, L., McKnew, D.H. & Bunney, W.E. (1980). Diagnosis of depression in children: A reassessment. *American Journal of Psychiatry,* 137:22–25.

Diagnostic and statistical manual of mental disorders (3rd edition, revised). DSM–III–R. (1987). Washington, DC: American Psychiatric Association.

Doherty, M.B., Mandansky, D., Kraft, J. Carter-Ake, L.L., Rosenthal, P.A., & Coughlin, B.F. (1986). Cortisol dynamics and test performance of dexamethasone suppression test in 97 psychiatrically hospitalized children aged 3–16 years. *Journal of the American Academy of Child Psychiatry,* 25:400–408.

Dreger, R.M. (1982). The classification of children and their emotional problems: An overview. II. *Clinical Psychology Review,* 2:349–385.

Egeland, J.A., Gerhard, D.S., & Pauls, D.L. (1987). Bipolar affective disorders linked to DNA markers on chromosome 2. *Nature,* 325:783–787.

Emslie, G.J., Rush, A.J., Weinberg, W.A., Rintelmann, J.W., & Roffearg, H.P. (1990). Children with major depression show rapid eye movement latencies. *Archives of General Psychiatry,* 47: 119–124.

Esquirol, J.E.D. (1838). *Des maladies mentales considerees sous les raports medical, hygienique et medico-legal.* Paris: Balliere.

Everitt, B.S., Gourlay, A.J., & Kendell, R.E. (1971). An attempt at validation of traditional psychiatric syndromes by cluster analysis. *British Journal of Psychiatry,* 119:399–412.

Finch, S. M. (1960). *Fundamentals of child psychiatry.* New York: Norton.

Finlay-Jones, R., & Brown, G.W. (1981). Types of stressful life events and the onset of anxiety and depressive disorders. *Psychological Medicine,* 11:803–816.

Freud, A., & Burlingham, D. (1944). *Infants without families.* New York: International Universities Press.

Garber, J., Kriss, M.R., Cock, M., & Lindholm, L. (1988). Recurrent depression in adolescents, a follow-up study. *Journal of the American Academy of Child and Adolescent Psychiatry,* 27:49–54.

Geller, B., Cooper, T.B., McCombs, H.G., Graham, D., & Wells, J. (1989). Double-blind placebo-controlled study of nortriptyline in depressed children using a "fixed plasma level" design. *Psychopharmacology Bulletin,* 25:101–108.

Geller, B. (1989). A double-blind placebo-controlled study of nortriptyline in adolescents with major depression. Annual Meeting of the New Clinical Drug Evaluation Unit, Washington, D.C.: National Institute of Mental Health.

Gershon, E., Bunney, W., & Leckman, J. (1976). The inheritance of affective disorders: A review of data and of hypotheses. *Behavioral Genetics,* 6:227–261.

Gillespie, R.D. (1929). The clinical differentiation of types of depression. *Guy's Hospital Report* 2: 306–344.

Glaser, K. (1967). Masked depression in children and adolescents. *American Journal of Psychotherapy*, 21:565–574.

Goetz, R.R., Puig-Antich, J., Ryan, N., Rabinovich, H., Ambrosini, P.J., Nelson, B., & Krawiec, V. (1987). Electroencephalographic sleep of adolescents with major depression and normal controls. *Archives of General Psychiatry*, 46:61–68.

Gold, P.W., Goodwin, F.K., & Chrousos, G.P. (1988). Clinical and biochemical manifestations of depression. II. Relation to the neurobiology of stress. *New England Journal of Medicine*, 319:413–420.

Gold, P.W., Goodwin, F.K., & Chrousos, G.P. (1988). Clinical and biochemical manifestations of depression I: Relation to the neurobiology of stress. *New England Journal of Medicine*, 319:348–353.

Grayson, D. (1986). Assessment of evidence for a categorical view of schizophrenia. *Archives of General Psychiatry*, 43:712–713.

Griesinger, W. (1861). *Die Pathologie und Therapie des psychischen Krankheiten.* Stuttgart: Krabbbe, 2nd edition.

Grof, P., Angst, J., & Haimes, T. (1974). The clinical course of depression: Practical issues. In J. Angst (ed.), *Classification and prediction of outcome of depression.* (pp. 104–130). Stuttgart: Schattauer Verlag.

Grove, W.M. & Andreasen, N.C. (1986). Multivariate statistical analysis in psychopathology. In T. Millon & G.L. Klerman (eds.), *Contemporary directions in psychopathology: Toward the DSM–IV.* (pp. 153–168). New York: Guilford.

Grove, W.M., Andreasen, N.C., Young, M., Endicott, J., Keller, M.B., Hirschfeld, R.M.A., & Reich, T. (1987). Isolation and characterization of a nuclear depressive syndrome. *Psychological Medicine*, 17:471–484.

Harrington, R., Fudge, H., Rutter, M., Pickles, A., & Hill, J. (1990). Adult outcomes of childhood and adolescent depressions. I. Psychiatric status. *Archives of General Psychiatry*, 47:465–473.

Hasselblad, V. (1966). Estimation of parameters for a mixture of normal distributions. *Technometrics*, 8:431–444.

Herjanic, B., & Campbell, W. (1977). Differentiating psychiatrically disturbed children on the basis of a structured interview. *Journal of Abnormal Child Psychology*, 5:127–134.

Hodges, K., Klien, J., Stern, L., Cytryn, L., & McKnew, D. (1982). The development of a child assessment interview for research and clinical use. *Journal of Abnormal Child Psychology*, 10:173–189.

Kahlbaum, K. (1863). *Die Gruppierung der psychischen Krankheiten und die Enteilung der Seelenstoerungen.* Danzig: Kaufman.

Kashani, J.H., McGee, R.D., Clarkson, S.E., Anderson, J.C., Walton, L.E., William, S., Silver, P.A., Robins, A.J., Cytryn, L., & McKnew, D.H. (1983). Depression in a sample of nine-year-old children: Prevalence and associated characteristics. *Archives of General Psychiatry*, 40:1217–1227.

Kashani, J.H., & Simonds, J.F. (1979). The incidence of depression in children. *American Journal of Psychiatry*, 136:1203–1205.

Kendell, R.E., & Gourlay, J. (1970). The clinical distinction between psychotic and neurotic depressions. *British Journal of Psychiatry*, 117:257–266.

Kendell, R.E. (1976). *The role of diagnosis in psychiatry.* Oxford: Blackwell.

Kiloh, L.G., Andrews, G., Neilson, M., & Bianchi, G.N. (1972). The relationship of the syndromes called endogenous and neurotic depression. *British Journal of Psychiatry*, 121:183–196.

Kiloh, L.G., & Garside, R.F. (1977). Depression: A multivariate study of Sir Aubrey Lewis's data on melancholia. *Australian and New Zealand Journal of Psychiatry*, 11:149–156.

Kiloh, L.G., & Garside, R.F. (1963). The independence of neurotic depression and endogenous depression. *British Journal of Psychiatry*, 109:451–463.

Klein, M. (1948). *Contributions to psychoanalysis 1921–1945*. London: Hogarth.

Klein, M. (1949). *The psychoanalysis of children*. London: Hogarth.

Kovacs, M. (1986). A developmental perspective on methods and measures in the assessment of depressive disorders: The clinical interview. In M. Rutter, C.E. Izard, & P.B. Read (eds.), *Depression in young people. Developmental and clinical perspectives*. (pp. 435–468). New York: Guilford.

Kovacs, M. (1985). The children's depression inventory. *Psychopharmacology Bulletin*, 21:995–998.

Kovacs, M., Finberg, T.L., Crose-Novak, M.A., Paulauskas, S.L., & Finkelstein, R. (1984a). Depressive disorders in childhood. I. A longitudinal prospective study of characteristics and recovery. *Archives of General Psychiatry*, 41:229–237.

Kovacs, M., Finberg, T.L., Crose-Novak, M.A., Paulauskas, S.L., Pollack, M., & Finkelstein, R. (1984b). Depressive disorders in childhood. II. A longitudinal study of the risk for a subsequent major depression. *Archives of General Psychiatry*, 41:643–649.

Kovacs, M. (1982). *The interview schedule for children (ISC)*. Unpublished manuscript. Pittsburgh: Department of Psychiatry, University of Pittsburgh.

Kraepelin, E. (1986). *Lehrbuch der Psychiatrie*. Leipzig: Barth, 5 Auflage.

Kramer, A.D., & Feiguine, R.J. (1981). Clinical effects of amitriptyline in adolescent depression: A pilot study. *Journal of the American Academy of Child Psychiatry*, 20: 636–644.

Kuhn, R. (1963). Über kindlichen Depressionen und ihre Behändlung. *Schweizer Medizinische Wochenschrift*, 93: 86–90.

Lahmeyer, H.W., Poznanski, E.O., & Beller, S.N. (1983). EEG sleep in depressed adolescents. *American Journal of Psychiatry*, 140:1150–1153.

Lehmann, H.E. (1971). The impact of the therapeutic revolution on nosology. In P. Doucet & C. Laurin (eds.), *Problems of psychoses*. (pp. 69–86). Amsterdam: Excerpta Medica, Excerta Medica Congress Series No. 194.

Leonhard, K. (1957). *Aufteilung der endogenen Psychosen*. Berlin: Akademie-Verlag.

Lessing, E.E., Williams, V., & Revelle, W. (1981). Parallel forms of the IJR behavior checklist for parents, teachers, and clinicians. *Journal of Consulting and Clinical Psychology*, 49:34–50.

Ling, W., Oftedal, G., & Weinberg, W. (1970). Depressive illness in children presenting as severe headaches. *American Journal of Diseases of Children*, 120:122–128.

Lord, F.M. (1958). Multimodal score distributions on the Myers-Briggs Type Indicator-I (ETS RM 58–8). Princeton, NJ: Education Testing Service.

Malmquist, C.P. (1971). Depressions in childhood and adolescence. *New England Journal of Medicine*, 284: 887–893.

Matthysse, S., & Kidd, K.K. (1981). Evidence of HLA linkage in depressive disorders. *New England Journal of Medicine*, 305:1340–1341.

Matussek, P., Soldner, M.L., & Nagel, D. (1982). Neurotic depression: Results of cluster analyses. *Journal of Nervous and Mental Diseases*, 170:588–597.

McConville, B.J., Boag, L.C., & Purohit, A.P. (1973). Three types of childhood depression. *Canadian Psychiatric Association Journal*, 18:133–138.

Meehl, P.E. (1979). A funny happened thing happened to us on the way to latent entities. *Journal of Personality Assessment*, 43:563–581.

Meehl, P.E. (1973). MAXCOV-HITMAX: A taxonomic search for loose genetic syndromes. In *Psychodiagnosis: selected papers*. Minneapolis: University of Minnesota Press.

Mendlewicz, J., Fleiss, J., & Fieve, R. (1972). Polymorphic DNA marker on X-chromosome and manic depression. *Journal of the American Medical Association*, 222:1624–1627.

Moebius, J.P. (1893). *Abriss der Lehre von den Nervenkrankheiten.* Leipzig: Deuticke.

Morel, B.A. (1857). *Traite des degenerescences physiques, intellectuelles et morales de l'espece humaine.* Paris: Balliere.

Mullaney, J.A. (1984). The relationship between anxiety and depression: A review of some principal component analytic studies. *Journal of Affective Disorders,* 7:139–148.

Ni Bhrolchain, M. (1979). Psychotic and neurotic depression. I. Some points of method. *British Journal of Psychiatry,* 134:87–93.

Nurcombe, B., Seifer, R., Scioli, A., Tramontana, M.G., Grapentine, W.L., & Beauchesne, H.C. (1989). Is major depressive disorder in adolescence a distinct diagnostic entity? *Journal of the American Academy of Child and Adolescent Psychiatry,* 28:333–342.

Parker, G., Hadzi-Pavlovic, D., Boyce, P., Wilhelm, K., Brodaty, H., Mitchell, P., Hickie, I., & Eyers, K. (1990). *British Journal of Psychiatry,* 157:55–65.

Paykel, E.S. (1971). Classification of depressed patients: A cluster analysis derived grouping. *British Journal of Psychiatry,* 118:275–288.

Pearce, J. (1978). The recognition of depressive disorder in children. *Journal of the Royal Society of Medicine,* 71:494–500.

Perris, C. (1966). A study of bipolar (manic-depressive) and unipolar recurrent depressive psychoses. *Acta Psychiatrica Scandinavica,* 194 (supplement): 1–189.

Pilowski, I., Levine, S., & Boulton, D.M. (1969). The classification of depression by numerical taxonomy. *British Journal of Psychiatry,* 115:937–945.

Poznanski, E., & Zrull, J. (1970). Child depression: Clinical characteristics of overtly depressed children. *Archives of General Psychiatry,* 23:8–15.

Puig-Antich, J., Dahl, R., Ryan, N., Novacenko, H., Goetz, D., Goetz, R., Toomey, J., & Kleper, T. (1989). Cortisol secretion in prepubertal children with major depressive disorder. *Archives of General Psychiatry,* 46:801–809.

Puig-Antich, J. (1983). Neuroendocrine and sleep correlates of prepubertal major depressive disorder: Current status of the evidence. In D.P. Cantwell & G.A. Carlson (eds), *Affective disorders in childhood and adolescence — An update.* (pp. 211–228). New York: Spectrum.

Puig-Antich, J., Novacenko, H., Davies, M., Chambers, W.J., Tabrizi, M.A., Krawiec, V., Ambrosini, P.J., & Sachar, E.J. (1984). Growth hormone secretion in prepubertal major depressive children. I. Sleep-related plasma concentrations during a depressive episode. *Archives of General Psychiatry,* 41:455–460.

Puig-Antich, J. (1986). Psychobiological markers: Effects of age and puberty. In M. Rutter, C.E., Izard, & P.B. Read (eds.), *Depression in young people: Developmental and clinical perspectives.* (pp. 341–382). New York: Guilford.

Puig-Antich, J., Goetz, D., Davies, M., Kaplan, T., Davies, S., Ostrow, L., Asnis, L., Toomey, J., Iyengar, S., & Ryan, N. (1989). A controlled family history study of prepubertal major depressive disorder, *Archives of General Psychiatry,* 46:406–418.

Puig-Antich, J. Chambers, W., Halpern, F., Hanlon, C., & Sachar, E.J. (1979). Cortisol hypersecretion in prepubertal depressive illness: A preliminary report. *Psychoneuroendocrinology,* 4:191–197.

Puig-Antich, J., & Chambers, W. (1978). *The schedule for affective disorders and schizophrenia for school-aged children.* New York: New York State Psychiatry Institute, Unpublished interview schedule.

Puig-Antich, J., Perel, J.M., Lupatkin, W., Chambers, W.J., Tabrizi, M.A., King, J., Goetz, R., Davies, M., & Stiller, R.L. (1987). Imipramine in prepubertal major depressive disorders. *Archives of General Psychiatry,* 44:81–89.

Puig-Antich, J., Goetz, R., Hanlon, C., Tabrizi, M.A., Davies, M., & Weitzman, E. (1982). Sleep architecture and REM sleep measures in prepubertal major depressives during an episode. *Archives of General Psychiatry,* 39:932–939.

Puig-Antich, J. (1982). Major depression and conduct disorder in pre-puberty. *Journal of the American Academy of Child Psychiatry*, 21:118–128.

Puig-Antich, J. (1987). Affective disorders in children and adolescents: Diagnostic validity and psychobiology. In H.Y. Meltzer (ed.), *Psychopharmacology: The third generation of progress*. (pp. 843–860). New York: Raven.

Puig-Antich, J., Tabrizi, M.A., Davies, M., Chambers, W., Halpern, F., & Sachar, E.J. (1981). Prepubertal endogenous major depressives hyposecrete growth hormone in response to insulin-induced hypoglycemia. *Journal of Biological Psychiatry*, 16:801–818.

Quay, H.C. (1986). Classification. In H.C. Quay & J.S. Werry (eds.), *Psychopathological disorders of childhood*. (Third Edition). (pp. 1–34). New York: Wiley & Son.

Rice, J.P., & McGuffin, P. (1986). Genetic etiology of schizophrenia and affective disorders. In J.E. Helzer, & S.B. Guze (eds.), *Psychiatry. Volume II. Psychoses, affective disorders and dementia.* (pp. 147–170). New York: Basic Books.

Richards, M.P.M., & Dyson, M. (1982). *Separation, divorce and the development of children: A review.* London: Department of Health and Social Security.

Rie, H.E. (1966). Depression in childhood: A survey of some pertinent contributions. *Journal of the American Academy of Child Psychiatry*, 5: 653–685.

Rochlin, G. (1959). The loss complex. *Journal of the American Psychoanalytic Association*, 7: 299–316.

Rutter, M. (1986). The developmental psychopathology of depression. In M. Rutter, C.E. Izard, & P.B. Read (eds.), *Depression in young people: Developmental and clinical perspectives.* (pp. 3–32). New York Guilford.

Rutter, M., Tizard, J., & Whitmore, K. (1970). *Education, health and behavior.* London: Longmans.

Ryan, N.D., Puig-Antich, J., Ambrosini, P., Rabinovich, H., Robinson, D., Neilson, B., Iyengar, S., & Toomey, J. (1987). The clinical picture of major depression in children and adolescents. *Archives of General Psychiatry*, 44:854–861.

Santostefano, S. (1978). *A biodevelopmental approach to clinical child psychology.* New York: Wiley.

Seifer, R., Nurcombe, B., Scioli, A., & Grapentine, W.L. (1989). Is major depressive disorder in childhood a distinct diagnostic entity? *Journal of the Academy of Child and Adolescent Psychiatry*, 28:935–941.

Slater, E. (1936). Inheritance of manic-depressive insanity. *Lancet* 1:429–431.

Spitz, R.A., & Wolf, K.M. (1946). Anaclitic depression: An inquiry into the genesis of psychiatric conditions in early childhood. *Psychoanalytic Study of the Child*, 2: 313–342.

Sroufe, L.A., & Rutter, M. (1984). The domain of developmental Psychopathology. *Child Development*, 55:17–29.

Tennant, C., & Bebbington, B. (1978). The social causation of depression: A critique of the work of Brown and his colleagues. *Psychological Medicine*, 8: 565–575.

Toolan, J.M. (1962). Depression in children and adolescence. *American Journal of Orthopsychiatry*, 32:404–414.

Trull, T.J., Widiger, T.A. & Guthrie, P. (1990). Categorical versus dimensional status of borderline personality disorder. *Journal of Abnormal Psychology*, 99:40–48.

Tsuang, M.T. (1978). Suicide in schizophrenics, manics, depressives, and surgical controls. A comparison with general population suicide mortality. *Archives of General Psychiatry*, 135:153–155.

Wagner, K.D., Saeed, M.A., Skyiepal, B., & Meyer, W.J. (1991). Thyrotrophin and growth hormone responses to TRH stimulation are normal in 6–12 year-old children with major depression. *Journal of Child & Adolescent Psychopharmacology*, 1: 199–206.

Wainer, H. (1978). Gapping. *Psychometrika*, 43:203–212.

Wehr, T.A., & Goodwin, F.K. (1981). Biological rhythms and psychiatry. In S.H. Arieti, & K.H. Brodie (eds.), *The American Handbook of Psychiatry. Volume II.* (pp. 251–271). New York: Basic Books, second edition.

Weinberg, W.A., Rutman, J., Sullivan, L., Penick, E.C., & Deitz, S.G. (1973). Depression in children referred to an educational diagnostic center: Diagnosis and treatment. *Behavioral Pediatrics*, 83:1065–1072.

Weller, E.B., Weller, R.A., Fristad, M.A., Preskorn, S.H., & Teare, M. (1985). The dexamethasone suppression test in prepubertal depressed children. *Journal of Clinical Psychiatry*, 46:511–513.

Winokur, G., & Tanna, V.L. (1969). Possible role of X-linked dominant factor in manic-depressive disease. *Diseases of the Nervous System*, 30:89–95.

Young, W., Knowles, J.B., MacLean, A.W., Boag, L., & McConville, B.J. (1982). The sleep of childhood depressives: Comparison with age-matched controls. *Biological Psychiatry*, 17:1163–1168.

Zeitlin, H. (1985). *The natural history of psychiatric disorder in children*. Institute of Psychiatry, Maudsley Monograph. London: Oxford University Press.

Zeitlin, H. (1972). A study of patients who attended the children's department and later the adults' department of the same psychiatric hospital. Unpublished M. Phil. dissertation, University of London.

Zis, A.P., Grof, P., & Goodwin, F.K. (1979). The natural course of affective disorders: Implications for lithium prophylaxis. In T.B. Cooper, S. Gershon, N.S. Klime, & M. Schou (eds.), *Lithium: Controversies and unresolved issues*. (pp. 181–196). Amsterdam: Excerpa Medica.

Zis, A.P., & Goodwin, F.K. (1979). Major affective disorders as a recurrent illness: A critical review. *Archives of General Psychiatry*, 36:835–839.

II A Neurobehavioral Systems Approach to Developmental Psychopathology: Implications for Disorders of Affect

PAUL F. COLLINS & RICHARD A. DEPUE *

Neurobehavioral systems represent a newly emerging approach to the study of human behavior. This approach involves an integration of the rapidly expanding database in behavioral neuroscience within the behavioral system framework of ethology. Accordingly, neurobehavioral systems organize a coherent domain of behavior, an underlying circuit of neuroanatomical and neurochemical pathways, and a set of neurobehavioral functions that account for brain-behavior relations within the system. As in ethology, these systems address the structure of human behavior, i.e., the small number of higher-order dimensions that arise from a larger group of interrelated behavioral traits. At this level of analysis, the theoretical objective is to explain how widely distributed neurobiological systems modulate broad patterns of behavior, such as approach versus inhibition or constraint, rather than to detail the neural mediation of specific behaviors. Because humans and related species overlap considerably with respect to the neurobiological modulation of behavior, neurobehavioral systems typically are formulated within an explicit evolutionary context. Consequently, these systems suggest a basis for universal features of human behavior preserved throughout mammalian phylogeny. Although such systems show qualitative consistency within and across species, the mechanisms that produce quantitative variation, i.e., individual differences, are preserved as well, and serve as the basis for microevolutionary changes. Thus, put simply, neurobehavioral systems provide one approach to understanding why humans share a limited number of general behavioral features, but vary considerably in their expression of these features.

Although a neurobehavioral systems approach has been applied primarily to adult behavior (e.g., Depue & Iacono, 1989; Gray, 1982; Panksepp, 1982),

* This work was supported by NIMH Research Grants MH37195 and MH48114, and by NIMH Research Training Grant MH17069 awarded to Dr Depue

it holds considerable promise for developmental psychology. Perhaps the clearest potential benefit is that neurobehavioral systems are incorporated within age-free psychological constructs. For example, our discussion in this chapter will focus upon the Behavioral Facilitation System, which modulates feelings of incentive-reward motivation and expression of approach behavior in response to cues of reward (Depue & Iacono, 1989). Obviously, the behaviors that indicate incentive-reward motivation in an infant, e.g., crawling toward the mother, will differ from those of an adult, e.g., finding some way to compliment a prospective sex partner. Nevertheless, the stimulus context (potential reward), the type of behavior (approach), and the motivational state (incentive-reward) remain qualitatively consistent across ages. In addition, the underlying neurobiological mechanisms that modulate incentive-reward motivation and approach behavior are qualitatively similar in infant and adult, since neural systems do not undergo major reorganizations after basic patterns of connectivity are established. Thus, neurobehavioral systems are defined with respect to basic brain-behavior functions that may be tested at any age, provided that developmentally appropriate measures are employed to assess relevant brain and behavioral processes.

An additional potential benefit to developmental work is that neurobehavioral systems possess specific neurobiological avenues through which genetic and environmental factors may exert influence during development. Both sources of influence must be considered within a comprehensive developmental construct, since forms of human social behavior that are influenced strongly by environmental experience during ontogeny are likely to be under strong quantitative genetic influence as well (Cairns, Gariepy, & Hood, 1990). In the young infant, converging influences from genetic and environmental factors are best illustrated by neural sensitive periods, in which genetic controls over the timing of large-scale neuronal modifications interact with environmental controls over the functional consequences of the neural modifications.

Perhaps as a complementary approach to developmental behavior genetics, neurobehavioral systems indicate how, rather than how much, genetic and environmental factors produce variation in behavior across individuals. An important consequence is that a developmental model of a neurobehavioral system will support hypotheses regarding the nature and timing of environmental determinants of developing behavioral traits. That is, although empirical tests of similar hypotheses may be found in the behavioral genetics literature, the neurobehavioral systems approach may facilitate the study of genetic and environmental factors by indicating how and when they exert maximal influence during development.

Neurobehavioral Systems as Emotional Systems

Ethologists and psychologists have long been concerned with the structure of behavior, that is, the manner in which behavior may be categorized into coherent patterns or systems (Fonberg 1986; Fowles, 1980; Gray, 1973, 1982; MacLean, 1986, 1990; Panksepp, 1982, 1986; Ploog, 1986; Rolls, 1986; Schneirla, 1959). From an evolutionary biology perspective, such systems represent neurobehavioral mechanisms that have evolved as a means of adapting to stimuli that are critical to the organism's survival and to the preservation of the species (Fonberg, 1986; Levi, 1975; Gray, 1973; MacLean, 1986). For instance, defensive aggression serves as an adaptive neurobehavioral response to pain and potential destruction, whereas in the case of appetitive behaviors such as sex and feeding, specific olfactory cues serve as critical stimuli in signaling a suitable mate or appropriate food. As is evident in these examples, a system is defined by the class of stimuli that engages it, as well as by the response patterns expressed by it. The importance of delineating such systems at the behavioral level is that they provide a framework for discovering the neurobiological systems that mediate the interface between classes of stimuli and specific response patterns.

Because their development has been closely tied to critical stimulus conditions, behavioral systems must be tightly linked with brain structures responsible for recognition of stimulus significance, on the one hand, and for subsequent activation of effector systems, on the other. Collectively, this group of interrelated brain functions has been referred to as emotion, or emotional evaluation and emotional expression, respectively (Depue, in press; LeDoux, 1987). Thus, adaptive behavioral systems, in the broadest sense, are really emotional systems that motivate and, in a general way, guide behavior in response to critical stimuli. Indeed, *emotion* derives from the latin verb *emovere*: to move, to push. Emotional systems, then, not only elicit certain patterns of behavior to particular stimuli, but they also provide a motivational state and subjective emotional experience that is concordant with the affective nature or reinforcement qualities of critical stimuli (Fonberg, 1986; Gray, 1973, 1982; MacLean, 1986; Ploog, 1986; Rolls, 1986). Concordant with this view, analyses of the basic types of emotion (Levi, 1975; Plutchik, 1980; Plutchik & Kellerman, 1986), combined with ethological descriptions of mammalian behavioral systems (MacLean, 1969, 1970, 1990), suggest that the emotions of desire, anger, fear, sorrow, joy, and affection are elicited by particular classes of stimuli and subsequently motivate six main forms of behavior, including searching, aggressive, protective, dejected, gratulant, and caressive, respectively (MacLean, 1986). Gray (1973, 1982) has added to this list a system of behavior inhibition that is associated with anxiety and that is activated by conditioned signals of punishment, nonreward, and novelty. Thus, a particular class of stimuli. the emotion generated, and the behavior patterns expressed all form integral components of a coherent emotional system.

The importance of this perspective for understanding the structure of *human* behavior has not been generally recognized. However, as Gray (1973) and others (Fonberg, 1986; Zuckerman, 1983) have cogently argued, behavioral systems that are closely linked to emotional mechanisms are largely unchanged along the pathway of mammalian evolution and, hence, are probably subject to strong genetic influence in our own species. Such systems are likely, therefore, to provide a foundation for individual differences in human emotional patterns (Plutchik 1980). When viewed from a broad temporal perspective, emotional systems may be conceptualized not simply as phasic response patterns, but rather as emotional dispositions with respect to particular classes of stimuli. That is, humans have individual differences in their sensitivity to particular classes of stimuli, and these differences are evident as trait variation both in subjective emotional experience and in overt patterns of emotional expression. Thus, it is possible to view emotional systems as major components of the structure of human personality (Ervin & Martin, 1986; Gray, 1973; Plutchik 1980; Tellegen, 1985; Zuckerman 1983).

Our goal is to outline the phenomenological, neurobiological, and neurochemical nature of one emotional system that has received relatively little attention in relation to the structure of human behavior or personality. We hypothesize that this system forms the basis of a major component of human personality structure, and we offer recently obtained data to support the hypothesis. With respect to developmental issues, we present a discussion of the ontological sources of individual differences in this emotional system, which includes genetic and experiential effects on the neurobiology of the system. Finally, we discuss the implications of the emotional system for conceptualizing various forms of affective disorder and for longitudinal analysis of affective disorder within a high-risk paradigm.

Phenomenology of the Behavioral Facilitation System

The focus of our discussion concerns an emotional system that has been consistently described in all animals across phylogenetic levels (Hebb, 1949; Schneirla, 1959). It has been described variously as a search system (MacLean, 1986; Ploog, 1986), a foraging-expectancy system (Panksepp, 1986), an approach system (Gray 1973; Schneirla, 1959), a preparatory system (Blackburn, Philips, Jakobovic & Fibiger, 1989), and a behavioral activation system (Fowles, 1980). For reasons that become evident later, we integrate these terms into one notion of a *behavioral facilitation system* or BFS. All of these descriptions, with minor variations, converge on the same basic themes. The BFS is an emotional system that has evolved to motivate forward locomotion and search behavior as a means of satisfying an animal's need for food, a sex partner, social interaction, a nesting place, etc. That is, the BFS serves to bring the animal into contact with positive rewarding stimuli when such stimuli are not within close proximity. Thus, the BFS is a generalized or nonspecific emotional system that is activated by a host of positive rewarding stimuli.

An important behavioral distinction should be recognized. The final purpose of BFS-facilitated, goal-oriented behavior is to perform a multitude of specific fixed action patterns involved in the consummation of specific rewarding stimuli (Ploog, 1986). Thus in keeping with distinctions long held in ethology (Eibl-Eibesfeldt, 1975; Tinbergen, 1951), the BFS promotes exploration and approach to goal stimuli but plays only a minimal, if any, role in the mediation of consummatory fixed action patterns (Blackburn et al., 1989). Approach and consummatory components of appetitive behavior appear to be neurobiologically, neurochemically, and neurophysiologically distinct (Blackburn et al., 1989; Konorski, 1967; Schultz, 1986; Wilson & Soltysik, 1985). Indeed, performance of consummatory behavior may inhibit activity in the BFS (Panksepp, 1986).

There is general agreement on the class of stimuli that elicit activity in the BFS. Stimuli that elicit consummatory responses are primary positive reinforcers. These same stimuli, when perceived at a distance by the animal, may be referred to as primary incentive stimuli, because they facilitate forward locomotion, alertness, and goal-oriented approach to the primary positive reinforcer. That is, the occurrence of the latter behavior suggests the existence of an internal state of incentive motivation (an intervening variable), and activation of this internal state appears to be inherently rewarding, as indicated by the occurrence of facilitated behavior in sated animals in the presence of incentive stimuli (Blackburn et al., 1989; Konorski, 1967; Stewart, de Wit, & Eikelboom, 1984). Neutral stimuli occurring in close temporal contiguity with primary incentive stimuli can become conditioned incentive stimuli and thereby can activate the BFS (Beninger, 1983; Bindra, 1968; Bolles, 1972; Panksepp, 1986; Stewart et al., 1984). The role of the BFS in determining an enduring emotional disposition in humans is most relevant in relation to conditioned incentive stimuli, because of the generally predominant influence of symbolic processes in guiding human behavior in the absence of unconditioned stimuli.

Several important distinctions with respect to stimulus control of the BFS are noteworthy. First, conditioned incentive stimuli apparently do not gain their power to activate the BFS simply through the process of association with primary incentive stimuli (i.e., via stimulus-stimulus [reinforcement] association), since the association of stimulus aspects of reinforcement with environmental stimuli can occur without those stimuli acquiring the ability to facilitate responding (Beninger, 1983; Fibiger & Philips, 1987). Rather, their association with the internal state of incentive motivation generated by primary incentive stimuli is required. We return to the neurobiologic basis of this issue later. Second, conditioned incentive stimuli may be established in two ways: (a) as a result of association with the internal state of incentive motivation generated by a primary incentive stimulus, as discussed above, or (b) by association with cues occuring in close proximity to the *termination* of a primary negative reinforcer. An example of the latter case is active avoidance learning in animals, where the conditioned incentive stimuli established by association with shock termination may be conceived of as cues denoting the reward of safety (Gray, 1973, 1982). These cues induce incentive motivation, and facilitated approach to safety subsequently occurs. Third, the BFS appears to facilitate (but not mediate) behavior in stimulus conditions associated with aggressive interaction. The opportunity to engage in affective attack is associated with goal-oriented behavior that is rewarding (Valzelli, 1981). Moreover, under conditions where reward acquisition is blocked, the BFS may facilitate aggressive behavior whose goal is removal of stimuli associated with frustrative nonreward. It may be that the BFS is elicited in this latter case by expectations of the reward acquisition that will result from removal of the obstacle to reward. Thus, whereas the BFS is activated by a broad array of stimulus contexts, these contexts share an incentive-reward component.

All of these stimulus conditions could be viewed as activating at least three major processes. First, incentive motivation, and its inherently rewarding nature, is a core element of the BFS. Whereas in animals the incentive construct is difficult to assess other than by behavioral responding, in humans subjective emotional experience can be assessed by self-report methods that are used to delineate the emotional structure of personality (Tellegen, 1985). Therefore, in contrast to animal work, for humans the emotional nature of the BFS is critical to define. A large body of research on human subjects suggests that conditions of novelty (i.e., mild levels of BFS activation) are associated with the emotional experience of curiosity. Indeed, Hebb (1949) argued that curiosity is a drive state found in all species. Under conditions of vigorous reward acquisition (i.e., at higher BFS activity levels), the emotion is desire, and this is accompanied by a general sense of positive affect (Stewart et al., 1984; Tellegen, 1985; Watson & Tellegen, 1985). When BFS activity is activated by conditioned incentive stimuli, strong anticipatory eagerness or expectancy characterizes the desire. Thus, incentive-reward motivation is a positive emotional state that activates goal acquisition. The emotional experience of gratification, on the other hand, is more closely associated with fulfillment of curiosity and desire and brings behavior to a satisfying termination (Bozarth, 1987; Fibiger & Phillips, 1987; Stein 1983).

With respect to the specificity of incentive and desire to the BFS system, one view of emotional systems posits that the emotion associated with a system is distinct in quality from other forms of emotional experience — that is, the intrinsic attributes of fluctuating activities of the system mediate a specific emotion (MacLean, 1986; Panksepp, 1986; Ploog, 1986). Indeed, MacLean (1986) suggested that the inherent mechanisms underlying emotions and their conscious experience may be analogous to fixed action patterns, i.e., stimulation of inherent neural circuitry evokes fixed *affect* patterns that have a specificity independent of peripheral feedback. Of importance, desire, or one of its variant expressions, is cited as one of the primary emotions in most classificatory systems of emotion (MacLean, 1986; Ploog, 1986; Plutchik, 1980; Plutchik & Kellerman, 1986), and is one of the few distinct emotional feelings that is reported with direct stimulation of the amygdala in conscious patients and by temporal lobe epileptics during the aura at the beginning of the epileptic storm (Ervin & Martin, 1986; MacLean, 1986).

A second core process involved in BFS activity is the initiation of locomotor activity as a means of supporting goal acquisition. This would be consistent with the fact that locomotor activity is the most reliable indicator of an animal's incentive state (Iversen, 1978). This suggests that neural structures associated with the BFS provide a link or interface between emotional evaluation processes, on the one hand, and the motor system, on the other. Put differently, the BFS may provide a mechanism for communicating the emotional state of incentive motivation to the initiatory structures of the motor system.

Third, active goal-seeking facilitated by the BFS will increase interaction with, and hence the need to evaluate, the environment. To assure that approach behavior is adaptively related to stimulus events, there will be an increased need to construct maps of extrapersonal space, to identify objects in space, to organize behavioral strategies, and to evaluate the emotional significance of objects and the outcomes of those behavioral strategies. These are complex cognitive functions. Their functional integrity requires the passage of information among distinct brain regions which serve as processing nodes in neural networks devoted to cognitive functions (Goldman-Rakic, 1987, 1988; Kosslyn, 1988; Mesulam, 1984, 1990; Posner, Petersen, Fox, & Raichle, 1988). Although a role for the BFS in cognitive processes has not been emphasized previously, Plutchik (1980) has argued compellingly that cognitive systems evolved for the purpose of increasing the adaptability of emotional behavior in complex environments. We suggest, and offer neurobiological support below, that the BFS plays a critical facilitatory role in these processes.

Stimulus control of the BFS may be viewed within a hierarchical framework that very generally reflects phylogenetic development of brain functions. The hierarchical nature of the system relates to the specificity of the eliciting stimuli. At the lowest level of the hierarchy, interoceptive stimuli signaling many distinct physiologic states (or what Gray (1973) and other learning theorists refer to as *drives*, such as hunger, thirst, cold, discomfort, and libido) have access to the BFS in order to effect exploratory locomotion in search of the specific primary positive reinforcers which satisfy these states (or in order to facilitate avoidance of damaging negative states; Blackburn et al., 1989; Gray, 1973; Panksepp, 1986). In this case, the BFS plays an intervening facilitatory role within a preprogrammed response system relating (a) specific, critical eliciting stimuli to (b) specific, invariant fixed action patterns associated with satisfaction of internal states (Panksepp, 1986; Ploog, 1986). At high levels of control (i.e., requiring cortical sensory processing and more neurally complex emotional evaluation processes), exteroceptive *unconditioned* incentive stimuli engage the BFS. These stimuli are, by definition, critical stimuli that have a specific, invariant relation to consummatory patterns of behavior. Hence, in this case as well, the BFS plays a relatively limited (albeit, important) role in the overall appetitive behavior sequence.

The rapid development of symbolic associative processes in mammals has permitted the process of emotional evaluation of stimuli to be based on the comparison of sensory information with acquired knowledge (i.e., knowledge that has attained significance through conditioning; LeDoux, 1987). This development has expanded the nature of the BFS in that the system is no longer yoked to serving specific goal-directed activities. Rather, the BFS can now be engaged by a broad range of *conditioned* incentive stimuli that may apply to individuals, situations, and things. And, owing to mentation, it may be activated by central representations of conditioned incentives far removed in time from primary positive reinforcers. Thus, control of the BFS by central representations of incentives may be a critical component of the neural processes that provide the foundation for long-term, delayed- gratification, goal-directed behavior in humans. This level of stimulus control of the BFS is more complex in that it is dependent on the evolution of brain processes that associate exteroceptive conditioned stimuli with emotional meaning, and that convey this association to BFS circuitry. Thus, comprehensive neurobiological models of the BFS as an emotional system must integrate this system with brain processes devoted not only to emotional evaluation, but also to emotional expression, since the BFS modulates but one form of emotional expression occurring under certain stimulus conditions.

A final perspective on the BFS is that it can be viewed not simply as a passive response system to stimuli, but rather as a dynamic system that influences emotional evaluation of incentive stimuli. There is evidence suggesting that responsivity of the BFS to incentive stimuli is dependent on the current state of BFS activity (Beninger, 1983; Beninger, Hanson, & Phillips, 1980; Blackburn et al., 1989; Hill, 1970; Panksepp, 1986; Robbins, 1975). That is, the effective incentive value of a stimulus is a relative function of stimulus intensity and current BFS activity. As noted above, it may also be supposed that the BFS is in reciprocal interaction with brain mechanisms that elaborate cognitive functions and central representations of incentives. The implication of these points for human personality is that variation in trait levels of BFS activity may influence sensitivity to incentive stimuli. This would have the effect of modulating the emotional evaluation of incentive stimuli (i.e., their perceived intensity), as well as the threshold for stimulus elicitation of subsequent responses.

Neurobiology of Emotional Processes

To understand the BFS as an emotional system, it is necessary to locate it at the neurobiological level within the network of neural structures devoted to emotional processes. Because goal-directed behavior in humans is predominantly influenced by conditioned incentive stimuli, it is particularly important to delineate the manner in which conditioned stimuli are associated with emotional meaning, and how this meaning comes to elicit BFS activity. The former refers to the process of emotional evaluation, the latter to the process of emotional expression, of which BFS activation is but one form. The neurobiological organization of these processes will be discussed next in highly condensed form; interested readers are referred to LeDoux (1987) for a more detailed review.

The Basolateral Limbic Forebrain and Emotion

Research over the past fifty years has indicated that all of the subcortical and cortical areas that came to be associated with the concept of the limbic system could not be viewed as an integrated system from a functional standpoint. Accordingly, Livingston and Escobar (1971) and Mesulam and Mufson (1982a,b) have extended Yakovlev's (1948, 1959) proposal that the limbic lobe be divided into two divisions. The division that is associated most closely with emotional functions is referred to as the basolateral limbic division, and its location in the brain is illustrated as the less regularly stipled areas in Figure 1. This division encompasses forebrain areas that evolved phylogenetically around very old olfactory cortex located at the posterior end of the olfactory bulb, which, since Broca's (1878) initial emphasis on the olfactory bulb as an integral part of the limbic lobe, indicates a central role for olfaction in the evolution of vertebrate emotional processes (Fonberg, 1986; Kling, 1986; MacLean, 1975; Papez, 1937).

The forebrain areas evolving around olfactory cortex and comprising the basolateral limbic division include the insula, temporal pole (TP), and orbital frontal cortex (OFC), areas which Mesulam and Mufson (1982a,b) refer to as paralimbic regions to distinguish them from core limbic structures such as the amygdala and hippocampus. The basolateral paralimbic regions evolved as a neural bridge to integrate unimodel sensory information into polymodel sensory representations that are then communicated to core limbic structures for emotional evaluation. For instance, the temporopolar cortex integrates visual and auditory sensory representations of an event, constructed in their respective temporal lobe regions, with olfactory information, while the insular cortex integrates autonomic, gustatory, and somatosensory input.

The amygdala, which is closely located to this olfactory core (see Figure 1), plays a central role in the basolateral limbic division. Sensory information from all unimodel sensory pathways and from polymodal paralimbic regions of

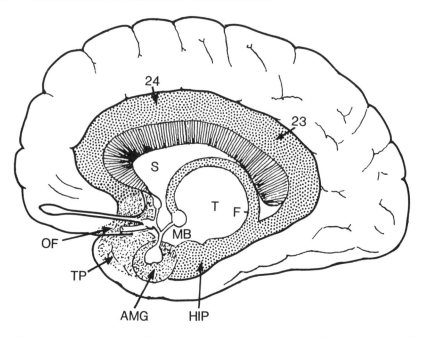

Figure 1. Medial view of brain showing two divisions of the limbic forebrain. The basolateral limbic division, which is most closely associated with emotional functions, is illustrated as the less regularly stipled areas. The dorsomedial division is illustrated as the regularly stipled areas. See text for discussion. AMG, amygdala; F, fornix; HIP, hippocampus; MB, mammillary bodies; OF, orbital frontal cortex; S, septal area; T, temporal lobe; TP, temporopolar cortex; 24, 23, Brodmann's designations for the anterior and posterior cingulate cortex, respectively.

the TP, OFC, and insular cortices converge in topographical order on the amygdala in the rhesus monkey (Aggleton, Burton & Passingham, 1980; Herzog & Van Hoesen, 1976; Jones & Powell, 1970; Kemp & Powell, 1970; Turner et al., 1980; Whitlock & Nauta, 1956). It has also been demonstrated that there are thalamic sensory neurons which project *directly* to the amygdala. Whereas the corticoamygdala pathways provide precise, highly processed information at the level of perceptual configurations (Aggleton & Mishkin, 1986; Turner et al., 1980), the thalamoamygdala projections appear to provide a rapid, crude representation of the sensory event (LeDoux, 1987). Since most sensory events in the natural environment are complex in character, perhaps the thalamoamygdala projections rapidly convey only essential features of critical events to which quick reaction is required.

The amygdala has a critical role in classical stimulus-reinforcement conditioning. That is, the process whereby neutral stimuli are associated with the reinforcing properties of primary positive and negative reinforcers, as well as the process of modifying such associations when environmental conditions vary, appear to depend on intact amygdalar function (see Aggleton &

Mishkin, 1986, for review). Thus, when specific central sensory representations of an event are activated, the amygdala (a) through a process of associative recall, apparently activates an emotional representation of the event, (b) generates a subjective emotional experience appropriate to the emotional significance of the event (such as desire or anger), and (c) elicits neural, hormonal, and behavioral patterns that comprise the emotional response (Mishkin, 1982).

The OFC represents the highest level of hierarchical control within the basolateral limbic forebrain. It receives multimodal, integrated extero- and interoceptive sensory information (Chavis & Pandya, 1976; Jones & Powell, 1970; LeDoux, 1987; Rolls, 1986; Van Hoesen, Pandya, & Butters, 1975), as well as emotional associations formed by the amygdala with respect to contemporaneous and recalled sensory events (Aggleton & Mishkin, 1986; Porrino, Crane, & Goldman-Rakic, 1981). The OFC holds these associations on-line in representational memory (Goldman-Rakic, 1987), and incorporates them into a larger, integrated structure of appetitive and aversive behavioral contingencies abstracted from the ongoing environment. Through its efferent projections, the OFC may initiate or inhibit motor, autonomic, and neurohumoral responses to specific sensory events (Kemp & Powell, 1970; Nauta, 1986, 1971, 1964; Rolls, 1986; Rosenkilde, 1979), depending upon the previous consequences of responses to similar events. When behavioral responses evoke unexpected reinforcement outcomes, the OFC actively encodes the new contingencies to avoid continued responding to nonrewarding or irrelevant events (Rolls, 1986, 1989; Thorpe, Rolls, & Maddison, 1983).

Integral to the capacity of the OFC to exert high-level regulation over behavioral responding is it connectivity with virtually all thalamic nuclei (Malakhova, Popovkin, & Gudina, 1989), and with the magnocellular basal forebrain cholinergic projection nuclei (Mesulam & Mufson, 1984; Russchen, Amaral, & Price, 1985). Through these connections, the OFC "ochestrates" a pattern of selective activation of cortical regions, against a background of signal-sharpening inhibition (Marczynski, 1986). By activating these modulatory feedback patterns, the OFC facilitates selection and initiation of appropriate behavioral responses within cortical nodes of neural networks devoted to emotional expression (Rolls, 1986, 1989).

An Antomical-Functional Circuit Modulating Emotional Expression

Once the process of emotional evaluation has determined the significance of an event, complex neural processing must occur to determine (a) where in space and toward which objects a behavioral response is to be made, and (b) whether such a response should be performed given the expected outcome of the response under this particular set of environmental circumstances. As shown in Figure 2, these determinations are accomplished via partially closed "loops" that extend from frontal and other regions of the cortex, through

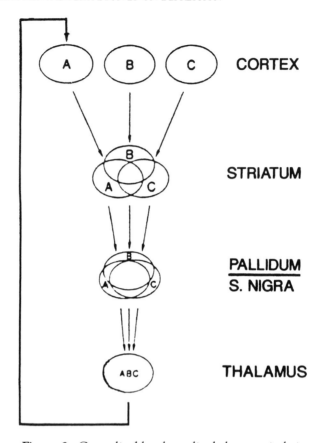

Figure 2. Generalized basal ganglia-thalamocortical circuit. "Skeleton" diagram of the proposed basal ganglia-thalamocortical circuits. Each circuit receives output from several functionally related cortical areas (A, B, C) that send partially overlapping projections to a restricted portion of the striatum. These striatal regions send further converging projections to the globus pallidus and substantia nigra, which in turn project to a specific region of the thalamus. Each thalamic region projects back to one of the cortical areas that feeds into the circuit, thereby completing the "closed loop" portion of the circuit. From Alexander & DeLong, 1986.

striatal structures, midbrain dopamine areas, pallidal regions, thalamus, and back to the frontal cortex (Alexander, DeLong, & Strick, 1986). For example, the formulation of a program of motor movement (i.e., selection of motor movements required in making an emotional response) is accomplished in a motor circuit (see Figure 3) that begins in motor (Broadmann's areas 8, 6, 4) and somatosensory (areas 3, 1, 2, 5) cortical regions, both of which are somatotopically organized precisely and can project information about specific body parts (e.g., the wrist) or specific movement of a body part (e.g., flexion of the wrist). This information, which is clustered into leg, face, and arm fiber bundles, is projected to the putamen. In the putamen, there are somatotopically organized matrices of cell clusters located within leg, face, and arm sectors that represent specific movements of body parts. Thus, the matrices allow for specific representations of movements to be formed and activated, while irrelevant movements are inhibited. Only the relevant matrices or movements are activated by the putamen's excitation of somatotopically relevant areas of the substantia nigra, which sends back dopamine projections to the relevant putamen matrices to switch this information through to the globus pallidus. Also somatotopically organized, the globus pallidus integrates the input from the putamen in relation to body parts, e.g., all facial inputs are integrated to represent the facial expression that is relevant to the emotional response. This information is then passed on to several nuclei in the thalamus, which direct the information to the somatotopically organized supplimentary motor area (SMA), which sequences and initiates the now programmed motor patterns by activating cortical motor regions that project to the spinal cord. The circuit is looped or partially closed so that a motor pattern can be maintained and/or updated (around the loop) for as long as is necessary.

Other, similarly organized circuits determine (a) a program for eye movements (the oculomotor circuit), (b) where in space the eyes and the above formulated motor patterns should be directed (the dorsolateral prefrontal cortical loop), and (c) toward which particular objects in that space movements should be directed (the lateral orbital prefrontal cortical circuit). All of this information converges on the SMA for exact sequencing and initiation of movement.

This picture is incomplete in that a circuit is needed to determine whether, under current emotional outcome expectations, the formulated motor programs *should* be released to activate the musculature. This is apparently the role of the neural network underlying the BFS, which we refer to as the medial orbital prefrontal circuit. The fundamental loop originates in the reciprocally interconnected triad of medial OFC, temporal pole, and amygdala. Upon detection of an incentive stimulus, information regarding its appetitive associations is transmitted by the amygdala and temporal pole to the OFC. The OFC encodes this information within its ongoing representation of the structure of environmental reinforcement, which may be augmented by input organized by hippocampal formation regarding similar stimuli experienced in the past. Assuming for the moment that an appropriate motor response is to be initiated in response to the incentive stimulus, the OFC transmits information regarding initiation or alteration of locomotor activity to the ventral striatum, which includes the nucleus accumbens (NAS). The NAS, like other striatal structures (e.g., putamen and caudate), may be a repository of phylogenetically old, species-specific response tendencies. The NAS, however, apparently does not formulate the actual motor program for these response tendencies, as in the

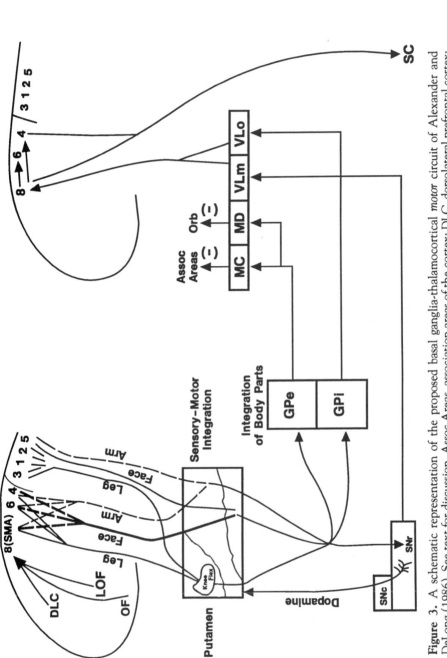

Figure 3. A schematic representation of the proposed basal ganglia-thalamocortical *motor* circuit of Alexander and DeLong (1986). See text for discussion. Assoc Areas, association areas of the cortex; DLC, dorsolateral prefrontal cortex; GPe, external segment of globus pallidus; GPi, internal segment of globus pallidus; LOF, lateral orbital prefrontal cortex; MC, MD, VLm, VLo, specific thalamic nuclei; OF and Orb, orbital frontal cortex; SC, spinal cord; SMA, supplementary motor area; SNc, substantia nigra, pars compacta; SNr, substantia nigra, pars reticulata. Numbers refer to Brodmann's

motor circuit described above. Rather, it apparently transmits information regarding whether the motor program should be initiated at all, and with what
degree of vigor it should be performed. That is, the NAS integrates the motivational imperative associated with the current environmental conditions and
transmits this imperative to the motor system. Thus, the NAS sends topo-
graphically organized inputs to the ventral tegmental area's (VTA) dopaminergic projections (as the putamen does to the substantia nigra), which
return, in part, to the NAS. These VTA dopamine projections, in like manner
to those of the substantia nigra in the motor circuit, (a) initiate the release of
specific NAS information, and (b) apparently code the relative vigor that each
motor movement should have. The NAS information is passed to the ventral
pallidum, which in turn relays output through the thalamus to the SMA,
premotor, and motor cortices. In this way, the SMA not only receives the
motor program but also information on the go-no go status of the motor program, and on the relative vigor with which specific movements should be
made. The ventral pallidum also initiates a descending projection to the me-
sencephalic motor area that eventually terminates on motor pattern gener-
ators in the spinal cord that mediate, for instance, motor patterns that support
forward locomotion, a major component of BFS behavior.

Dopamine Innervation of the Basolateral Limbic Forebrain: Implications for Behavioral Facilitation System Function

The above discussion on neural circuits involved in motor behavior indicates that dopamine (DA) plays a critical role in the functioning of the
circuits. In both the motor circuit and the medial orbital prefrontal loop, DA
projections to the striatum (putamen and NAS, respectively) provide a means
of facilitating the flow of specific information from striatal to pallidal structures. That DA's facilitatory role in these circuits is critical is dramatically
illustrated in the retarded motor behavior of Parkinson's disease, where the
deterioration of DA cells in the substantia nigra result in a loss of DA
facilitation in the putamen in the motor circuit.

DA neurons of the mesencephalon appear to have the general function of
facilitating neural processes in brain regions they innervate. This functional
principle of DA activity is manifested generally in motivational-emotional,
goal-directed behavior, where the general effects of DA agonists in rats and
monkeys are to facilitate locomotor activity, incentive-reward motivation,
exploratory behavior (when applied particularly to the NAS and perhaps
certain areas of prefrontal cortex), aggressive behavior (when applied particularly to the amygdala), formulation of behavioral strategies, and acquisition
and maintenance of approach and active avoidance behavior (Depue, in
press; Louilot et al., 1987; Oades, 1985). Conversely, bilateral 6-hydroxydo-
pamine (6OHDA) lesions in rats and monkeys resulting in DA reductions of
90% or more in the VTA or NAS produce major deficits in the initiation of
behavior associated with incentive motivation, including social interaction,

sexual behavior, food-hoarding, maternal nursing behavior, approach and active avoidance responses, exploratory activity in novel environments, and locomotor activity. Thus, as in the lack of facilitation of sensorimotor integration in Parkinson's disease due to DA deficiency, lesions of DA cells in the VTA appear to result in a generalized lack of facilitation of motivated, emotional behavior. This suggests that DA may play a critical modulatory role in the function of the BFS in motivational processes, and in the organization and initiation of goal-directed behavior.

The underlying neural network of the BFS, i.e., the basolateral limbic forebrain including the ventral striatum, is, indeed, strongly innervated by projections arising from the VTA A10 DA cells. We shall briefly describe selective behavioral functions of two VTA DA ascending systems that innervate BFS structures, referred to as the mesolimbic and mesocortical systems (see Figure 4 for the location of structures described below).

Selected BFS Functions of the Mesolimbic
Dopamine Projection System

Perhaps the largest VTA mesolimbic DA projection is to the ventral striatum, i.e., the NAS, olfactory tubercle, and ventromedial caudate. There is substantial evidence that these structures, and in particular the NAS, serve as a functional interface between limbic structures, which integrate motivational processes, and the extrapyramidal motor system, which integrates motor responses (Mogenson, Jones, & Yim, 1980; Oades & Halliday, 1987; Nauta, 1986). As noted above in the discussion of the medial orbital circuit, VTA DA projections to the NAS facilitate the flow of motivational information to the motor system, which informs the motor program as to the imperative value of the current situation. DA release in the NAS appears to be associated with two major BFS functions, i.e., incentive-reward motivation as a means of motivating approach to a goal, and initiation of forward locomotion which provides the means to reach a goal, while DA release in the amygdala may be related to the threshold for emotional expression.

Incentive-reward motivation. Several recent reviews have concluded that DA is integral to rewarding stimulation of mes- and diencephalic loci, although a lesser role for norepinephrine has not been ruled out (Bozarth, 1987; Fibiger & Phillips, 1987; Mason, 1984). Although the initial activation during intracranial self-stimulation (ICSS) occurs in non-DA, myelinated, fast-conducting neurons, at least some of which are cholinergic (Gallistel, Shizgal, & Yeomans, 1981), these first-stage fibers descend to trans-synaptically activate a second-stage fiber system consisting of ascending mesolimbic DA projections (Bozarth, 1987). Fibiger and Phillips (1987) reported increased DA metabolism during VTA-ICSS confined to the structures of the ventral striatum (NAS, olfactory tubercle, ventromedial caudate) ipsilateral to the

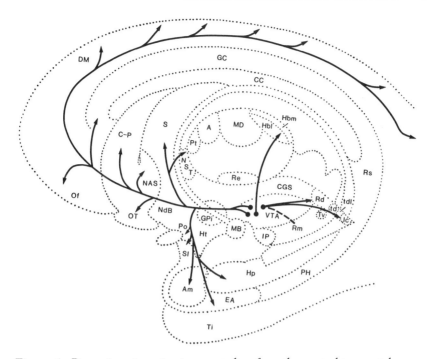

Figure 4. Dopaminergic projections ascending from the ventral tegmental area (shown as one mesolimbic-mesocortical bundle for clarity), as described in the text. A: nucleus anterior thalami; Am: amygdala; CC: corpus callosum, CGS: Central grey substance; C-P: caudatoputamen; EA: entorhinal area; GC: gyrus cinguli; GPi: globus pallidus, internal segment; Hbl: lateral habenular nucleus; Hbm: medial habenular nucleus; Hp: hippocampal formation; Ht: hypothalamus; IP: interpeduncular nucleus; lc: locus coeruleus; MB: mammillary body; MD: nucleus mediodorsalis thalami; Nacc: nucleus accumbens; NdB: nucleus of the diagonal band of Broca; NST: bed-nucleus of stria terminalis; OF: orbitofrontal cortex; OT: olfactory tubercle; PH: parahippocampal gyrus; Po: preoptic area; Pt: nucleus parataenialis thalami; Rd: dorsal raphe nucleus; Re: nucleus reuniens thalami; Rm: median raphe nucleus; Rs: retrosplenial cortex; SI: substantia innominata; td: dorsal tegmental nucleus of Gudden; tdl: nucleus tegmenti dorsalis lateralis; Ti: inferior temporal cortex. (Adapted from Nauta & Domesick 1981).

stimulating electrode. Furthermore, direct pharmacological evidence for specific DA involvement in VTA-ICSS was obtained in a study employing unilateral microinjections of the DA receptor antagonist spiroperidol into the NAS (Mogenson, Takigawa, Robertson, & Wu, 1979). Microinjections into either the ipsilateral or contralateral prefrontal cortex did not affect VTA-ICSS, suggesting that DA mediation of rewarding VTA stimulation does not require activation of telencephalic DA receptors.

In a related line of research, psychomotor stimulants such as amphetamine and cocaine have been shown to enhance responding during ICSS (Bozarth, 1987). Both drugs potentiate DA activity by blocking the reuptake process that normally terminates synaptic DA actions, while amphetamine may also increase DA release (Koob & Bloom, 1988). Moreover, humans, other primates, and rats perform operant responses to receive intravenous administrations or microinjections of the drugs (stimulant self-administration or SSA; Wise, 1978). Wise (1982) proposed that the VTA-NAS pathway is activated by all forms of rewarding stimuli, and DA lesioning studies have indicated that an intact VTA-NAS pathway is necessary for the rewarding effects of stimulants (Lyness, Friedle, & Moore, 1979; Roberts, Corcoran, & Fibiger, 1977; Roberts, Koob, Klonoff, & Fibiger, 1980). In contrast, lesions of other DA terminal fields, e.g., in the caudate, or of NE projections do not affect SSA (Roberts & Zito, 1987). Furthermore, studies using both ICSS and SSA have revealed an overlapping pattern of regional alterations in subcortical DA metabolism (Porrino, 1987; Porrino, Esposito, Crane, Sullivan, & Pert, 1984), leading Porrino (1987) to conclude that rewarding self-administration of electrical stimulation and psychomotor stimulants produce converging activation of VTA mesolimbic DA pathways. Thus, it seems clear that a neurobiological substrate for the mediation of reward, and presumably the generation of incentive motivation, is represented within BFS circuitry by the dopaminergic VTA-NAS pathway. It is interesting to note in this context that while the OFC plays an integral role in emotional evaluation and expression within the BFS, it does not directly participate in the mediation of the intervening state of incentive motivation (Mogenson et al., 1979).

Initiation of Locomotor Activity (LA). Processes involved in the generation of volitional locomotion can be divided into three useful, albeit oversimplified, phases: initiation, programming, and execution. Processes involved in LA initiation have received comparatively least attention, but it is specifically this phase of locomotor generation that relates to the facilitation construct of the BFS because the initiation process is closely tied to affective/motivational input to the motor system.

There is a vast literature demonstrating that DA (but not norepinephrine, NE) is the primary neurotransmitter in the initiation of LA (see reviews by Fishman, Feigenbaum, Yanaiz, & Klawans, 1983; Iversen, 1978; Kelly, 1978; Oades, 1985). Importantly, LA initiation occurs via the action of DA and its agonists in the mesolimbic DA system, in general, and in the VTA A10 DA projection to the NAS, in particular. A recent review concluded that, although some role for the striatum in LA appears likely (as some role for the NAS in stereotypy may exist), "a formidable number of studies have demonstrated that DA and its agonists injected into the NAS induce a greater arousal of LA than equivalent injections in the striatum; there are virtually no studies in the literature to the contrary" (Fishman et al., 1983, p. 61). Moreover, the quantity of spontaneous exploratory LA and magnitude of amphetamine-induced LA are both positively related to number of DA neurons (including those of the VTA cell group), the relative density of innervation of DA terminals in target fields, and DA content in the NAS in inbred mouse strains, effects perhaps related to the proportionately greater synthesis and release of DA in high-DA neuron mouse strains (Fink & Reiss, 1981; Oades, 1985, Sved, Baker, & Reis, 1984, 1985). Mesolimbic DA projections to the amygdala and olfactory tubercle do not account in a significant way for initiation of LA (Oades, 1985; Oades, Taghzouti, Rivet, Simon, & Le Moal, 1986).

Threshold of emotional expression. The VTA projects strongly to the amygdala. Indeed, approximately 90% of the DA in the amygdala is derived from VTA projections, which terminate in several nuclei of the amygdala, including the central, anterior lateral, posterior lateral, medial, and basal (Moore & Bloom, 1978; Oades & Halliday, 1987). The basolateral, medial, and central nuclei receive the densest DA innervation. The DA projections to the central and medial nuclei of the amygdala may have significance for BFS facilitation of emotional behavior, since these nuclei serve as important centers for output from the amygdala to brainstem and hypothalamic areas involved in the activation of vocal, gross motor, facial, hormonal, and autonomic aspects of emotional behavior. DA apparently influences the threshold for output from the amygdala, since increased DA activity in the central nuclei, for instance, facilitates remarkably the expression of aggressive behavior (Depue & Iacono, 1989).

Summary. Thus, activation of VTA DA projections to the limbic striatum and amygdala appears to facilitate behavioral functions that support emotional engagement of the animal with environmental goals. These functions include incentive motivation, forward locomotion, and enhanced emotional expression, and as such, they define core functions proposed for the BFS construct.

Selected BFS Functions of the Mesocortical Dopamine Projection System

Active goal-seeking facilitated by the BFS will increase interaction with, and hence the need to evaluate, the environment. To assure that approach behavior is adaptively related to stimulus events, there will be an increased need to design maps of extrapersonal space, to identify objects in space, to organize behavior strategies, and to evaluate the emotional significance of objects and the outcomes of those behavioral strategies. We suggest that the BFS, via the mesocortical DA projection system, plays a critical facilitatory role in these processes. An expansion of neocortical DA projections ascending from the VTA has paralleled the expansion of the neocortex itself in mammalian evolution. This connectivity can be observed in rat brain (Berger, Verney, Alvarez, Vigny, & Helle, 1985), but it is particularly extensive in primate brain, in which virtually all neocortical regions are innervated by VTA DA projections (Lewis, Campbell, Foots, & Morrison, 1986). In relative terms, DA density is lowest in primary visual, auditory, and somatosensory regions, and highest in motor, premotor, and supplemental motor cortices. DA density is intermediate but variable within the temporal and parietal cortices. In the temporal lobe, DA density is low in the caudal portion of the superior gyrus (which includes primary auditory cortex), high in the rostral portion (auditory association cortex), and intermediate in the inferior gyrus (visual association cortex). In the parietal lobe, DA density is significantly higher in the inferior lobule.

The concentration of DA in prefrontal cortex (PFC) is among the highest of all cortical areas in monkeys (Brown, Crane, & Goldman 1979), and both DA-containing terminals and DA receptors are prominent in the PFC of primates (Berger, Trottier, Verney, Gaspar, & Alvarez 1988; Gaspar, Berger, Febvret, Vigny, & Henry 1989; Levitt, Rakic, & Goldman-Rakic 1984a,b; Lewis, Campbell, Foote, Goldstein, & Morrison 1987; Lewis, Foote, Goldstein, & Morrison 1988; Lidow, Goldman-Rakic, Rakic, & Innis 1989) and humans (Camps, Cortes, Gueye, Probst, & Palacios 1989; Cortes, Gueye, Pazos, Probst, & Palacios 1989). More specific innervation patterns were reported by Porrino and Goldman-Rakic (1982), where prefrontal areas on the ventral surface of the frontal lobe (inferior convexity, medial and lateral orbital cortex, frontal pole) were innervated preferentially by midline VTA nuclei. Dorsolateral and dorsomedial prefrontal areas were innervated by a band of cells that extends laterally from the midline VTA to the medial region of the substantia nigra.

In recent years there has been increasing interest in the neurobiology of higher-order cognitive function. Much of this interest has focused specifically on the ability of the PFC to provide an association between events separated in time: that is, between environmental stimuli that occur sequentially and together signal the appropriateness of particular motor responses (Funahashi, Bruce, & Goldman-Rakic 1989; Fuster 1973, 1980; Kubota & Niki 1971; Niki 1974a,b,c; Sawaguchi, Matsumura, & Kubota 1988, 1990a,b; Watanabe & Niki 1985). Goldman-Rakic (1987, 1988) has suggested that a critical prefrontal process for spanning the time period between stimuli and response is a special form of short-term memory, referred to as working memory. Working memory refers to the mnemonic process(es) by which information relevant for an appropriate response is temporarily maintained or held "on line," to be reevaluated or updated on a trial-by-trial basis (Baddeley 1986; Baddeley & Hitch 1974; Friedman, Janas, & Goldman-Rakic 1990; Olton, Becker, & Handelmann 1979; Roitblat 1987).

The functional importance of DA to one form of cognition, spatial mnemonic processing, has been demonstrated by several findings. First, 6-hydroxydopamine lesions of the dorsolateral convexity of the PFC have produced impaired spatial delayed alternation performance in rhesus monkeys, an effect reversed by DA agonists (Brozoski, Brown, Rosvold, & Goldman 1979). Second, DA enhances the activity of PFC neurons of monkeys that is correlated with events related to mnemonic processes, including the spatial visual cue, the delay, and/or the response during the performance of delayed response tasks (Sawaguchi et al., 1988, 1990a,b). Third, DA enhances spatial delayed performance in humans (Luciana, Depue, Arbisi, & Leon, 1992). Fourth, pharmacological blockade of DA receptors in monkeys has been shown to cause a reversible decrement in accuracy and latency of an oculomotor spatial delayed response task (Sawaguchi & Goldman-Rakic 1991). In accordance with the BFS construct, Sawaguchi et al. (1988, 1990a,b) concluded that "dopamine plays a role in the neuronal processes of facilitating . . . goal-directed behaviors associated with spatial cues of memory traces, as well as those associated with non-spatial cues used for environmental adaptation" (1988, p. 472).

Recent conceptualizations of the neurobiologic basis of cognition have emphasized a network approach (Goldman-Rakic 1987, 1988; Kosslyn 1988; Mesulam 1984, 1990; Posner, Petersen, Fox, & Raichle 1988). The proposal is that complex cognitive functions are composed of many elementary operations, and each operation is localized in distinct, yet interconnected, cortical and subcortical regions. Collectively, these brain regions and their connections constitute an integrated network for that function. Coordination of such an integrated network would require communication between the distinct brain regions involved, as well as facilitation of neural processes within nodes of the network (Goldman-Rakic 1987, 1988). As discussed above, mesocortical DA projections appear to facilitate or enhance task- related processes within nodes of such a network (Sawaguchi & Goldman-Rakic 1991; Sawaguchi et al., 1988, 1990a,b). They may also initiate or gate the transfer of information across the different brain regions of a network, as suggested by Oades' review (1985), by facilitating long corticocortical, corticostriatal, and corticotectal projection neurons.

In general, then, mesocortical DA projections may serve to facilitate goal-directed activity, as do mesolimbic DA projections, but they would facilitate neocortical, rather than limbic, processes that underlie cognitive functions necessary for behavior flexibility. A similar conclusion was reached by others based on extensive reviews of DA's role in behaviors that require higher-order cognitive functioning, i.e., behavioral responses to changing environmental contingencies, as in alternation, reversal, and extinction paradigms, and in tasks requiring changes in cognitive behavioral strategies (Cools 1980; Louilot, Taghzouti, Deminiere, Simon, & LeMoal 1987; Oades 1985).

VTA DA Coordination of the BFS Neural Network

When an appropriate response to an incentive cue involves motor activity, the OFC activates the NAS. Physiologically, however, this OFC projection appears to hold the NAS under tonic inhibition (Glowinski, Tassin, & Thierry, 1984), and activation of VTA DA projections to both the OFC and the NAS is required if a motor response is to occur. Thus, DA activation may be divided into three components: first, the OFC activates an excitatory projection to the VTA (Thierry, Deniau, & Feger, 1979; Thierry et al., 1984); second, the VTA activates an excitatory projection to the NAS (Reibaud, Blanc, Studler, Glowinski, & Tassin, 1984; Tassin, Simon, Glowinski, & Bockaert, 1982); and third, the VTA may activate an inhibitory backprojection to the OFC (Reader, Ferron, Descarries, & Jasper, 1979; Stone, 1976; Stone & Bailay, 1975), which temporarily removes the tonic inhibition of the OFC over the NAS.

Essentially, then, the OFC recruits both its own inhibition and excitation of the NAS, and the amygdala as well, by activating specific nuclei in the VTA. This pattern is consistent with a general model of prefrontal cortical functioning (Goldman-Rakic, 1987), in which specific prefrontal areas tonically inhibit a diverse network of cortical and subcortical structures that subserve a particular behavioral function. By activating a subset of VTA nuclei, a prefrontal area may initiate coordinated excitation of DA pathways to other structures in its circuit that, in turn, ultimately execute the behavioral function organized in the prefrontal area. This may occur, for instance, in the medial orbital prefrontal circuit described above. In addition, recruitment of inhibitory VTA DA backprojections to prefrontal cortex may influence activity in other behaviorally relevant cortical regions, since part of the mesocortical DA innervation consistently terminates in cortical layers containing reciprocal corticocortical projections (Lewis et al., 1986).

Thus, core DA influences in the initiation of motor and emotional responses to incentive stimuli occur within the OFC-VTA-NAS pathways, and the importance of this subcircuit is reflected in its neuroanatomical connectivity. These innervations themselves overlap, in that ascending VTA projections to the prefrontal cortex terminate in the same regions that originate descending projections to the NAS and amygdala, and the projections of the VTA, the amygdala, and the OFC converge on the same terminal zones in the NAS (Beckstead, 1979; Phillipson & Griffiths, 1985). The full pattern of VTA innervation of BFS structures, however, extends to the temporal pole in terms of incentive stimulus evaluation, and to the motor, premotor, and supplemental motor cortices in terms of execution of behavioral responses.

Overall, DA activity may be conceptualized as facilitating the OFC "orchestration" of neural excitation and inhibition within other cortical and subcortical structures, at least within environmental contexts that elicit incentive motivation. At the behavioral level, the VTA DA systems would facilitate emotional evaluation of rapidly occuring incentive events, particularly when such sequences signal a change in previous reward contingencies. Moreover, DA would facilitate continuous adaptation of motor sequences to ensure that the energizing influence of incentive motivation results in positive behavioral engagement. At the cognitive level, DA would facilitate the construction and serial testing of alternative strategies to obtain perceived, but initially distant, rewards. In humans, DA facilitation may be essential for goal-oriented behavior that requires delay of gratification, since central representations of the ultimate reward must be continuously adapted to sequential revisions in long-term planning, presumably mediated by the PFC (Goldman-Rakic, 1987); moreover, DA activity would appear to be critical in maintaining incentive motivation throughout the period of delayed gratification.

Dopamine, the BFS, and the Structure of Personality

The BFS can be viewed not simply as a passive response system to stimuli, but rather as a dynamic system that influences emotional evaluation of incentive stimuli. There is evidence suggesting that responsivity of the BFS to incentive stimuli is dependent on the current state of BFS activity (Beninger, 1983; Beninger, Hanson, & Phillips, 1980; Blackburn et al., 1989; Hill, 1970; Panksepp, 1986; Robbins, 1975). That is, the effective incentive value of a stimulus is a relative function of stimulus intensity and current BFS activity, which implies that variation in trait levels of BFS activity may influence sensitivity to incentive stimuli. Such trait differences would have the effect of modulating: (a) percieved intensity of incentive stimuli; (b) intensity and frequency of subjective experience of desire, incentive, and positive feelings; and (c) the threshold for stimulus-elicitation of overt emotional responses.

Variation in DA functioning could underly individual differences in BFS activity. In a 33 year old man, there are approximately 450,000 cells in the VTA-substantia nigra complex, and this number may vary across individuals by as much as ± 20,000 cells (Oades & Halliday, 1987). Importantly, variation in DA cell number does affect BFS behaviors. As noted above, the quantity of spontaneous exploratory locomotion and magnitude of amphetamine-induced locomotion are both positively related to number of DA neurons (including those of the VTA cell group), the relative density of innervation of DA terminals in target fields, and to DA content in the NAS in inbred mouse strains (Fink & Reiss, 1981; Oades, 1985; Sved, Baker, & Reis, 1984, 1985).

This conceptualization of a DA-BFS trait resembles existing personality "supertraits" or "superfactors", which represent common influences across a number of individual, lower-order traits, just as the BFS is viewed as influencing a number of lower-order behaviors. Almost every trait theory of personality includes a dimension that encompasses positive affect, desire, incentive motivation, and a sense of personal efficacy. Numerous labels have been used, including extraversion (e.g., Eysenck & Eysenck, 1985), but because of the emotional aspects of the trait, we prefer positive emotionality.

In developing his Multidimensional Personality Questionnaire (MPQ), Tellegen has proposed an emotional systems approach to the structure of personality (see review by Tellegen & Waller, in press). This structure includes a superfactor, labelled positive emotionality (PE), that corresponds to the BFS construct, correlates strongly (.62 – .01) with Eysenck's EPQ Extraversion scale, and is subject to significant genetic influence. Tellegen systematically incorporated many subdomains into the item pool that comprises the emotional experience associated with the BFS, including sociability, social potency or dominance, positive emotional feelings, incentive or achievement motivation and its subjective sense of desire and excitement, level of energy and activity, etc. The affective interpretation of higher order MPQ PE is supported by its convergent-discriminant relations to the state dimensions of Positive and Negative Affect, respectively, which dominate measures of current mood. Importantly, there is a strong emphasis on effectance motivation; for example, amount of socialization is less relevant than one's perceived effectiveness and "power" in social interaction. This emphasis is more in keeping with the motivational aspect of the BFS construct.

A Preliminary Study of Dopamine Activity and Human Positive Emotionality

The validity of drawing comparisons between the personality construct of PE and the construct of the BFS developed from animal research may be addressed by assessing similarities in their neurobiology. To this end, we measured the effects of a specific DA receptor agonist on two indices of central DA activity in subjects widely distributed along the dimension of MPQ PE (Depue, Luciana, Arbisi, Collins, & Leon, submitted). Two indices of DA response, prolactin and spontaneous eye blinking, served as a within-study replication of a PE-DA association, since they are innervated by separate DA projection systems.

The experimental manipulation involved administration of bromocriptine mesylate, a potent and specific agonist at D_2 receptor sites. Bromocriptine has a time-dependent biphasic effect, in which its initial agonist effect on presynaptic D_2 autoreceptors is inhibitory to DA function, while its subsequent postsynaptic D_2 effect accompanying rising concentrations in blood activates DA function. Behaviorally, the biphasic effect may be seen in an initial dose-dependent immobility or hypomotility in rats, followed some time later, depending on dose, by hyperlocomotion. The latter effect suggests that bromocriptine activates DA terminals involved in initiating processes relevant to the BFS construct (i.e., forward locomotion and incentive-reward motivation).

Subjects were caucasian premenopausal females (n=11) ranging in age from 20–36 years (M±SD = 28.3±3.1) who were sampled evenly along the full dimension of MPQ PE. The protocol ran from 11 AM to 6 PM, beginning with the insertion into the firearm of an indwelling intravenous catheter with heparin lock. In a randomized, crossover design under double-blind conditions, identical bromocriptine (2.5 mg) or placebo (2.5 mg lactose) capsules were ingested at 12 noon. The two drug condition were separated by no less than three days.

Our first DA indicator, prolactin (PRL) secretion, was assessed because DA is the primary substance of hypothalamic origin involved in the tonic inhibition of PRL secretion. In humans, PRL secretion is reliably and markedly inhibited by bromocriptine in a dose-dependent fashion, with strong correlations between inhibition of PRL secretion and bromocriptine dose and serum concentration [$r = -.93$, $p = 0.001$; $r = -.76$, $p = 0.02$, respectively]. Time-dependent biphasic effects of bromocriptine on PRL have been observed. Pre-drug samples for baseline serum PRL were obtained at 11:45 AM and 11:55 AM and averaged; 10 post-drug samples were obtained every 30 minutes from 1:00–5:30 PM.

Each bromocriptine-inhibited PRL value was corrected for daily variation in pre-drug PRL baseline, and for natural diurnal variation reflected in the series of placebo values. Using these adjusted PRL values, we first assessed the presynaptic D_2 receptor effects of bromocriptine on PRL secretion. We reasoned that two variables, each reflecting the time to bromocriptine's postsynaptic inhibition of PRL secretion, would assess the efficacy of presynaptic activation: (a) time until the first consistent drug-induced reduction in PRL values (PRL Descent), and (b) time until the point of maximum inhibition of PRL secretion (PRL TMax). Both PRL Descent and PRL TMax were strongly related to MPQ PE (Fig. 5, C and B), suggesting the MPQ PE is related to the "sensitivity" of presynaptic D_2 autoreceptors to bromocriptine's agonist effects. These relations were specific to MPQ PE, as shown by the absence of significant correlations with MPQ Negative Emotionality (NE, r's = .33, .43, respectively, p's>0.25) and MPQ Constraint (C, r's = $-.18$, $-.11$, respectively, p's>0.50).

We assessed postsynaptic D_2 receptor effects of bromocriptine by measuring the maximum inhibitory effect of the drug on PRL secretion (PRL Max). PRL Max was strongly related to MPQ PE (Fig. 5A), but not to MPQ NE (r = .39, p<0.25) or MPQ C (r = .02, p>0.50). Moreover, bromocriptine's postsynaptic receptor index (PRL Max) was significantly related to both presynaptic receptor indices (PRL TMax, r = .88, p<0.0004; PRL Descent, r = .68, p.< 0.02). Thus, pre- and postsynaptic PRL indices of bromocriptine's D_2 receptor effects were highly correlated, and both types of synaptic indices were specifically related to MPQ PE.

To provide a replication of a PE-DA association, we measured spontaneous eye blinking. Central DA activity modulates the rate of spontaneous blinking in nonhuman primates and man. The neurocircuitry of spontaneous blinking is complex, but the importance of nigrostriatal projections has been demonstrated, which are distinctly different from the hypothalamic DA projections involved in the control of PRL secretion.

Two-minute epochs of spontaneous eye blink rate (EBR) were video taped just prior to all PRL samples. Time to reach a maximum rate of drug-induced blinking (Blink TMax) was strongly related to MPQ PE (Fig. 5E), and again

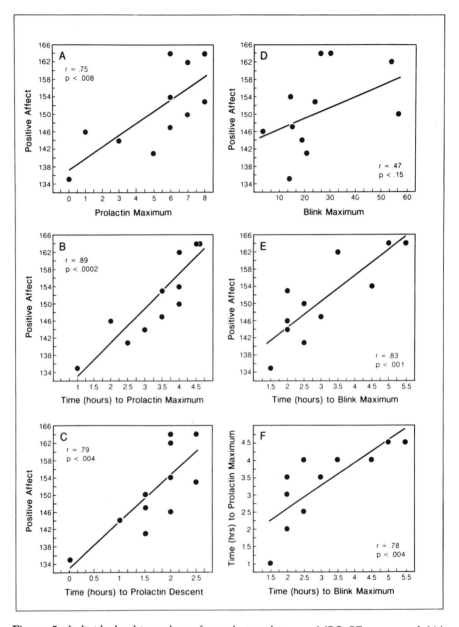

Figure 5. Individual subject plots of correlations between MPQ PE scores and (A) maximum inhibitory effect of bromocriptine on prolactin secretion, (B) time to reach the maximum inhibition of prolactin secretion by bromocriptine, (C) time to reach initial point of consistent reduction in prolactin secretion due to bromocriptine, (D) maximum augmenting effect of bromocriptine on spontaneous eye-blinking rate, and (E) time to reach the maximum augmentation of spontaneous eye-blinking rate by bromocriptine. (F) represents the correlation between Time to Prolactin Maximum (B) and Time to Blink Maximum (E).

specificity was indicated by the absence of significant associations between Blink TMax and MPQ NE (r = .21, p>0.30) and MPQ C (r = −.24, p>0.30). In addition, Blink TMax and PRL TMax values were strongly related (Fig. 5F), which suggests that the temporal effects of bromocriptine are similar, and are similarly related to MPQ PE (Fig. 5, B and E), across two variables that are influenced by separate DA systems.

Several points concerning interpretation of results are noted. First, because the sample was selected along the diagonal of greatest behavioral variation between MPQ PE and MPQ C, the correlations between MPQ PE and DA response indices may be smaller in unrestricted samples. The goal of the current study, however, was not to estimate the PE-DA relation in the population, but rather to demonstrate a specific and potentially important relation between PE and DA, if such existed. Second, because PRL and EBR are regulated by a variety of neurotransmitters and neuropeptides, associations between DA indices and PE may be obscured under *basal* conditions, as indicated in our data by the lack of association between MPQ PE and baseline PRL (r = .21, p>0.30), baseline EBR (r = .19, p>0.30), and pre-Descent PRL (r = −0.15, p>0.30) values. Interpretative clarity is increased in this study because the response to a DA receptor agonist was assessed. Thus, a PE-DA association emerged only after reactivity of DA systems was induced. Third, interpretation of the effects of bromocriptine on PRL and EBR as due solely to nonspecific processes unrelated to DA functioning seems unlikely. We have observed no significant magnitude or temporal effects (p's>0.30) of bromocriptine on biletter cancellation (attention) and spatial location (memory) tasks, or on blood pressure (general arousal).

Taken together, the current findings suggest that the trait structure of personality is related to the responsivity of central DA projection systems. What is intriguing is that PRL and EBR variables, reflecting the action of DA in the hypothalamic and nigrostriatal DA systems, respectively, were so strongly related to a set of personality behaviors that most likely reflect DA function in ascending projections arising from VTA DA cells. It is known that DA cell groups, including those in the substantia nigra, VTA, and hypothalamus, can manifest a common genetic influence that is reflected in their functional properties. For instance, DA agonist effects are correlated across PRL secretion, exploratory behavior, and locomotor activity in inbred strains of mice that differ in DA cell number within all DA cell groups. It is possible, therefore, that the heritability of MPQ PE is related to genetic influences on DA cell groups, and that unmeasured genetic variance in our subjects contributed substantially to the observed correlations between MPQ PE and drug response indices controlled by separate DA projection systems. In any case, the consistently strong and specific PE-DA associations indicate that the emotional-behavioral functions of DA derived from animal research may hold for humans as well.

Neural and Behavioral Development within the BFS

If the BFS underlies or contributes to a major emotional trait dimension in humans, it must be subject to sources of variation that ultimately produce stable individual differences in levels of BFS responsivity. Whether genetic or environmental, these influences will converge within the adaptive neural circuitry of the BFS to produce functional variations, such as individual differences in DA responsivity, that correspond to variation in behavioral trait levels. Thus, one approach to understanding the developmental origins of individual differences within the BFS is to examine genetic and environmental processes as they shape the development of its underlying neural system, i.e., to focus upon a neurobiological interface between genotype and environment. At present, this approach is constrained by the relative paucity of neurodevelopmental data beyond the early postnatal period, but several sources of influence over mammalian neural system development have been studied in detail. Although this work has been applied primarily to perceptual and cognitive development, an extension to the development of emotional systems, if valid, would provide an organizational structure for future study of the origins of BFS trait levels. Accordingly, we will outline these neurodevelopmental influences, and describe how they might apply to neural and behavioral development within the BFS.

Sources of Influence in Structural and Functional Brain Development

Within the developmental neurobiology literature, Greenough and colleagues (e.g., Black & Greenough, 1986; Greenough & Black, in press; Greenough, Black, & Wallace, 1987) have proposed a framework in which three basic sources of input to the developing brain induce functional specialization across a variety of information processing pathways. First, "genotype driven" processes influence the basic structure and function of neuron populations in a manner that is largely insensitive to experiential input. These processes are most prominent during embryological development, although the rapidly expanding field of behavioral teratology is beginning to document the effects of nongenetic influences, e.g., drugs or alcohol, within the intrauterine environment. Second, "experience-expectant" processes occur within sensitive periods in brain development, and they involve widespread overproduction of neuronal synapses that preceeds environmental experience. Through selective preservation and strengthening of a subset of these synapses, species-typical patterns of neuronal cytoarchitecture are established during exposure to phylogenetically predictable forms of environmental experience. This type of development is regulated rather than driven to genotype, i.e., the timing and regional location of experience-expectant synaptic overproduction are determined by genotypic influences, but the functional relations encoded by the preserved synapses vary in response to environmental experience. Third, "experience-dependent" processes modify neuronal cytoarchitecture to encode environmental experience that is unique to the individual, and thus unpredictable on the basis of phylogeny. In contrast to experience-expectant development, experience-dependent processes involve localized synapse production that is initiated during the encoding of information arising from any significant form of experience, including mentation; thus, the timing and location of experience-dependent modifications are not influenced by genotype. Although the three types of processes undoubtedly overlap during the development of neural systems, it is useful to consider them separately in terms of their possible application to individual differences within the BFS.

Genotype-Driven Development

The technical features of genotype-driven processes during pre- and perinatal brain development, e.g., differentiation and specification of neuronal cell types, are not directly relevant to discussion of neurobehavioral systems of emotion. However, one outcome of genotype-driven development is of obvious importance to individual differences in BFS responsivity: variation across individuals in DA cell number. In animals, variation in DA cell number is related strongly to differences in DA-regulated behaviors, such as locomotor reactivity to novel environments (Fink & Reis, 1981; Sved, Baker, & Reis, 1984, 1985). It is likely that differences in DA cell number will have similar functional consequences in humans; for example, variation in DA cell number may have contributed to the strong association between bromocriptine-induced DA responsivity and PEM scores, as described above. Thus, one simple but important source of individual differences in BFS responsivity may be genotype-driven variation in the number of DA cells produced during prenatal development.

As with any early emerging source of neurobiological variation, behavioral correlates of differences in DA cell number would likely bear some relation to traditional classifications of "temperamental" qualities in infants. For example, an individual born with a relatively large number of DA cells would be expected to respond strongly to cues for pleasurable social interaction during early infancy, because the subjective emotional experience related to this form of reward would be relatively intense; at least within Plomin's (1986) framework, such an infant would be described with reference to a temperamental dimension of "sociability." However, we would prefer to avoid longstanding debates in the literature on infant temperament (see Goldsmith, Buss, Plomin, Rothbart, Thomas, & Chess, 1987, for discussion), and suggest instead that DA cell number at birth may represent a strong genetic contribution to a single neurobehavioral dimension of emotional development, structured by the BFS, that extends into adult personality.

Experience-Expectant Development

In contrast to genotype-driven processes, discussion of some of the technical features of experience-expectant and -dependent processes will provide a basis for their application to neurodevelopment within the BFS. A primary feature of experience-expectant processes is widespread cortical synapse overproduction, which defines sensitive periods in brain development. The magnitude of synaptic overproduction at the cortical level is striking, as juvenile synaptic density values are 75–95% above adult values in nonhuman primates (O'Kusky & Colonnier, 1982; Rakic, Bourgeois, Eckenhoff, Zecevic, & Goldman-Rakic, 1986). Following overproduction, excess cortical synapses are "pruned back" gradually in response to stimulation provided by the environment; in simple terms, a particular synapse is eliminated, or regresses, if activity at an adjacent synapse is driven more strongly by environmental stimuli. This regressive competition among synapses occurs within a relatively discrete period of time, and establishes a specific and organized pattern of functional synaptic connections within a developing cortical region. Clearly, such powerful neurodevelopmental processes are adaptive only if they are restricted to early experiences with both a predictable content and a relatively consistent timing for all young members of a species. As Greenough and Black (in press) suggested, the reliable occurrence of such experience through phylogeny may have supported the eventual emergence of animals with the capacity to encode it reliably, and with considerable specificity, during experience-expectant sensitive periods. The resulting increase in the sensitivity of neural system adaptation to local sensory environments would appear to confer a substantial competitive advantage over animals with species-typical neuroarchitecture that is fixed at birth. Furthermore, experience-expectant processes may represent one important component of a larger neurobehavioral adaptation, since the vastly expanded human neocortex is associated with both the prolongation of fetal rates of brain development into the postnatal period (see Gould, 1977), and at least a partial release from genotype-driven processes (see Killackey, 1990).

It should be noted that similar processes occur at subcortical levels, but they involve the overproduction and subsequent elimination of entire cells. The phenomenon of cell death during nervous system development has been observed in a wide variety of vertebrate species, but it appears to be less prominent in species with complex nervous systems (Huttenlocher, 1990). Conversely, cortical synapse overproduction and elimination appear to occur only in mammals, and with greatest prominence in primates (Huttenlocher,

1990; Killackey, 1990). Accordingly, the remainder of this section will focus upon experience-expectant processes as they apply to the functional development of information processing pathways within mammalian cortex.

The functional consequences of regressive synaptic competition are best illustrated by the development of stereoscopic depth perception, which emerges as specific synaptic relations are established among a set of visual cortex neurons that receive overlapping input from ocular dominance columns. Normally, these binocular neurons mediate stereoscopic depth perception by integrating inputs from separate dominance columns driven primarily by the left or right eye. If one eye is occluded, or merely forced out of alignment, during an early sensitive period in visual development, impaired depth perception will emerge as an irreversible condition (e.g., von Noorden & Dowling, 1970; Weisel & Hubel, 1963). An aberration in regressive development underlies the impairment in depth perception: the terminal fields of axons within columns corresponding to the occluded eye regress much more than those from columns corresponding to the open eye, yielding a permanently asymmetrical synaptic overlap that distorts subsequent information processing in binocular neurons (LeVay, Wiesel, & Hubel, 1980). This finding illustrates two defining characteristics of experience-expectant development: (a) it occurs within a relatively discrete temporal window; and (b) functional relations among synapses established within the window are resistant to large scale modification by later experience.

At a gross level, several cortical regions appear to undergo regressive development along a staggered time schedule (Huttenlocher, 1990, 1979; Huttenlocher, de Courten, Garey, & Van der Loos, 1982). Interestingly, Turkewitz and Kenny (1982; see also Greenough & Black, in press) have speculated that this scheduled competition may represent a mechanism similar to Piaget's "disequilibration." More specifically, early developing cortical regions may drive subsequent functional specialization in other regions by transmitting information that demands more complex integration. For example, the development of visuomotor regions may be structured by the demand to integrate an initially disruptive convergence of information, which arises as precise stimulation from early maturing proprioceptive pathways overlaps with less refined input from the relatively immature visual system. In this manner, temporally staggered regressive development may organize functional specializations within and across neural systems, so that later refinements can be accomplished efficiently in response to more complex, and less predictable, environmental stimulation (Greenough & Black, in press). The concept of a coherent "neural system" is fundamental to this formulation, because regressive synaptic events in a particular cortical region typically are accompanied by some form of alteration in associated subcortical structures (see Killackey, 1990). Greenough and Black (in press) stressed that multiple regressive periods can occur across the distributed components of a neural system, as well as within separate layers of a single cortical structure. In this context, constructing a schematic circuit of cortical and subcortical BFS structures facilitates consideration of neurodevelopmental sensitive periods with respect to BFS functional processes. The basic implication of experience-expectant processes for the development of individual differences in neural system functioning is shown schematically in Figure 6. During a period of experience-expectant development, individuals exposed to a stimulation-rich environment ("experienced" curve) will encode that experience by retaining a large number of functional synaptic connections within relevant neural system pathways. In contrast, individuals exposed to a stimulation-impoverished environment ("inexperienced" curve) will retain a relatively small number of functional synaptic connections. As a lasting consequence, individual differences will be established in the functional capacity of the neural system to respond to subsequent environmental stimulation. Similar patterns of synaptic development may occur within the BFS. For example, if experience-expectant development were to occur within the reciprocal pathways connecting the amygdala and temporal pole, an individual exposed to a reward-rich environment may establish functional synaptic relations that provide an enhanced capacity to respond to conditioned signals of reward in the future. A degree of ecological validity may be incorporated into this scenario by considering the overlap between genotype-driven and experience-expectant processes: an individual born with a relatively large number of VTA-DA cells would seek engagement with potentially rewarding stimuli, and thereby contribute actively to the development of enhanced synaptic connectivity among BFS structures during an experience-expectant sensitive period.

Experience-Dependent Development

While experience-expectant development may provide an early foundation for future neural system refinements, experience-dependent processes may mediate smaller scale synaptic modifications throughout the lifespan. Since the pioneering work of Hebb (1949), stimulation-induced changes in functional connectivity among neurons has become a tenet of neuroscientific approaches to learning and memory. Nevertheless, neuronal activity has many sources of intrinsic and extrinsic modulation, and there are a variety of potential mechanisms for functional alterations, including changes in non-neuronal elements such as the surrounding arborizations of capillary or glial cells. One of the primary contributions of Greenough and colleagues is their empirical documentation of the production of new synapses, on demand, as a fundamental component of experience-dependent processes in postweanling animals. (Of course, new synapses require corresponding non-neuronal alterations, such as changes in capillary branching; see Sirevaag, Black, Shafron & Greenough, 1988.) The most direct data is derived from studies in

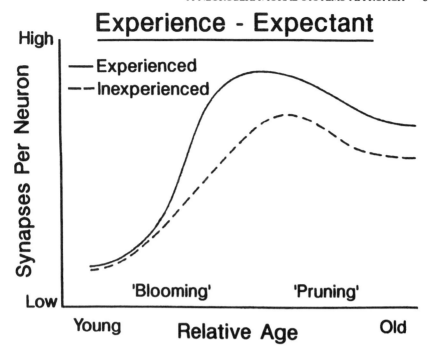

Figure 6. Schematic diagram of synapse overproduction ("blooming") and deletion ("pruning") during an experience-expectant process. From Black & Greenough (1986).

which differences in synaptic number were recorded in groups of postweanling animals (usually rats) after extended exposure to three different environments: (1) group housing in cages filled with toys that were changed daily ("environmental complexity" or EC condition), usually accompanied by daily exploration of a separate, toy-filled playbox; (2) paired housing in standard laboratory cages ("social" or SC condition); and (3) individual housing in standard cages (IC condition). Although many researchers describe EC animals as housed within an "enriched" environment, Greenough and Black (in press) emphasized that all three conditions actually are impoverished relative to the feral environment, albeit in varying degrees. The distinction is not trivial, since synaptic phenomena observed under the EC condition should be viewed as experimental analogs of what occurs in natural settings, rather than the unnatural products of laboratory manipulation.

At the behavioral level, EC animals have demonstrated consistently superior learning ability in many types of complex tasks involving potential rewards or punishers (e.g., Brown, 1968; Freeman & Ray, 1972; Greenough, Fulcher, Yuwiler, & Geller, 1970; Greenough, Wood, & Madden, 1972; Greenough, Yuwiler, & Dollinger, 1973; Morgan, 1973). At the neural level, several studies have described enhancement of various morphological features of EC animals, including a thicker visual cortex with enlarged cell bodies (Diamond, 1967) and a higher ratio of RNA and protein to DNA (i.e., altered gene expression; Rosenzweig & Bennett, 1978). Empirical data also suggest that preexisting synaptic connections may be strengthened in EC animals (e.g., Greenough, West, & De Voogd, 1978; Sirevaag & Greenough, 1985; West & Greenough, 1972). However, the most illuminating data are found in studies that reported a greater number of synapses within samples of brain tissue from EC animals. In visual cortex, EC rats have demonstrated approximately 20–25% more synapses per neuron than IC rats, with SC rats intermediate but somewhat closer to IC values (Bhide & Bedi, 1984; Greenough, 1972; Greenough & Volkmar, 1973; Turner & Greenough, 1983, 1985; Volmar & Greenough, 1972). Similar results have been reported in cats and monkeys (Beaulieu & Colonnier, 1987; Floeter & Greenough, 1979), as well as in other cortical regions, the hippocampus, and the cerebellum (Greenough, Volkmar, & Juraska, 1973; Juraska, Fitch, Henderson, & Rivers, 1985; Juraska, Fitch & Washburne, 1989; Pysh & Weiss, 1979), although effect sizes have been smaller outside of the visual cortex. Experience-dependent synapse production has no discernable association with sensitive periods, as it demonstrates a similar pattern (EC>SC>IC) and a nearly equivalent magnitude in adult or even middle-aged rats (Green, Greenough, & Schlumpf, 1983; Juraska, Greenough, Elliott, Mack, & Berkowitz, 1980; Uylings, Kuypers, & Veltman, 1978). Moreover, the synaptic patterns appear to have a specific association with learning and memory, since they do not reliably covary with generalized hormonal or metabolic alterations related to differential housing or training (see Greenough & Black, in press; Greenough et al., 1987).

In recent reviews, Greenough and Black (in press; Greenough et al., 1987) have emphasized the importance of moving beyond experimental designs in which the effects of environmental manipulations are examined in only one brain region. Obviously, such designs are difficult to interpret with respect to complex tasks employed in developmental psychology research, but they also lack clear relevance for emerging models of parallel distributed pathways or networks in neural processing. As described earlier, Goldman-Rakic (1987) has outlined a general model in which specific areas of the prefrontal cortex modulate neural activity within diverse networks of cortical and subcortical structures, each subserving a separate class of complex behavioral functions. At a more detailed level, Rolls (in press; 1989) has described task-specific correlations of single-unit activity across subsets of neurons in multimodal cortical regions, the hippocampal formation, and the amygdala. Rolls has extended these findings to a general computational model of neural networks, in which competitive learning contributes to the establishment of "ensemble encoded" associative memories, i.e., information that is stored in a distributed fashion across subsets of neurons in task-relevant brain structures. With respect to this model, Greenough and Black (in press) suggested that

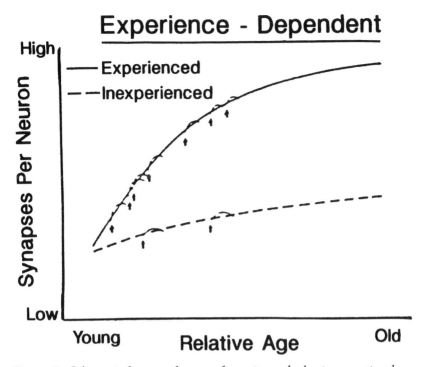

Figure 7. Schematic diagram of synapse formation and selective retention during an experience-dependent process. The arrowheads mark salient experiences that generate local synaptic overproduction and deletion (small curves). The cumulative effect of such synaptic blooms and prunes is a smooth increase in synapses per neuron, which is greater for the animals with more experience. From Black & Greenough (1986).

experience-dependent processes may continuously modify the pattern of synaptic connectivity within neural networks in response to new learning experiences.

These theoretical motions may be applied to the type of learning and memory that occurs in the BFS. Specifically, associative memories of positive behavioral engagements may be formed within the interconnected neural structures of the BFS, as they encode relations among the perceived incentive value of a stimulus, the incentive motivation experienced, and the rewarding consequences of the behavior expressed. Experience-dependent synaptic processes may mediate this ensemble encoding of emotional evaluation, experience, and expression, and thereby contribute over time to learning-related modifications in BFS responsivity. In this manner, experience-dependent processes may contribute substantially to individual differences in BFS responsivity, but unlike experience-expectant development, changes in neural system responsivity will accrue in a gradual, step-wise manner (see Figure 7).

Neurobiological Control of Synapse Production and Elimination

Although the synaptic alterations associated with experience-expectant and experience-dependent processes have been well documented, the underlying control of synaptic events remains poorly understood. By definition, the timing and magnitude of experience-expectant overproduction of synapses are controlled by specific, but largely unknown, genetic mechanisms. More data exist with respect to extrinsic neurochemical modulation of new synapses, which appears to follow a similar form in both experience-expectant and experience-dependent development. During early sensitive periods, the development of functional synaptic connections may be initiated and/or regulated by levels of thyroid and coticosteroid hormones, neurotrophic factors such as nerve growth factor, and classical neurotransmitters (reviewed by Greenough & Black, in press; see also Lauder & Krebs, 1986). More generally, the specific patterns of neuronal cyctoarchitecture produced by experience- expectant and experience-dependent processes appear to be regulated by local interactions with diffuse neurotransmitter projection systems. As described recently by Mattson (1988), these local interactions may represent modulatory processes by which projection systems contribute to the organization of input-output relations within neural systems that they innervate. Accordingly, we will outline a possible neurodevelopmental role for diffuse neurotransmitter systems, such as the projections arising from VTA DA cells, that may be related inherently to their role in modulating the functonal activity levels within neurobehavioral systems.

After axons have stopped their primary growth, a sequence of events occurs that leads to stabilization of functional synaptic contacts. During pre- and early postnatal periods, this sequence features stages of neurite outgrowth (i.e., fine, hair-like processes that extend from the tip of the developing axon, referred to as the growth cone), cessation of outgrowth, and synaptogenesis. As described previously, a stage of regressive competition completes the sequence and provides a foundation for neural systems underlying the species-typical behavioral repertoire. Particularly at higher levels of the neuraxis, e.g., allocortex, cortex, and neocortex, the release of various neurotransmitters regulates the expression of each stage in the sequence, perhaps by altering metabolic activity within neurons through second messengers such as calcium (Mattson, 1988). As a distributed form of this regulation, activity within diffuse neurotransmitter systems may guide the development of basic patterns of synaptic connectivity (see Figure 8), and thereby elevate neural system development to a level of functional fine-tuning beyond the scope of genotype-driven process (Mattson, 1988; see also Greenough & Black, in press). The developmental influence of diffuse neurotransmitter systems may be organized by intrinsic controls over the timing of specific neurochemical interactions, since receptors on developing dendrites appear to follow a staggered schedule of sensitivity to particular neurotransmitters. For example, outgrowing hippocampal dendrites are sensitive to glutamate significantly earlier than to acetylcholine (Anderson, 1979; Mattson, Dou, & Kater, 1988), and this temporal staggering may contribute to the development of segregated glutamate and acetylcholine innervation layers in the hippocampus (see Mattson, 1988).

Thus, mechanisms may exist within the growth cone for transducing the release of various neurotransmitters into signals that guide neurodevelopment at the synaptic level. Through these mechanisms, activity in neurotransmitter projection systems may regulate patterns of functional synaptic connectivity within the distributed structures of a particular neural system; for example, the activity of VTA DA cells during development may influence synaptic relations within critical neural pathways of the BFS, such as the OFC-VTA-NAS loop. In addition, alterations in neurotransmitter levels may mediate regression of dendritic terminals (Mattson, 1988), perhaps as a tightly regulated and adaptive expression of the capacity of some neurotransmitters, such as excitatory amino acids, to produce selective cell death (Watkins & Evans, 1981) or dendritic loss (Mattson et al., 1988). As Mattson (1988) noted, the potential is obvious for applying these cell-level neurotransmitter actions to the encoding of early sensory experience within neuronal cyctoarchitecture, since variation in the early sensory environment will be reflected, ultimately, in alterations of neurochemical transmission at cortical synapses. Furthermore, there is direct empirical evidence of the persistence of neurotransmitter modulation of neuronal cytoarchitecture throughout the lifespan. Put simply, the transition of nerve cell endings from growth cones to presynaptic terminals appears to be a two-way street, and reversions to growth cone mode may occur in the adult brain when locally altered neural activity levels demand changes in dendritic fields (Mattson, 1988).

From this perspective, neurotransmitter projection systems may be viewed as modulators of synaptic structure as well as function, i.e., as sources of influence over both cytoarchitectural and chemical encoding of information within neural pathways. In terms of the framework of Greenough and colleagues, neurotransmitter activity likely modulates dendritic outgrowth, synaptogenesis, and synaptic regression during both experience-expectant and experience-dependent development. Moreover, the regulation of neuroarchitecture by neurotransmitters may be one avenue for collaboration among all three forms of neurodevelopmental processes. As an illustration, consider the earlier suggestion that individual differences in the number of VTA DA cells may be viewed as an outcome of genotype-driven processes. If the number of cells is relatively large, an individual will possess the structural capacity to release high levels of DA at the terminals of VTA projections during experience-expectant sensitive periods. Such an individual would be predisposed to stabilize, and thereby retain, a large number of synaptic contacts within BFS structures, provided that a sufficient level of activity were maintained in the VTA source cells. Although this functional outcome would not occur if environmental experience were reward-impoverished, empirical findings in animal behavior genetics suggest that an individual with a rich genetic

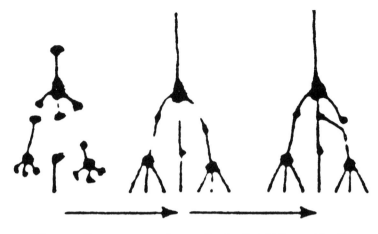

Development   Adult Plasticity

Figure 8. Neurotransmitter involvement in brain development and adult plasticity. As neurons extend axons and dendrites during development, axons releasing neurotransmitter stabilize the outgrowth of the dendritic fields that they invade, and synapses form, establishing a functional circuitry. Throughout adult life, changes in neuronal circuitry may be mediated by the activity of neurotransmitters. From Mattson (1988).

endowment of DA cells would actively explore the environment in search of rewarding stimulation (Fink & Reis, 1981; Sved, Baker, & Reis, 1984, 1985). Thus, the likely (but not inevitable) outcome of the sensitive period would be the emergence of a strong functional capacity in the VTA DA system to motivate and guide emotional responses to signals of reward, and this foundation for BFS responsivity would be resistant to large scale modification in the future. As neural system development proceeds, experience-dependent processes would likely provide incremental increases in the synaptic connectivity within BFS structures, since an enduring predisposition to engage potentially rewarding stimuli would entail frequent demands for additional synapses in the terminal fields of VTA DA projections. By adulthood, the extensive synaptic arborization within BFS circuitry would consistently amplify responses of the VTA DA system to signals of reward, and the individual would exhibit a high and stable level of BFS responsivity.

Despite its simplicity, this hypothetical example illustrates how fundamentally distinct neurodevelopmental processes, i.e., genotype-driven, experience-expectant, and experience-dependent, may exert overlapping influences upon the development of neural systems by converging upon modulatory neurochemical systems. To the extent that modulatory neurotransmitters form an integral component of neurobehavioral systems, they will incorporate these developmental influences within basic parameters of neural functioning, such as synaptic connectivity, that underlie variation in neurobehavioral traits. With respect to the developmental origins of individual differences in the BFS, trends in the level of BFS responsivity will emerge as individuals experience stimulus contexts that modify earlier neurodevelopmental outcomes involving the structural and functional capacities of the VTA DA projection system. In view of the potential for collaboration among neurodevelopmental processes, it is likely that individuals will exhibit progressively discrepant outcome trajectories that ultimately stabilize as trait level variation in BFS responsivity. However, it is important to emphasize that retention of mechanisms for functional alterations during later development is an inherent property of adaptive neural systems; through these mechanisms, developmental discontinuities in the BFS will be expressed over time if individuals are guided toward, or subjected to, a significantly altered reward environment.

Infant-Mother Attachment as Expected Emotional Experience

At this point, it will be helpful to anchor the discussion of neurodevelopmental influences within a specific application involving a content area familiar to many developmental psychologists: infant-mother attachment. The attachment relationship is a sound theoretical starting point for a developmental analysis of the BFS in humans, since it has been portrayed for some time as a sensitive period in human emotional development (e.g., Bowlby, 1969). From the perspective of neurobehavioral systems, reformulating infant-mother attachment as an experience-expectant period in BFS development provides at least three potential benefits. First, emotional experience within the attachment relationship will emerge more clearly as a sensitive period phenomenon, i.e., as contributing to a foundation for later experience, when it is viewed as coherent input stimulation to a major neurobehavioral system undergoing experience-expectant development. Second, the potential for collaboration among the various sources of neurodevelopmental influences indicates a position for infant-mother attachment along a temporal continuum of BFS development from the prenatal period to adulthood. This extended dimension of neurobehavioral development reflects the capacity of the BFS construct to incorporate both preattachment influences, perhaps in terms of genotype-driven components of "temperament," and developmental consequences of attachment, perhaps as experience-dependent refinements of an early neurobiological foundation for positive emotionality. Third, characterizing both infant and mother in terms of the origins of their trait levels of BFS responsivity will produce a simple framework for considering how, rather than how much, genetic and environmental factors jointly influence early emotional development.

Overall, these potential benefits share a common basis in the structure of the BFS construct, which organizes a domain of relevant behavior and suggests avenues of developmental influence upon the neurobiological system that underlies the behavior. In this context, discussion of infant-mother attachment in terms of BFS development will provide support for the application of cell-level theory from developmental neurobiology to the study of human emotional behavior. As noted previously, empirical neurodevelopmental research has focused upon neural systems involved in perception and cognition, rather than emotion. The most immediate consequence of this empirical focus is that key structures in emotional information processing, e.g., the amygdala, have not been studies with regard to either experience-expectant or experience-dependent processes. However, there is little doubt that emotional neural systems participate in most empirical paradigms that examine effects of environmental manipulations on learning and memory, since the experimental stimuli typically are designed to elicit motivated rather than passive responding. For example, the EC condition of the paradigm employed by Greenough and colleagues clearly is designed to elicit high levels of spontaneous exploration, which involves mild levels of BFS activation corresponding to relatively unstructured reward-seeking behavior. Similarly, the superiority of EC animals in the performance of appetitive tasks likely involves enhanced BFS responsivity, since the BFS modulates directed (approach) behavior rather than general levels of arousal or global "emotionality." At the synaptic level, it would be predicted that changes in functional connectivity within and across BFS structures accompany observed differences in approach behavior. In any case, it seems unlikely that emotional neural systems develop without engaging genotype-driven, experience-expectant, and experience-dependent processes, although the specific cellular products associated with these processes need not be formally similar to those in perceptual or cognitive systems.

Attachment from a Neurobehavioral Systems Perspective

As described earlier, a period of experience-expectant neural development is associated with the highly predictable occurence of a particular environmental context for all young members of a species. The context of infant-mother attachment clearly meets this criterion, since some form of attachment occurs in humans and many other mammalian species under natural environmental conditions. We will assume that the mother is the primary participant in the attachment relationship, simply to facilitate comparisons with findings from animal research. In humans, the primary caregiver may be male or female, and the infant may form multiple attachments if infant care is distributed across several members of a social group (see Tronick, Winn, & Morelli, 1985). However, these alternative arrangements have been studied primarily with observational methods, and little data exists with regard to possible differences in underlying neurobehavioral processes. Adopting an ethological perspective, Bowlby (1969) characterized infant-mother attachment as a behavioral system that evolved to increase the likelihood of survival of infants born highly underdeveloped and relatively helpless. He noted that during the second half of the first year of life, human infants gradually acquire the capacity for independent locomotion, which entails a progressively greater risk of wandering into potentially harmful of even life-threatening situations. Three basic components of the behavioral repertoire emerge at this time as well, and together they reduce the risk associated with increased mobility. First, the infant begins to freeze and show fear when approaching unstable or uneven surfaces, such as a steeply descending staircase. Second, the infant begins to show wariness to strangers, usually involving sobered or negative affect and a tendency to turn away when a stranger approaches. Third, the wariness to strangers is accompanied by increasing selectivity in positive emotional responses to familiar figures, which typically includes a clear preference for engagement with the primary caregiver (here assumed to be the mother). During the second year of life, further development occurs in all three behavioral components as well as in locomotor ability, and the infant relies on active approach as well as signaling behavior for maintaining proximity to the mother. Additionally, the infant develops more fully the cognitive capacity to form mental representatives of absent objects, including the object of attachment, and the attachment relationship remains stable over brief separations of infant and mother. It is at this point in development, roughly the first half of the second year, that the infant is truly "attached" to the mother, since the attachment is maintained at a high level of specificity without constant behavioral reinforcement (Bowlby, 1969).

A variety of specific behaviors occur reliably within the attachment relationship, including smiling, vocalizing, reaching, locomotion toward the mother, and visual checking of the mother's location during exploration or play. Bowlby (1969) argued that these various behaviors form a coherent behavioral system, with the primary function of maintaining proximity to the mother to insure protection from predators and satisfaction of basic biological needs. Accordingly, he emphasized the proximity-seeking behaviors of infants when signals of danger or internal disequilibrium (e.g., hunger) are present. Later theorists have emphasized the salience of attachment behaviors within contexts that lack obviously aversive stimuli, such as exploratory play, and have stressed that infants approach caregivers for affection as well as for comfort; consequently, the primary function of the behavioral system has been redefined in terms of "felt security" rather than proximity (e.g., Ainsworth, 1973; Sroufe, 1979; Waters, 1981). Nevertheless, it is possible to expand Bowlby's (1969) forulation without discarding the original neurobehavioral systems perspective. Infant behavior associated with attachment occurs during forms of environmental engagement facilitated by the BFS, namely approach to reward stimuli and active avoidance of potential punishers. Within the attachment relationship, the mother is a source of many discrete forms of reward, some of which are based on biological needs, e.g., nursing, rocking, and vocal soothing, while others are primarily social in nature, e.g., pleasurably modulated affective interchanges such as reciprocal smiling or babbling. Many physical characteristics of the mother, including facial features, skin texture, scent, and vocal patterns, become powerful conditioned incentive cues for the infant, and she also represents the reward of safety or security to be obtained through locomotion in active avoidance contexts. Accordingly, proximity-seeking behavior may be viewed as a general consequence of the potency of the mother to elicit strong levels of BFS activation, and hence strong incentive motivation for approach, in the infant.

Although Bowlby emphasized the context of active avoidance, i.e., approach to the mother to obtain safety and comforting, it is clear that infants frequently approach to obtain physical affection, such as cuddling or caressing, when no threat is present in the environment. Perhaps as a neurobehavioral correlate of "felt security," the outcome produced by both types of infant approach may be an increase in brain opioid levels within the system described by Panksepp (1982; Panksepp, Siviy, & Normansell, 1985). In brief, social isolation may elicit activity in the same opiate system that responds to visceral pain, possibly by stimulating a common input pathway associated with affective distress. In Panksepp's model, an absence of social contact eventually leads to a reduction in opioid levels and an affectively aversive state of internal distress or disequilibrium. When the infant approaches the mother after a period of separation, the resulting tactile stimulation from maternal stroking and caressing may induce an increase in the infant's opioid levels, which will restore internal equilibrium and generate a more comfortable affective state. Similar opiate mechanisms may operate when an external stimulus, e.g., the approach of a stranger, generates acute affective distress that the infant seeks to relieve through maternal contact. In this manner, the opiate system may participate in the formation of a strong social bond between the infant and mother, as maternal contact becomes associated with sensations of comfort and pleasure produced by opioid release in the infant.

Thus, proximity-seeking and felt security may reflect the activity of separate neurobehavioral systems within the infant. The interaction of these two systems may contribute to the development of the level of "security" that characterizes individual attachments. For example, activation of the BFS, associated with proximity-seeking infant behavior, may be followed reliably by increased opioid levels, associated with comforting or affectionate maternal behavior. When the infant forms a mental representation of this relation, s/he will derive a form of pleasurable emotional security from the attachment relationship, and the need for constant behavioral reinforcement will be diminished. On the other hand, no such relation will be encoded if maternal behavior is emotionally inconsistent, e.g., if the mother frequently rejects or simply ignores the infant's approach for comfort or affection. In this case, the infant may continue to approach consistently if maternal behavior is occasionally appropriate to the infant's needs, since the opiate system can support social bonds (as well as self-administration of narcotics) under conditions of partial reinforcement (Panksepp et al., 1985). However, the infant will not derive emotional security from this type of attachment due to the absence of a highly predictable relation between his or her approach behavior and subsequent relief from affective distress and internal disequilibrium. Because the need for constant behavioral reinforcement has not been diminished, the infant's behavior will continue to be dominated by proximity-seeking, at the cost of development in other domains such as exploratory play. Finally, if approach is consistently met with rejection or indifference by the mother and no other attachment figures are present, the infant may turn to asocial behaviors that elicit activity in the opiate system, i.e., self-stimulation such as rocking or other repetitive movements. Based on the findings from research with nonhuman primates (e.g., Kraemer, 1985), this form of early social isolation would be expected to produce significant retardation in social and emotional development.

Although the interaction between the BFS and the opiate system may contribute to the various behaviors and emotions observed in attachment relationships, neither system contains a theoretical mechanism that could account for the ubiquity of infant attachment within and across a variety of mammalian species. From a neurobehavioral perspective, the concept of psychobiological synchrony or "attunement" possesses substantial explanatory potential as an underlying mechanism of attachment. As detailed elsewhere (see Reite & Field, 1985), infants and mothers within many mammalian species demonstrate considerable coherence in responses (attunement) at both behavioral and biological levels within the attachment relationship. For example, Hofer (1987) has described what he refers to as "hidden regulators" within infant-mother attachment in the rat, i.e., multiple maternal influences over infant homeostatic systems that become obvious when they are globally disrupted by involuntary separation. As shown in Table 1, these regulators are numerous and widely distributed across the behavioral and biological systems of the rat, and presumably an even more complex regulation occurs within primates (Hofer, 1987). Moreover, much of the homeostatic regulation is reciprocal within the infant-mother attachment, as Hofer (1987) noted in his analysis of "hidden" interactive components, such as induction of mutual slow-wave sleep, during nursing. Homeostatic regulation emerges reliably within the first 6 months of human infancy, a period to which Bowlby (1969) applied the conceptually barren label of "preattachment;" as suggested by Hofer (1987) and others (e.g., Pipp & Harmon, 1987), a continuous progression from early attunement to formal attachment may emerge as the infant begins to construct mental representations of maternal regulators, presumably within associative neural networks in developing higher-level cortical regions. The internalization of homeostatic regulators provides a measure of freedom for the infant, who begins to explore a wider range of environmental stimulation within the more flexibly structured attachment. In turn, the expansion of environmental experience confers a considerable advantage with respect to the fine-tuning of neural system development during an early sensitive period. Thus, a more basic evolutionary function of attachment, as compared to protection from predators and promotion of an early social bond,

Table 1. Regulators Hidden Within the Mother-Infant Interaction

Infant Systems	Direction	Maternal Regulators
Behavioral		
activity level	increased	bodywarmth
	decreased	tactile and olfactory
sucking		
nutritive	decreased	milk (distention)
nonnutritive	decreased	tactile (perioral)
Neurochemical (central nervous system)		
norepinephrine, dopamine	increased	body warmth
ODC	increased	tactile (dorsal)
Metabolic		
oxygen consumption	increased	milk (sugar)
Sleep-wake states		
REM sleep	increased	periodicity, milk, tactile
arousal	decreased	periodicity, milk, tactile
Cardiovascular		
heart rate (β-adrenergic)	increased	milk (interoreceptors)
resistance (a-adrenergic)	decreased	milk (interoreceptors)
Endocrine		
growth hormone	increased	tactile (dorsal)

ODC = ornithine decarboxylase, a rate-limiting enzyme important in growth of brain and most other tissues; resistance = arterial resistance, the constriction of peripheral blood vessels; REM = rapid eye movement sleep.

may be to provide reliably structured environmental interactions that adaptively modulate the timing of gene expression for both somatic and neural development (Hofer, 1987).

Attachment and Experience-Expectant Development within the BFS

If infant-mother attachment represents expected emotional experience, it may be associated with a sensitive period in which a neurobiological foundation for BFS responsivity is established through experience-expectant processes. However, the BFS is but one of several qualitatively and neurobiologically distinct emotional systems, and during a sensitive period its input will compete with input from other emotional systems as the entire range of emotional experience is encoded. At the neural level, competition among these systems may establish enduring patterns of behavioral modulation, i.e., a trait structure of emotion, by stabilizing highly active synapses within emotion-processing structures. Consider, for example, a hypothetical analog of the development of binocular vision during an early sensitive period. Rather than competing visual input from two eyes, we might envision competing emotional input derived from (1) approach behavior, which is modulated by the VTA DA projection system; and (2) behavioral inhibition or constraint, which may be modulated by the serotonin (5-HT) projection system (Depue & Spoont, 1986; Soubrie, 1986). As elimination of excess subcortical cells and cortical synapses proceeds during infancy, the strength of input arising from behavioral approach versus inhibition may determine which modulatory system, VTA DA or 5-HT, retains greater influence over distributed neural networks of emotion. At one extreme, a high frequency of rewarding infant-mother engagements would be associated with strong activation of the VTA projection system, and the release of DA at projection terminals would be expected to stabilize (and thereby retain) a large number of synapses within target structures. Conversely, a high frequency of unpredictable maternal behavior, e.g., responding to the infant's approach with affection on one occasion and anger on another, gradually would weaken the infant's prepotent tendency to approach the attachment figure. Over time, the infant would learn to inhibit approach when the mother unexpectedly displays negative affect, and this increase in the frequency of behavioral inhibition would be associated with increased neurotransmitter release, and retention of more synapses, at the terminals of the 5-HT projection system.

In terms of BFS responsivity, the neurodevelopmental impact of individual differences in attachment experience may be illustrated with reference to the amygdala, in which VTA DA and 5-HT projections overlap at output nuclei. A high frequency of rewarding infant-mother engagements ultimately would yield strong modulation of amygdala output nuclei by VTA-DA projections, and this experience-expectant outcome would be resistant to large-scale modifications during later development. Accordingly, a foundation would be established for a low threshold of BFS responsivity to incentive stimuli, since the amygdala is a critical neural structure for processing the emotional valence of stimuli. In a similar manner, a high frequency of unpredictable maternal behavior would establish the foundation for a higher threshold of BFS responsivity, as well as a lower threshold for behavioral inhibition or constraint.

Of course, the neurobiological substrates of both forms of emotional behavior are not localized to the amygdala, and the full competition among emotional systems likely extends to many of the structures involved in emotional processes. With respect to individual differences in BFS responsivity, the most influential neurodevelopmental outcome of the attachment period may be the relative magnitude of functional VTA DA innervation, distributed across these various structures, that is established by experience-expectant processes. For each infant, the range of potential functional outcomes will be constrained by genetic influences over structural DA parameters, such as the number of DA cells. To some extent, variation in the number of DA cells will determine the modulatory strength of VTA projections, simply by introducing individual differences in the amount of DA release at terminal synapses. However, it is likely that this genotype-driven source of variation will collaborate with experience-expectant processes during development, since DA cell number will influence the vigor with which the infant explores the environment for potential rewards. For example, an infant born with a high number of DA cells would be expected to initiate a high frequency of rewarding engagements with the mother, as well as to respond strongly to the mother's attempts at engagement. The likely outcome of attachment for this infant would be the development of extensive functional innervation of BFS structures by VTA DA projections, as well as a behavioral progression from temperamental "sociability" to more far ranging positive emotionality associated with high levels of BFS activity. In this manner, genotype-driven processes may create a bias toward a particular trait level of BFS responsivity, and this bias may be expressed at both the behavioral and neurobiological levels as it influences the nature of emotional experience during attachment.

Finally, variation in maternal trait levels of BFS responsivity must be considered, since it represents the primary source of influence over individual differences in neurobehavioral development during attachment. Over the course of attachment, the mother's trait level of BFS responsivity will modulate her sensitivity to the array of incentive cues that the infant provides, and thereby provide another biasing influence over the emotional quality of attachment. For example, a mother with traitwise low BFS responsivity may predispose the attachment relationship to a relatively low frequency of rewarding engagements, since she would lack the sensitivity to incentive stimuli necessary to generate and sustain reward responding over prolonged periods of time. A mother at the opposite end of the BFS trait dimension would seem well suited to initiate rewarding engagements at a relatively high frequency, although she may have some difficulty in adapting her high level of behavioral facilitation to the infant's limited capacity for modulating arousal.

Thus, both infant and mother approach the attachment relationship with preexisting neurobehavioral features that influence the specific nature of emotional experience to be encoded by experience-expectant processes. These features are not likely to represent independent sources of influence, since biologically related infant-mother pairs would share quantitative variance in genotype-driven processes; for example, DA cell number is likely to be more similar in mother and infant than in a biologically unrelated pair of individuals. Nevertheless, a considerable range of disparity is possible with respect to maternal BFS responsivity and infant DA cell number, albeit along a continuum of decreasing probability of occurrence. If experience-expectant processes are active during attachment, the interaction between these preexisting neurobehavioral features may exert a lasting directional influence over developing trait levels of BFS responsivity in the infant, as shown schematically in Figure 9. In this figure, the relative frequency of rewarding engagements during attachment is derived largely from an interaction between infant DA cell number and maternal traitwise BFS responsivity. Over time, individual differences in the modulatory strength of VTA DA projections may be amplified or diminished as rewarding experience during attachment is encoded by experience-expectant processes. For instance, when maternal BFS responsivity is relatively high (Figure 9, solid line), the effect of differences in infant DA cell number will be amplified, since the number of terminal synapses retained is likely to have a multiplicative, rather than one-to-one, relation with the number of DA cells. Accordingly, when high maternal BFS responsivity increases the probability of rewarding infant-mother engagements, an infant born with a relatively high number of DA cells would be expected to establish strong functional DA modulation of emotion-processing structures. In contrast, an infant born with a relatively low number of DA cells will have a more limited capacity to encode rewarding experience during attachment within the cytoarchitecture of VTA DA innervation pathways. By the end of the sensitive period of attachment, the initial difference between the two infants in DA cell number will be amplified, as shown in Figure 9, across a widely distributed neurobiological threshold for BFS responsivity. The same underlying mechanics may produce a dampening of the effect of differences in infant DA cell number when maternal levels of BFS responsivity are relatively low (dashed line), since the infant with a high DA cell number may lose a relatively greater proportion of potential functional DA modulation at terminal synapses. Finally, it should be noted that the figure displays a range of possible functional outcomes in developing trait levels of BFS responsivity that is substantially smaller for the infant born with a low DA cell number, and that does not extend into the outcome range of the infant born with a high DA cell number. This hypothetical separation of outcome ranges provides a simple illustration of the manner in which genetic influences may constrain experience-expectant neurodevelopment within the BFS, i.e., through exerting overlapping influences upon the functional development of the VTA DA projection system.

Later Development

The primary limitation of a neurobehavioral systems approach to emotional development is the paucity of existing neurodevelopmental data beyond the period of infancy in humans. Undoubtedly, the neurobiological foundation of individual differences in levels of BFS responsivity will be refined and extended at least through adolescence, and perhaps throughout adulthood. It is highly probable as well that alterations in neuroarchitecture primarily will involve localized, experience-dependent synaptic processes within the existing VTA-DA terminal innervation of BFS structures. While there may be a cummulative trend in the experience-dependent synaptic modification (see Figure 7), it is likely that the neurobiological foundations established during experience-expectant development will continue to exert a directional influence upon developing trait levels of BFS responsivity. For example, a young

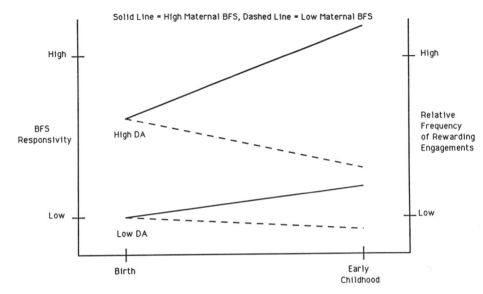

Figure 9. Schematic representation of the relation between behavioral facilitation system (BFS) responsivity as a function of variation in ventral tegmental area dopamine cell number, maternal BFS level, and rewarding environmental engagements. See text for discussion.

child emerging from the attachment period with a very high level of BFS responsivity (uppermost line in Figure 9) would be expected to participate actively in the maintenance of a high frequency of rewarding environmental engagements, e.g., by approaching the development of peer relations with great vigor and relatively little anxiety or inhibition. Conversely, a child entering this developmental phase with a very low level of BFS responsivity (lowermost line) may appear relatively sluggish or disengaged during play with peers, and thereby contribute to a continuation of relatively low frequency and intensity of rewarding engagements.

In addition to continuity in neurobehavioral development, a complete developmental model of trait-level variation within the BFS would have to address the tendency of discrete alterations in mood, including affective disorders, to emerge during adolescence. The fundamental neurodevelopmental issue involves the impact of emotional experience during adolescence, which (a) may be encoded within some type of hormonally regulated burst of synaptic remodeling, i.e., within a neural sensitive period linked to reproductive maturation; or (b) may simply challenge the functional integrity of smoothly developing neurobehavioral systems. While a clear context of phylogenetically predictable environmental experience is lacking, it is possible that hormonal mechanisms of rapid bodily changes at puberty trigger a neural sensitive period as well. For example, increased levels of gonadal steriod hormones may induce a reversion to growth cone mode and subsequent neurite outgrowth (Mattson, 1988) within late-maturing neocortical regions. In view of the retarded emergence of highly self-regulated behavioral processes, such as planning of long-term reward acquisition and prolonged delay of gratification, synaptic modification at puberty may be most prominent within the prefrontal cortex. At odds with this speculation is current empirical evidence that synaptic density in human frontal cortex decreases slowly toward adult levels in the period from 7–16 years (Huttenlocher, 1990); accordingly, if any localized but relatively exuberant production of synapses were to occur during puberty, e.g., within the OFC, it apparently would be masked by the magnitude of ongoing competitive synaptic elimination. As Greenough and Black (in press) noted, new experimental techniques will be required to detect patterns of simultaneous synaptic production and elimination that may underlie stable overall trends in synapse number.

Alternatively, it is possible that the emergence of highly self-regulated behavioral processes during adolescence simply reflects the endpoint of a smooth maturational trend in the higher cortical regions. From this perspective, abnormalities in adolescent outcome would arise as the final consequences of disruptions in earlier neurodevelopmental processes. For example, Clark and Goldman-Rakic (1989) reported behavioral effects of early prenatal exposure to androgen that became apparent only after subsequent maturation of the OFC. Moreover, several findings from research on attachment in rhesus monkeys appear to conform to this developmental pattern as well. It is well established that rhesus monkeys develop an array of behavioral deficits after social deprivation during infancy, and that this "isolation syndrome" can be reversed through subsequent housing with younger, normally developing monkeys (see Kraemer, 1985). However, several somewhat overlooked studies have shown that isolation deficits persist in latent form, which may be observed when rehabilitated monkeys are exposed to socially complex or stressful situations (Anderson & Mason, 1974, 1978; Sackett Bowman, Meyer, Tripp, & Grady, 1973). A possible linkage with latent abnormalities in catecholamine functioning was indicated by a study in which rehabilitated preadolescent monkeys exhibited a primary symptom of the isolation syndrome (hyperaggression) in response to low doses of amphetamine, a nonselective DA agonist (Kraemer, Ebert, Lake, & McKinney, 1984).

Thus, the complex social and emotional experience associated with adolescence may be encoded within a hormonally regulated neural sensitive period, perhaps largely restricted to the prefrontal cortex, or it may simply challenge the functional integrity of smoothly developing neurobehavioral systems. This issue may prove difficult to resolve on the basis of animal studies, since the timing of bursts of cortical synaptogenesis appears to be different in humans and nonhuman primates. Specifically, research with nonhuman primates suggests that synaptic overproduction occurs in temporal synchrony across diverse cortical regions (Rakic, Bourgeois, Eckenhoff, Zecevic, & Goldman-Rakic, 1986), while data from human autopsy studies indicate that significant asynchronies occur along an anterior-posterior axis from visual to prefrontal cortex (see Greenough et al., 1987; Huttenlocher, 1990). Although Greenough and Black (in press) suggested plausible measurement confounds that may account for the empirical discrepancy, direct comparisons using clearly interpretable methodologies will be required to facilitate analysis of the larger issue regarding the continuity of neurodevelopmental processes after infancy.

Implications for Disorders of Affect

A natural extension of the BFS into the domain of psychopathology emerges upon examination of the symptoms associated with disturbances of positive emotionality, i.e., affective disorders. When core affective symptoms are considered, they fall primarily within the locomotor, incentive-reward, and mood dimensions (Depue & Iacono, 1989), and the relevance of the BFS construct becomes obvious. Space limitations preclude a full discussion of this issue, and many of the points have been discussed elsewhere (Depue et al., 1987; Depue & Iacono, 1989). However, any BFS framework for disorders of affect needs to consider the following conditions.

Extreme BFS State Levels and Affective Disorders

As illustrated in Figure 10, symptoms of bipolar depression and hypomania/mania appear to represent opposite extremes of normal behavioral dimensions (Depue & Iacono, 1989; Post & Uhde, 1982) that describe extreme states of engagement (and disengagement) with both interpersonal and achievement-related environments. The poles of the core behavioral dimensions may be viewed as the products of extreme variations in the probability that incentive stimuli of all forms, e.g., interoceptive or cognitive, will initiate or facilitate motor and affective responses. In these terms, the probability of initiating emotional behavior is excessively low in depression and excessively high in hypomania or mania. Both states, then, may be viewed along a single dimension representing the propensity to behavioral and affective reactivity to incentive stimuli (Depue & Iacono, 1989).

In the case of bipolar depression, low reactivity encompasses familiar behavioral features such as psychomotor retardation, as well as typical subjective features involving the lack of usual interest or enthusiasm for engagement in social, sexual, vocational, or recreational activities (Depue & Monroe, 1978; Post & Uhde, 1982). In addition, bipolar depressives frequently display general affective poverty or blunting, and the absence of positive affect is typically a far more prominent clinical feature than the presence of negative affect. This observation is consistent with the higher-order structure of mood derived from research with normal subjects (Watson & Tellegen, 1985), which is modeled better by orthogonal positive and negative dimensions, each with "high" and "low" poles, than by a single positive vs. negative dimension. As noted previously, self-report ratings of positive affect (state) and positive emotionality (trait) correlate strongly (Tellegen & Waller, in press), which again raises the possibility of a direct relation between bipolar depressive episodes and extreme reductions in BFS responsivity. Thus, the essential features of bipolar depression may be modeled parsimoniously as an extreme state-wise reduction in the effective value of rewarding stimuli to elicit the primary components of BFS activation: incentive motivation, psychomotor activation, and positive mood.

The primary features of hypomania/mania may be viewed an analogous manifestations of excessively high BFS responsivity. In comparison with bipolar depression, however, the extreme state of behavioral facilitation is more transparent in hypomania/mania. Along with excessive levels of incentive motivation, locomotor activation, and positive mood, distractibility and mixed affect are typically observed during hypomanic/manic episodes (Post & Uhde, 1982; Secunda, Swann, Katz, Koslow, Crougnan, & Chang, 1987). Distractibility in hypomania/mania appears to represent excessive responsivity to stimuli that are rewarding or novel but task-irrelevant, rather than a generalized and affectively neutral attentional impairment (Depue & Iacono, 1989). At a more detailed level, this type of inappropriate reward responding reflects both attribution of exaggerated incentive value to stimuli during emotional evaluation, and an extremely low threshold for initiating approach-type responses. With such extreme amplification of these fundamental BFS processes, sustained and focused behavioral responding is difficult to maintain; thus, the hypomanic/manic exhibits high levels of incentive motivation in the context of apparently purposeless behavior. In sum, when hypomania/mania is viewed as an episode of extreme behavioral and affective reactivity to incentive stimuli, its core symptoms emerge as polar opposites of those in bipolar depression.

Extreme BFS Trait Levels and Disorders of Affect

When less extreme but enduring (i.e., trait rather than state) levels of BFS responsivity are postulated, the above formulation naturally extends to characterological expressions of affective disorder, such as hyperthymia and dysthymia. Consistent with their classification as characterological entities, some forms of dysthymia and hyperthymia may reflect levels of BFS responsivity that constitute minimum and maximum values, respectively, along a trait dimension underlying positive emotionality in the normal population.

One source of extreme BFS trait levels may be genotype-driven in terms of the number of neurons per DA cell group formed during the prenatal period. As noted above, this variation can be substantial in that, in a 33 year old man, there are 450,000 DA cells in the substantia nigra/VTA complex, but this number can vary across individuals by ±20,000 cells (Oades & Halliday, 1987). Such variation strongly influences the range of functional expression of DA-modulated behaviors in rodents. From a developmental perspective,

MOTOR			INCENTIVE-REWARD ACTIVATION		MOOD
Locomotion	Speech	Facies	Hedonia (Social, Sex, Food)	Desire for Excitement	
hyperactivity	rapid, pressured	expressive	excessive interest and pleasure	excessive, creates new activities	elation, euphoria reactive
| | | | | | |	| | | | | | |	| | | | | | |	| | | | | | |	| | | | | | |	| | | | | | |
retardation slowed delayed stupor	retardation slowed delayed mute	unchanging, unexpres-sive	no interest or pleasure (pervasive anhedonia)	avoidance of stimulation	devoid of emotion, depres-sion, lack reactivity

Figure 10. Extremes of normal behavioral dimensions associated with

this influence could become manifest in several ways, and these are summarized in Figure 11. Consider low (vs. high) VTA DA cell number as an example that is most relevant to depressive conditions (Person B vs. Person A, respectively, at the top of Figure 11). As shown across the first line of type in Figure 11, during experience-expectant emotional periods, a reduced number of VTA DA cells (i.e., genotype) would yield fewer possibilities for synapogenesis in the DA terminal fields of the NAS for Person B vs. Person A (A>B). Thus, even adequate environmental reward experiences at the expected time would have a reduced neurological substrate in Person B in terms of synaptic connections within the NAS. In this way, the development of sensitivity to reward stimuli in Person B may begin in a diminished fashion; or, as indicated in Figure 11, less intense incentive motivation would be encoded for Person B vs. Person A within the VTA DA-NAS pathway.

This differential sensitivity to reward stimuli could have at least two major effects. First, as shown in the second line in Figure 11, subsequent rewarding experiences would be modulated by differential incentive motivation, via VTA DA-NAS mechanisms, and involve differential approach to or engagement with reward. Second, differential engagement-induced DA activation, with Person B experiencing much less DA activation than Person A, would result in a decrease in DA synapse maintenance in the NAS for

NONSPECIFIC AROUSAL						COGNITIVE	
Appetite	Energy	Sleep/Wake	Thought	Attention	Sensory Vividness	Optimism	Self-Worth
decreased	excessive, boundless	< need for sleep	sharper, flight of ideas, witty, > decisional power	concrete, distractible	extremely vivid	> self-confidence, < estimation of negative outcomes, grandiosity	increased worth, grandiosity
> carbohydrate intake	easily fatigued, devoid of energy	hypersomnia, naps	< decisional power, thoughts "dead," mind dull	poor concentration	senses dull, food tastes bland	pessimistic, persistent gloom, brood about past, hopeless about future outcomes, suicidal ideation	totally worthless, delusional

ipolar affective disorder.

Person B, which would exacerbate an already diminished sensitivity to reward stimuli. That is, as shown on the third line of Figure 11, a progressively less active process of experience-dependent DA synaptic growth in the NAS might be expected in Person B relative to Person A. By adulthood, this experience-dependent trend of diminished DA release to reward stimuli, and hence of diminished synaptic growth in DA terminal areas, in Person B could result in significantly reduced synaptic arborization within BFS circuitry. Behaviorally, this outcome might appear as a quantitatively low trait level on the dimension of positive emotionality (à la Tellegen's model) — or, in psychiatric terms, as a form of characterological depression or pure dysthymia.

A more general effect of reduced sensitivity to reward stimuli in Person B is that other neurobiological systems that function *interactively* with DA in modulating emotional behavior would become dominant relative to BFS activity. For instance, a situation that presents signals of both reward and punishment may increasingly evoke constraint and behavioral inhibition, rather than exploration and goal acquisition. Subjectively, the cumulative effect of reduced behavioral facilitation and increased behavioral inhibition could be a sense of low self-efficacy in obtaining rewarding goals (a form of learned helplessness or passive avoidance?), and a persistent lack of positive affect, or persistent dysphoria, due to the low frequency of achieved rewards over time.

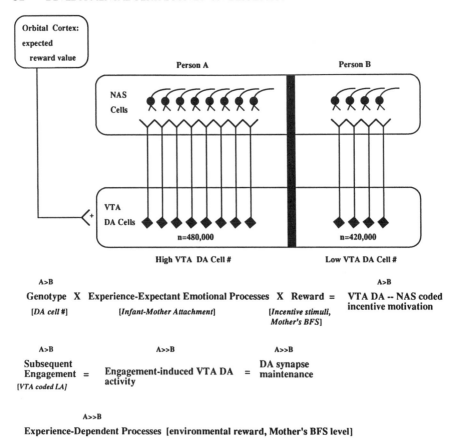

Figure 11. Schematic representation of how ventral tegmental area dopamine cell number (genotype) interacts with (a) experience-expectant processes during predictable environmental reward circumstances to determine the encoded incentive-reward value of stimuli (first line of type), (b) the subsequent level of engagement-induced dopamine activity (second line of type), and (c) experience-dependent processes during idiographic environmental reward circumstances (third line of type).

As suggested in the last line of Figure 11, the above view of the ontology of some forms of characterological depression would be modified by the quality and quantity of environmental reward experience, and perhaps by BFS trait levels of caregivers, who are predominantly responsible in early years for providing reward and for encouraging exploration and goal acquisition. However, the magnitude of effect of the interpersonal environment on the development of BFS trait levels will vary according to the individual's genotype-driven DA cell number, as illustrated in the discussion of Figure 11. At extreme ends of a dimension of DA responsivity, the effects of environmental reward are likely to be constrained in the direction of the extremity. For instance, in an individual at the low extreme of DA responsivity, a reward-rich environment may increase DA function over time, but the effects of rewarding stimuli will always be encoded within a restricted range of DA synaptic plasticity (see Figure 11). Moreover, the effects of a reward-poor environment may be diminished due to the already low level of DA reactivity. The opposite effects would be predicted at the extreme high end of DA responsivity. It is in the midrange values of DA cell number that variations in environmental reward would be predicted to have complementary effects on experience-dependent synaptic growth, since rich and poor environments will have equally strong, but opposite, effects. This leads to the intriguing possibility that the effects of variation in rewarding environments on DA, and hence BFS, responsivity may be most powerfully demonstrated within less extreme or midrange values of positive emotionality trait levels.

BFS Regulatory Strength as a Trait and Disorders of Affect

Unlike dysthymia and hyperthymia, bipolar and some forms of unipolar affective disorders cannot be modeled sufficiently with a single dimension of trait level of BFS responsivity, since the symptomatology of these disorders reflects extreme intraindividual alterations in BFS, and perhaps DA, functioning. Accordingly, we will describe briefly a second dimension of DA functioning that we refer to as regulatory strength, which is a summarizing construct for the variety of processes within a neurotransmitter system that modulate reactivity during functional challenge (Depue et el., 1987). Regulatory strength is viewed as a dimension that is etiologically orthogonal to trait level of DA responsivity. However, weak regulatory strength, which may involve weak negative feedback processes that result in positive feedback "snowball" effects, would possibly interact with trait-wise DA responsivity. Under weak regulatory conditions, at low and high extremes of the trait dimension of DA responsivity, strong functional challenges to the DA system may produce prolonged state DA levels that are sufficiently low or high, respectively, to be manifested as extreme BFS states, or simply as affective disorder.

The possibility that weak regulatory strength in some DA projection systems, leading to episodes of dysregulation, is present in bipolar disorders is supported by a growing literature reviewed elsewhere (Depue & Iacono, 1989). In comparison to normal controls, bipolar patients demonstrate qualitatively similar but quantitatively exaggerated BFS responsivity when functional activity in their DA system is challenged by either enhancement or antagonism (Depue & Iacono, 1989). Together with their naturally occurring fluctuation in extreme states of affective symptomatology, this biological characteristic suggests that bipolar patients possess a vulnerability to episodes of extreme engagement or disengagement (dysregulation) of DA-modulated processes within the BFS. Thus, a dimension of BFS regulatory strength may be conceptualized as independent of trait levels of BFS responsivity, since dysregulation of BFS activity may presumably occur at any trait level. With the introduction of a dysregulation threshold at the extreme, weak end of the

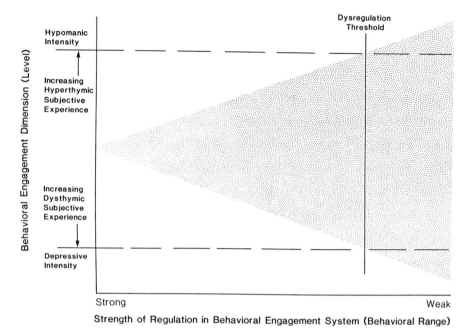

Figure 12. Schematic model of one form of bipolar affective disorder. Bipolar disorder is hypothesized to occur at the weak end of a trait dimension of regulatory strength in the behavioral facilitation system (BFS). Disorder is hypothesized to occur when BFS regulatory strength is so weak that a dysregulation threshold is approached or surpassed. See text for details. From Depue et al. (1987).

regulatory strength dimension, the full neurobehavioral model of bipolar disorder emerges (see also Depue et al., 1987). The dysregulation threshold is displayed schematically in Figure 12, which also illustrates the manner in which BFS regulatory strength can vary independently, while the level of traitwise BFS responsivity remains fixed. It should be emphasized that the positions along the regulatory dimension in Figure 12 represent the range of variation across, not within, individuals, i.e., the strength of BFS regulation is itself a stable, trait-like characteristic. As Tellegen (1988) noted, this model may be viewed as incorporating two basic parameters of interindividual measurement with respect to a dimensional personality trait, namely, the relative level and the relative consistency of trait expression (also referred to as "traitedness"). Accordingly, the model departs from the domain of normal personality only in that it includes a dyregulation threshold to account for distinctly pathological trait expression within the BFS.

BFS Trait Level and Modification of Clinical Course in Affective Disorders

Whereas the above model suggests that the vulnerability to bipolar disorder may be related to the level of BFS regulatory strength, the trait level of BFS responsivity may be a primary determinant of clinical course (Depue et al., 1987). In other words, a bipolar patient's traitwise BFS responsivity may determine which extreme of BFS state level is experienced most intensely at times of dysregulation. As shown in Figure 13, in which the strength of BFS regulation is held constant, descending trait levels of BFS responsivity are associated with a stepwise progression toward a predominantly depressive course of illness. For instance, individuals beyond the dysregulation threshold who have low trait levels of BFS responsivity would experience reductions of BFS activity during dysregulation as intense depression, whereas their experience of dysregulated increases in BFS activity would rarely, if ever, exceed the subjective intensity of normal positive emotionality. Indeed, dysthymics and chronic unipolar depressives often describe their normal states of positive emotionality as "high" mood periods. Corcordant with this hypothesis, we have recently found that MPQ PE, but not MPQ NE or C, correlates positively and significantly with the ratio (frequency) of hypomanic-depressive episodes in unipolar and bipolar affective disorder patients (Depue, Kraus, Spoont & Arbisi, 1989).

Developmental, Longitudinal Assessment of Risk for Affective Disorders

One of the major obstacles in longitudinal analysis of developmental phenomena, including risk for psychopathology, is the comparability of different measures of a construct used during different developmental periods — that is, to what extent do different measures validly represent the same construct. Often, this problem is exacerbated by the lack of a theoretical framework for the construct that would define the basic functional principle(s) to be assessed. In this respect, conceptualizing the structure of behavior in terms of neurobehavioral systems provides an advantage in approaching longitudinal measurement. All neurobehavioral systems attempt to define a specific class of eliciting stimuli, a specific set of behavioral responses, and an underlying neurobiology that mediates between stimulus and response. Thus, using the BFS as an example, one would be guided in the selection or development of tasks, independent of age, that assess the basic functional principle of the BFS: sensitivity to signals of reward.

Depending on the hypothesized alteration associated with risk for psychopathology, i.e., trait level of sensitivity to reward stimuli or trait level of regulatory strength within the BFS, the variables to be assessed within a reward-sensitivity task might differ. In the case where the trait level of sensitivity to reward stimuli is the focus, one can assess the customary

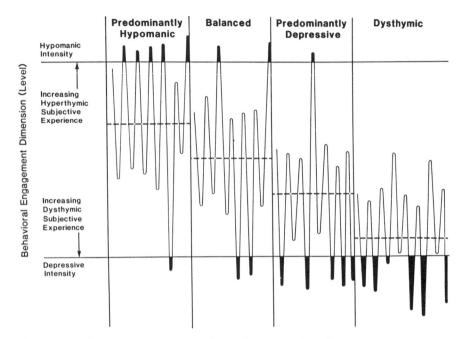

Figure 13. Phenotypic variation in the predominant clinical course as a function of trait level in the behavioral facilitation system. See text for discussion. From Depue et al. (1987).

variables of mean performance over several types of tasks or slope of performance in a "dose-response" design where several levels of reward are used. This type of assessment, however, would be less sensitive to variation in strength of regulation. Strength of regulation can be assessed most sensitively when the functioning of a system is challenged and, hence, is in a state of dynamic variation. In this case, level or mean performance is not informative of the process of adapting to challenges. Four variables, each reflecting the "tightness" of control or negative feedback processes, may be more sensitive: (a) peak level reached during the challenge, (b) slope (rate of change) from beginning of challenge to peak level, (c) magnitude of the variance of the variable during both rest and challenge, and (d) slope or rate of recovery from peak to pre-challenge baseline values.

A Developmental Vulnerability Model of Disorders of Affect

In summary, DA-related vulnerability to disorders of affect incorporates at least four parameters that, no doubt, interact in complex ways. Nevertheless, these parameters can be represented in the following, oversimplistic model:

vulnerability = f[DA trait responsivity +/× DA regulatory strength] × [Mother's BFS + other environmental reward]

The probability, type (characterological, unipolar, bipolar), and predominant course of affective disorder would depend more strongly on the value of the first two parameters, whereas the intensity (severity) of disorder would depend more strongly on the latter two parameters, since these will affect both experience-expectant and experience-dependent processes over the course of development. The challenge for developmental psychopathologists will be to operationalize these four parameters. DA trait responsivity presumably reflects, in part, genotype-driven DA cell number, but it can be estimated by reactivity of the DA system to agonist challenge, as in the DA-MPQ PE study described above. DA regulatory strength needs validation as a construct, but variance, peak, and recovery rate of DA levels under agonist challenge conditions may be a place to begin this validation. The mother's (or caregiver's) BFS level may be estimated by MPQ PE, if the results of the DA-MPQ PE study are replicated and extended. Finally, investigation of nonmaternal environmental reward will require the development of new assessment instruments. It is in relation to this last parameter that developmentalists ought to have special insights. In any case, assessment of these parameters within a multiple prediction model in a longitudinal, developmental study may suggest a host of interesting relations. As more is learned about the interaction of these parameters, more complex models may be entertained. For instance, other neurotransmitters (e.g., serotonin, which modulates DA activity) and enzymes (e.g., activity level of monoamine oxidase, which influences the degradation rate and storage levels of DA and other monoamines) will undoubtedly modify vulnerability via their effect on the functional properties of DA (Depue & Iacono, 1989).

In general, then, the powerful advantage of the neurobehavioral systems approach to developmental psychopathology is that it provides a framework for studying behavior-biology relations, since both domains are specified. This affords the exciting possibility of conducting concurrent, longitudinal assessment of biological reactivity and behavioral responses during development, thereby providing unique information on the interactive nature of behavior, biology, and environment, which is perhaps the ultimate goal of developmental research.

REFERENCES

Aggleton, J. P., Burton, M. J. & Passingham, R. E. (1980). Cortical and subcortical afferents to the amygdala of the rhesus monkey (*Macaca mulatta*). *Brain Research, 190,* 347–368.

Aggleton, J. P., & Mishkin, M. (1986). The amygdala: Sensory gateway to the emotions. In E. Plutchik & H. Kellerman (eds.), *Emotion: Theory, research, and experience. Volume 3: Biological foundations of emotion.* New York: Academic Press, pp. 281–299.

Ainsworth, M. D. S. (1973). The development of infant-mother attachment. In B. M. Caldwell & H. N. Ricciuti (eds.), *Child development and social policy (Review of child development research,* Volume 3). Chicago: University of Chicago Press, pp. 1–94.

Akiskal, H. S. (1984). Characterologic manifestations of affective disorders: Toward a new conceptualization. *Integrative Psychiatry, 2,* 83–96.

Alexander, G. E., DeLong, M. R., & Strick, P. L. (1986). Parallel organization of functionally segregated circuits linking basal ganglia and cortex. *Annual Review of Neuroscience, 9,* 357–381.

Anderson, P. (1979). Factors influencing functional connectivity during hippocampal development. *Progress in Brain Research, 51,* 139–147.

Anderson, C. O., & Mason, W. A. (1974). Early experience and complexity of social organization in groups of young rhesus monkeys (Macaca mulatta). *Journal of Comparative and Physiological Psychology, 87,* 681–690.

Anderson, C. O., & Mason, W. A. (1978). Competititve social strategies in groups of deprived and experienced rhesus monkeys. *Developmental Psychobiology, 11,* 289–299.

Antelman, S. M., & Caggiula, A. R. (1977). Norepinephrine-dopamine interactions and behavior. *Science, 195,* 646–651.

Arai, K., Kosaka, K., & Iizuka, R. (1984). Changes of biogenic amines and their metabolites in postmortem brains from patients of Alzheimer-type dementia. *Journal of Neurochemistry, 43,* 388–393.

Baddeley, A. D. (1986). *Working memory.* Oxford: Oxford University Press.

Baddeley, A. D., & Hitch, G. (1974). Working memory. In G. H. Bower (ed.), *The psychology of learning and motivation: Advances in research and theory.* New York: Academic Press, Vol. 8, pp. 47–89.

Beaulieu, C., & Colonnier, M. (1987). Effects of the richness of the environment on the cat visual cortex. *Journal of Comparative Neurology, 266,* 478–494.

Beckstead, R. M. (1979). An autoradiographic examination of corticocortical and subcortical projections of the mediodorsal-projection (prefrontal) cortex in the rat. *Journal of Comparative Neurology, 184,* 43–62.

Beninger, R. J. (1983). The role of dopamine in locomotor activity and learning. *Brain Research Reviews, 6,* 173–196.

Beninger, R. J., Hanson, D. R., & Phillips, A. G. (1980). The effects of pipradrol on the acquisition of responding with conditioned reinforcement: A role for sensory preconditioning. *Psychopharmacology, 69,* 235–242.

Berger, B., Trottier, S., Gaspar, P., Verney, C., & Alvarez, C. (1988). Regional and laminar distribution of dopamine and serotonin innervation in the cynomolgus cerebral cortex. Major differences of dopamine input in the granular and agranular cortices. A radioautographic study. *Journal of Comparative Neurology, 273,* 99–119.

Berger, B., Verney, C., Alvarez, C., Vigny, A., & Helle, K. B. (1985). New dopaminergic fields in the motor, visual (area 18b) and retrosplenial cortex in the young and adult rat: Immunocytochemical and catecholamine histochemical analyses. *Neuroscience, 15,* 983–998.

Bhide, R. G., & Bhide, K. S. (1984). The effects of a lengthy period of environmental diversity on well fed and previously undernourished rats. II. Synapse to neuron ratios. *Journal of Comparative Neurology, 227*, 305–310.

Bindra, D. (1986). Neuropsychological interpretation of the effects of drive and incentive-motivation on general activity and instrumental behavior. *Psychological Review, 75*, 1–22.

Black, J. E., & Greenough, W. T. (1986). Induction of pattern in neural structure by experience: Implications for cognitive development. In M. E. Lamb, A. L. Brown, & B. Rogoff (eds.), *Advances in developmental psychology, Volume 4.* New Jersey: Erlbaum, pp. 1–50.

Blackburn, J. R., Phillips, A. G., & Fibiger, H. C. (1987). Dopamine and preparatory behavior: I. Effects of pimozide. *Behavioral Neuroscience, 101*, 352–360.

Blackburn, J. R., Phillips, A. G., Jakubovic, A., & Fibiger, H. C. (1989). Dopamine and preparatory behavior: II. A neurochemical analysis. *Behavoral Neuroscience, 103*, 15–23.

Bolles, R. C. (1972). Reinforcement, expectancy, and learning. *Psychological Review, 79*, 394–409.

Bowlby, J. (1969). *Attachment and loss. Volume 1: Attachment.* New York: Basic Books.

Bozarth, M. A. (1987). Ventral tegmental reward system. In J. Engel & L. Oreland (eds.), *Brain reward systems and abuse.* New York: Raven Press, pp. 1–17.

Broca, P. (1878). Anatomie comparee des circonvolutions cerebrales. Le grand lobe limbique et la scissure limbique dans le serie des mammiferes. *Reviews in Anthropology, 1*, 385–498.

Brown, R. M., Crane, A. M., & Goldman, P. S. (1979). Regional distribution of monoamines in the cerebral cortex and subcortical structures of the rhesus monkey: Concentrations and in vitro synthesis rates. *Brain Research, 168*, 133–150.

Brown, R. M., & Goldman, P. S. (1977). Catecholamines in neocortex of rhesus monkeys: Regional distribution and ontogenetic development. *Brain Research, 124*, 576–580.

Brown, R. T. (1968). Early experience and problem solving ability. *Journal of Comparative and Physiological Psychology, 65*, 433–440.

Brozoski, T. J., Brown, R. M., Rosvold, H. E., & Goldman, P. S. (1979). Cognitive deficit caused by regional depletion of dopamine in prefrontal cortex of rhesus monkey. *Science, 205*, 929–931.

Bunney, W. E. (1978). Psycholpharmacology of the switch process in affective disorders. In *Psychopharmacology: A generation of progress.* M. A. Lipton, A. DiMascio, & K. F. Killam (eds.). New York: Raven, pp. 1249–1259.

Cairns, R. B., Gariepy, J-L, & Hood, K. E. (1990). Development, microevolution, and social behavior. *Psychological Review, 97*, 49–65.

Camps, M., Cortes, R., Gueye, B., Probst, A., & Palacios, J. M. (1989). Dopamine receptors in human brain: Autoradiographic distribution of D2 sites. *Neuroscience, 28*, 275–290.

Chavis, D. A., & Pandya, D. N. (1976). Further observations on corticofrontal connections in the rhesus monkey. *Brain Research, 117*, 369–386.

Clark, A. S., & Goldman-Rakic, P. S. (1989). Gonadal hormones influence the emergence of cortical function in nonhuman primates. *Behavioral Neuroscience, 103*, 1287–1295.

Cookson, J. C. (1985). The neuroendocrinology of mania. *Journal of Affective Disorders, 8*, 233–241.

Cools, A. R. (1980). The role of neostriatal dopaminergic activity in sequencing and selecting behavioral strategies: Facilitation of processes involved in selecting the best strategy in a stressful situation. *Behavioral Brain Research, 1*, 361–374.

Cortes, R., Gueye, B., Pazos, A., Probst, A., & Palacios, J. M. (1989). Dopamine receptors in human brain: Autoradiographic distribution of D1 sites. *Neuroscience, 28*, 263–273.

Crow, T. (1972). Catecholamine-containing neurons and electrical stimulation: I. A review of some data. *Psychological Medicine, 2*, 414–421.

Dahlstrom, A., & Fuxe, K. (1964). Evidence for the existence of monoamine-containing neurons in the central nervous system. *Acta Physilogica Scandinavica, 62*, 1–55.

Depue, R. S., & Iacono, W. G. (1989). Neurobehavioral aspects of affective disorders. *Annual Review of Psychology, 40*, 457–492.

Depue, R. A., Kraus, S., & Spoont, M. R. (1987). A two-dimensional threshold model of seasonal bipolar affective disorder. In D. Magnusson & A. Ohman (eds.), *Psychopathology: An interactional perspective.* New York: Academic Press, pp. 95–123.

Depue, R. A., Kraus, S., Spoont, M. R., & Arbisi, P. (1989). Identification of unipolar and bipolar affective conditions in a nonclinical university population with the General Behavior Inventory. *Journal of Abnormal Psychology, 88*, 117–126.

Depue, R. A., Luciana, M., Arbisi, P., Collins, P. F., & Leon, A. Relation of agonist-induced dopamine activity to personality. Unpublished manuscript.

Depue, R. A., & Monroe, S. M. (1978). The unipolar-bipolar distinction in the depressive disorders. *Psychological Bulletin, 85*, 1001–1029.

Depue, R. A., & Spoont, M. R. (1986). Conceptualizing a serotonin trait: A behavioral dimension of constraint. *Annals of the New York Academy of Sciences, 487*, 47–62.

Diamond, M. C. (1967). Extensive cortical depth measurements and neuron size increases in the cortex of environmentally enriched rats. *Journal of Comparative Neurology, 131*, 357–364.

Durkin, T. P., Hashem-Zadeh, H., Mandel, P., Kempf, J., & Ebel, A. (1983). Genotypic variation in the dopaminergic inhibitory control of striatal and hippocampal cholinergic activity in mice. *Pharmacology, Biochemistry, and Behavior, 19*, 63–71.

Eibl-Eibesfeldt, I. (1975). *Ethology: The biology of behavior.* New York: Holt, Rinehart, & Winston.

Ervin, F. R., & Martin, J. (1986). Neurophysiological bases of the primary emotions. In E. Plutchick & H. Kellerman (eds.), *Emotion: Theory, research, and experience. Volume 3; Biological foundations of emotion.* New York: Academic Press, pp. 145–170.

Evenden, J. L., & Robbins, T. W. (1983). Increased response switching, perseveration and perseverative switching following d-amphetamine in the rat. *Psychopharmacology, 80*, 67–73.

Eysenck, H. J., & Eysenck, M. W. (1985). *Personality and individual differences: A natural science approach.* New York: Plenum Press.

Fibiger, H. C., & Phillips, A. G. (1981). Increased intracranial self-stimulation in rats after long-term administration of desipramine. *Science, 214*, 683–685.

Fibiger, H. C., & Phillips, A. G. (1987). Role of catecholamine transmitters in brain reward systems: Implications of the neurobiology of affect. In J. Engel & L. Oreland (eds.), *Brain reward systems and abuse.* New York: Raven Press, pp. 61–74.

Fink, J. S. & Reis, D. J. (1981). Genetic variations in midbrain dopamine cell number: Parallel with differences in responses to dopaminergic agonists and in naturalistic behaviors mediated by dopaminergic systems. *Brain Research, 222*, 335–349.

Fishman, R., Feigenbaum, J., Yanaiz, J., & Klawans, H. (1983). The relative importance of dopamine and norepinephrine in mediating locomotor activity. *Progress in Neurobiology, 20*, 55–88.

Floeter, M. K., & Greenough, W. T. (1979). Cerebellar plasticity: Modification of Purkinje cell structure by differential rearing in monkeys. *Science, 206*, 227–229.

Fonberg, E. (1986). Amygdala, emotions, motivation, and depressive states. In E. Plutchik & H. Kellerman (eds.), *Emotion: Theory, research, and experience. Volume 3: Biological foundations of emotion.* New York: Academic Press, pp. 301–331.

Fowles, D. C. (1980). The three arousal model: Implications of Gray's two-factor learning theory for heart rate, electrodermal activity, and psychopathy. *Pyschophysiology*, *17*, 87–104.

Fowles, D. C. (1987). Application of a behavioral theory of motivation to the concepts of anxiety and impulsivity. *Journal of Research in Personality*, *21*, 417–435.

Fray, P. J., Sahakian, B. J., Robbins, T. W., Koob, G. F., & Iversen, S. D. (1980). An observational method for quantifying the behavioural effects of dopamine agonists: Contrasting effects of d-amphetamine and apomorphine. *Psychopharmacology*, *69*, 253–259.

Freeman, B. J., & Ray, O. S. (1972). Strain, sex, and environmental effects on appetitively and aversively motivated learning tasks. *Developmental Psychobiology*, *5*, 101–109.

Friedman, H. R., Janas, J. D., & Goldman-Rakic, P. S. (1990). Enhancement of metabolic activity in the diencephalon of monkeys performing working memory tasks: A 2-deoxyglucose study in behaving rhesus monkeys. *Journal of Cognitive Neuroscience*, *2*, 18–31.

Funahashi, S., Bruce, C. J., & Goldman-Rakic, P. S. (1989). Mnemomic coding of visual space in the monkey's dorsolateral prefrontal cortex. *Journal of Neurophysiology*, *61*, 331–349.

Fuster, J. M. (1973). Unit activity in prefrontal cortex during delayed-response performance: Neuronal correlates of transient memory. *Journal of Neurophysiology*, *36*, 61–78.

Fuster, J. M. (1980). *The prefrontal cortex*. New York: Raven Press.

Fuxe, K., Agnati, L. F., Kalia, M., Goldstein, M., Andersson, K., & Harfstrand, A. (1985). Dopaminergic systems in the brain and pituitary. In E. Fluckiger, E. E. Muller, & M. O. Thorner (eds.), *The dopaminergic system*. New York: Springer-Verlag, pp. 11–26.

Gallistel, C. R., Shizgal, P., & Yeomans, J. S. (1981). A portrait of the substrate for self-stimulation. *Psychological Review*, *88*, 228–273.

Gaspar, P., Berger, B., Febvret, A., Vigny, A., & Henry, J. P. (1989). Catecholamine innervation of the human cerebral cortex as revealed by comparative immunohistochemistry of tyrosine hydroxylase and dopamine-beta-hydroxylase. *Journal of Comparative Neurology*, *279*, 249–271.

Glowinski, J., Tassin, J. P., & Thierry, A.-M. (1984). The mesocortico-prefrontal dopaminergic neurons. *Trends in the Neurosciences, November*, 415–418.

Goldman-Rakic, P. S. (1987). Circuitry of the prefrontal cortex and the regulation of behavior by representational memory. *Handbook of physiology*, *5* (Part 1, Ch. 9). Washington DC: American Physiological Society, pp. 373–417.

Goldman-Rakic, P. S. (1988). Topography of cognition: Parallel distributed networks in primate association cortex. *Annual Review of Neuroscience*, *11*, 137–156.

Goldman-Rakic, P. S., & Brown, R. M. (1981). Regional changes of monoamines in cerebral cortex and subcortical structures of aging rhesus monkeys. *Neuroscience*, *6*, 177–187.

Goldsmith, H. H., Buss, A. H., Plomin, R., Rothbart, M. K., Thomas, A., Chess, S., Hinde, R. A., & McCall, R. B. (1987). Roundtable: What is temperament? Four approaches. *Child Development*, *58*, 505–529.

Gould, S. J. (1977). *Ontogeny and phylogeny*. Cambridge: Harvard University Press.

Gray, J. A. (1973). Causal theories of personality and how to test them. In J. R. Royce (ed.), *Multivariate analysis and psychological theory*. New York: Academic Press, pp. 409–463.

Gray, J. A. (1982). *The neuropsychology of anxiety*. New York: Oxford Press.

Green, E. J., Greenough, W. T., & Schlumpf, B. E. (1983). Effects of complex or isolated environments on cortical dendrites of middle-aged rats. *Brain Research*, *264*, 233–240.

Greenough, W. T., & Black, J. E. (in press). Induction of brain structure by experience: Substrates for cognitive development. To appear in M. R. Gunnar & C. A. Nelson (eds.), *Minnesota symposia on Child Psychology, Volume 24*.

Greenough, W. T., Black, J. E., & Wallace, C. S. (1987). Experience and brain development. *Child Development, 58*, 539–559.

Greenough, W. T., Fulcher, J. K., Yuwiler, A., & Geller, E. (1970). Enriched rearing and chronic electroshock: Effects on brain and behavior in mice. *Physiology and Behavior, 5*, 371–373.

Greenough, W. T., & Volkmar, F. R. (1973). Pattern of dendritic branching in rat occipital cortex after rearing in complex environments. *Experiental Neurology, 40*, 491–504.

Greenough, W. T., Volkmar, F. R., & Juraska, J. M. (1973). Effects of rearing complexity on dendritic branching in frontolateral and temporal cortex of the rat. *Experimental Neurology, 41*, 371–378.

Greenough, W. T., West, R. W., & DeVoogd, T. J. (1978). Subsynaptic plate perforations: Changes with age and experience in the rat. *Science, 202*, 1096–1098.

Greenough, W. T., Wood, W. E., & Madden, T. C. (1972). Possible memory storage differences among mice reared in environments varying in complexity. *Behavioral Biology, 7*, 717–722.

Greenough, W. T., Yuwiler, A., & Dollinger, M. (1973). Effects of post-trial eserine administration on learning in "enriched" and "impoverished" reared rats. *Behavioral Biology, 8*, 261–272.

Haas, H. L. (1983). Amine neurotransmitter actions in the hippocampus. In W. Seifert (ed.), *Neurobiology of the hippocampus*. New York: Academic Press, pp. 139–155.

Harris, J. P., & Phillipson, O. T. (1981). Chlorpromazine reduces the perceptual ambiguity of a reversible visual figure. *Neuropharmacology, 20*, 1337–1338.

Hebb, D. O. (1949). *The organization of behavior*. New York: Wiley.

Heimer, L. (1978). The olfactory cortex and the ventral striatum. In K. E. Livingston & O. Hornykiewicz (eds.), *Limbic mechanisms*. New York: Plenum Press, pp. 134–162.

Heimer, L., & Wilson, R. D. (1975). The subcortical projections of the allocortex: Similarities in the neural associations of the hippocampus, the piriform cortex and the neocortex. In M. Santini (ed.), *Golgi Centennial Symposium: Perspectives in neurobiology*. New York: Raven Press, pp. 177–193.

Herkenham, M., & Nauta, W. J. H. (1977). Afferent connections of the habenular nuclei in the rat. A horseradish peroxidase study, with a note on the fiber-of-passage problem. *Journal of Comparative Neurology, 173*, 123–146.

Herkenham, M., & Nauta, W. J. H. (1979). Efferent connections of the habenular nuclei in the rat. *Journal of Comparative Neurology, 187*, 19–48.

Herzog, A. G., & Van Hoesen, G. W. (1976). Temporal neocortical afferent connections to the amygdala in the rhesus monkey. *Brain Research, 115*, 57–69.

Hill, R. T. (1970). Facilitation of conditioned reinforcement as a mechanism of psychomotor stimulants. In E. Costa & S. Garattini (eds.), *Amphetamines and related compounds*. New York: Raven Press, 781–795.

Hofer, M. A. (1987). Early social relationships: A psychobiologist's view. *Child Development, 58*, 633–647.

Huttenlocher, P. R. (1979). Synaptic density in human frontal cortex: Developmental changes and effects of aging. *Brain Research, 163*, 195–205.

Huttenlocher, P. R. (1990). Morphometric study of human cerebral cortex development. *Neuropsychologia, 28*, 517–527.

Huttenlocher, P. R., de Courten, C., Garey, L. G., & van der Loos, H. (1982). Synaptogenesis in human visual cortex: Evidence for synapse elimination during normal development. *Neuroscience Letters, 33*, 247–252.

Iversen, S. D. (1978). Brain dopamine systems and behavior. In L. Iversen, S. Iversen, &

S. Snyder (eds.), *Handbook of psychopharmacology, Vol. 8*. New York: Plenum Press, pp. 333–384.

Iversen, S. D. (1984). Cortical monoamines and behavior. In L. Descarries, T. Reader, & H. H. Jasper (eds.), *Monoamine innervation of the cerebral cortex*. New York: Alan R. Liss, Inc., pp. 321–349.

Iversen, S. D., & Fray, P. J. (1982). Brain catecholamines in relation to affect. In A. Beckman (ed.), *The neural basis of behavior*. New York: Spectrum Publications, pp. 229–269.

Izard, C. E., & Saxton, P. M. (1988). Emotions. In R. C. Atkinson, R. J. Herrnstein, G. Lindzey, & R. D. Luce (eds.), *Stevens' handbook of experimental psychology, Volume 1: Perception and motivation*. New York: Wiley, pp. 627–676.

Jimerson, D. C., & Post, R. M. (1984). Psychomotor stimulants and dopamine agonists in depression. In R. M. Post & J. C. Ballenger (eds.), *Neurobiology of mood disorders*. Baltimore: Williams & Wilkins, pp. 619–628.

Jones, E. G., & Powell, T. P. S. (1970). An anatomical study of converging sensory pathways within the cerebral cortex of the monkey. *Brain, 93*, 793–820.

Juraska, J. M., Fitch, J., Henderson, C., & Rivers, N. (1985). Sex differences in the dendritic branching of dentate granule cells following differential housing experience. *Brain Research, 333*, 73–80.

Juraska, J. M., Fitch, J., & Washburne, D. L. (1989). The dendritic morphology of pyramidal neurons in the rat hippocampal CA3 area. II. Effects of gender and experience. *Brain Research 479*, 115–119.

Juraska, J. M., Greenough, W. T., Elliott, C., Mack, K. J., & Berkowitz, R. (1980). Plasticity in adult rat visual cortex: An examination of several cell populations after differential housing. *Behavioral and Neural Biology, 29*, 157–167.

Kelley, A. E., Stinus, L., & Iversen, S. D. (1979). Behavioral activation induced in the rat by substance P infusion into the ventral tegmental area: implication of dopaminergic A10 neurones. *Neuroscience Letters, 11*, 335–339.

Kelley, A. E., Stinus, L., & Iversen, S. D. (1980). Interactions between d-ala-met-enkephalin, A10 dopaminergic neurones, and spontaneous behavior in the rat. *Behavioral Brain Research, 1*, 3–24.

Kelley, P. (1978). Drug-induced behavior. In S. D. Iversen, L. L. Iversen, & S. Snyder (eds.), *Handbook of psychopharmacology, Vol. 8*. New York: Plenum Press, 295–331.

Kemp, J. M., & Powell, T. P. S. (1970). The cortico-striate projections in the monkey. *Brain, 93*, 525–546.

Killackey, H. P. (1990). Neocortical expansion: An attempt toward relating phylogeny and ontogeny. *Journal of Cognitive Neuroscience, 2*, 1–17.

Kling, A. S. (1986). The anatomy of aggression and affiliation. In E. Plutchik & H. Kellerman (eds.), *Emotion: Theory, research, and experience, Volume 3: Biological foundations of emotion*. New York: Academic Press, pp. 237–263.

Konorski, J. (1967). *Integrative activity of the brain: An interdisciplinary approach*. Chicago: University of Chicago Press.

Koob, G. F., & Bloom, F. E. (1988). Cellular and molecular mechanisms of drug dependence. *Science, 242*, 715–723.

Kosslyn, S. M. (1988). Aspects of a cognitive neuroscience of mental imagery. *Science, 240*, 1621–1626.

Kraemer, G. W. (1985). Effects of differences in early social experience on primate neurobiological-behavioral development. In M. Reite & T. Field (eds.), *The psychobiology of attachment and separation*. New York: Academic Press, pp. 135–161.

Kraemer, G. W., Ebert, M. H., Lake, C. R., & McKinney, W. T. (1984). Hypersensitivity to d-amphetamine several years after early social deprivation in rhesus monkeys. *Psychopharmacology, 82*, 266–271.

Kubota, K., & Niki, H. (1971). Prefrontal cortical unit activity and delayed alternation performance in monkeys. *Journal of Neurophysiology*, 34, 337–347.

Larson, J., & Lynch, G. (1986). Induction of synaptic potentiation in hippocampus by patterned stimulation involves two events. *Science*, 232, 985–988.

Lauder, J. M., & Krebs, H. (1986). Do neurotransmitters, neurohumors, and hormones specify critical periods? In W. T. Greenough & J. Juraska (eds.), *Developmental neuropsychobiology*. New York: Academic Press, pp. 120–174.

LeDoux, J. E. (1987). Emotion. *Handbook of physiology*, 5 (Part 1, Ch. 10). Washington DC: American Physiological Society, pp. 419–459.

LeVay, S., Wiesel, T. N., & Hubel, D. H. (1980). The development of ocular dominance columns in normal and visually deprived monkeys. *Journal of Comparative Neurology*, 191, 1–51.

Levi, L. (1975). *Emotions – their parameters and measurement*. New York: Raven Press.

Levitt, P., Rakic, P., & Goldman-Rakic, P. (1984a). Region-specific distribution of catecholamine afferents in primate cerebral cortex: A fluorescence histochemical analysis. *Journal of Comparative Neurology*, 227, 23–36.

Levitt, P., Rakic, P., & Goldman-Rakic, P. (1984b). Comparative assessment of monoamine afferents in mammalian cerebral cortex. In H. H. Jasper & N. van Gelder (eds.), *Monoamine innervation of the cerebral cortex*, New York: Alan Liss, Inc., pp. 41–59.

Lewis, D. A., Campbell, M. J., Foote, S. L., & Morrison, J. H. (1986). The monoaminergic innervation of primate neocortex. *Human Neurobiology*, 5, 181–188.

Lewis, D. A., Campbell, M. J., Foote, S. L., & Morrison, J. H. (1987). The distribution of tyrosine hydroxylase immunoreactive fibers in primate neocortex is widespread but regionally specific. *Journal of Neuroscience*, 7, 279–290.

Lewis, D. A., Foote, S. L., Goldstein, M., & Morrison, J. H. (1988). The dopaminergic innervation of monkey prefrontal cortex: A tyrosine hydroxylase immunohistochemical study. *Brain Research*, 449, 225–243.

Lidow, M. S., Goldman-Rakic, P. S., Rakic, P., & Innis, R. B. (1989). Dopamine D2 receptors in the cerebral cortex: Distribution and pharmacological characterization with [3H]raclopride. *Proceedings of the National Academy of Science*, 86, 6412–6416.

Livingston, K. E., & Escobar, A. (1971). Anatomical bias of the limbic systems concept. *Archives of Neurology*, 24, 17–21.

Louilot, A., Taghzouti, K., Deminiere, J. M., Simon, H., Le Moal, M. (1987). Dopamine and behavior: Functional and theoretical considerations. In M. Sandler, *Neurotransmitter interactions in the basal ganglia*. New York: Raven Press, pp. 193–204.

Luciana, M., Depue, R. A., Arbisi, P., & Leon, A. (1992). Facilitation of working memory in humans by a D2 dopamine receptor agonist. *Journal of Cognitive Neuroscience*, 4, 58–68.

Lyness, W. H., Friedle, N. M., & Moore, K. E. (1979). Destruction of dopaminergic nerve terminals in nucleus accumbens: Effect on d-amphetamine self-administration. *Pharmacology, Biochemistry, and Behavior*, 11, 553–556.

MacLean, P. D. (1969). The hypothalamus and emotional behavior. In W. Haymaker, E. Anderson, & W. J. H. Nauta (eds.), *The Hypothalamus*. Springfield: Thomas.

MacLean, P. D. (1970). The triune concept of the brain and behavior. In F. O. Schmitt (ed.), *The Neurosciences Second Study Program*. New York: Rockerfeller University Press.

MacLean, P. D. (1975). Sensory and perceptive factors in emotional functions of the triune brain. In L. Levi (ed.), *Emotions – their parameters and measurement*. New York: Raven Press, pp. 71–92.

MacLean, P. D. (1986). Ictal symptoms relating to the nature of affects and their cerebral substrate. In E. Plutchik & H. Kellerman (eds.), *Emotion: Theory, research, and* experience. Volume 3: Biological foundations of emotion. New York: Academic Press, pp. 61–90.

MacLean, P. D. (1990). The triune brain in evolution: Role in paleocerebral functions. New York: Plenum Press.

Malakhova, O. E., Popovkin, E. M., & Gudina, I. G. (1989). Efferent connections of various parts of the orbitofrontal cortex with the thalamic structures of the cat. Neuroscience and Behavioral Physiology, 19, 507–515.

Mandell, A. J., Knapp, S., Ehlers, C., & Russo, P. V. (1984). The stability of constrained randomness: Lithium prophylaxis at several neurobiological levels. In R. M. Post & J. C. Ballenger (eds.), Neurobiology of Mood Disorders. Baltimore: Williams & Wilkins, pp. 744–776.

Marczynski, T. J. (1986). A model of brain function. In W. C. McCallum, R. Zappoli, & F. Denoth (eds.), Cerebral psychophysiology: Studies in event-related potentials. (Electroencephalography and Clinical Neurophysiology suppl. 38), pp. 351–367.

Mason, S. T. (1984). Catecholamines and behavior. New York: Cambridge.

Mattson, M. P. (1988). Neurotransmitters in the regulation of neuronal cytoarchitecture. Brain Research Reviews, 13, 179–212.

Mattson, M. P., Dou, P., & Kater, S. B. (1988). Outgrowth-regulating actions of glutamate in isolated hippocampal pyramidal neurons. Journal of Neuroscience, 8, 2987–2100.

Mesulam, M.-M. (1984). A cortical network for directed attention and unilateral neglect. In A. Ardila & F. Ostrosky-Solis (eds.), The right hemisphere. New York: Gordon & Breach, pp. 61–96.

Mesulam, M.-M. (1985). Principles of behavioral neurology. Philadelphia: FA Davis Company.

Mesulam, M.-M. (1990). Large-scale neurocognitive networks and distributed processing for attention, language, and memory. Annals of Neurology, 28, 597–613.

Mesulam, M.-M., & Mufson, E. J. (1982a). Insula of the old world monkey. Part I. Architectonics in the insulo-orbito-temporal component of the paralimbic brain. Journal of Comparative Neurology, 212, 1–22.

Mesulam, M.-M., & Mufson, E. J. (1982b). Insula of the old world monkey. Part III. Efferent cortical output and comments on function. Journal of Comparative Neurology, 212, 38–52.

Mesulam, M.-M., & Mufson, E. J. (1984). Neural inputs into the nucleus basalis of the substantia innominata (CH4) in the rhesus monkey. Brain, 107, 253–274.

Milner, P. (1977). Theories of reinforcement, drive, and motivation. In L. Iversen, S. Iversen, & S. Snyder (eds.), Handbook of psychopharmacology, Vol. 7. New York: Plenum Press, pp. 181–200.

Mishkin, M. (1982). A memory system in the monkey. Philosophical Transactions of the Royal Society, B298, 85–95.

Mogenson, G. J., Jones, D. L., & Yim, C. Y. (1980). From motivation to action: Functional interface between the limbic system and the motor system. Progress in Neurobiology, 14, 69–97.

Mogenson, G. J., Takigawa, M., Robertson, A., & Wu, M. (1979). Self-stimulation of the nucleus accumbens and ventral tegmental area of Tsai attenuated by microinjections of spiroperidol into the nucleus accumbens. Brain Research, 171, 247–259.

Mogenson, G. J., Wu, M., & Manchanela, S. K. (1979). Locomotor activity initiated by microinfusions of picrotoxin in the ventral tegmental area. Brain Research, 161, 311–319.

Moore, R. Y., & Bloom, F. E. (1978). Central catecholamine neuron systems: Anatomy and physiology of the dopamine systems. Annual Review of Neuroscience, 1, 129–169.

Morgan, M. J. (1973). Effects of post-weaning environment on learning in the rat. Animal Behaviour, 21, 4429–4442.

Nauta, W. J. H. (1964). Some efferent connections of the prefrontal cortex in the monkey. In J. M. Warren & K. Akert (eds.), *The frontal granular cortex and behavior*. New York: McGraw-Hill, pp. 397–409.

Nauta, W. J. H. (1971). The problem of the frontal lobe: A reinterpretation. *Journal of Psychiatric Research, 8*, 167–187.

Nauta, W. J. H. (1986). Circuitous connections linking cerebral cortex, limbic system, and corpus striatum. In B. K. Doane & K. E. Livingston (eds.), *The limbic system: functional organization and clinical disorders*. New York: Raven Press, pp. 43–54.

Nauta, W. J. H., & Domesick, V. B. (1981). Ramifications of the limbic system. In S. Matthysse (ed.), *Psychiatry and the biology of the human brain*. Amsterdam: Elsevier North Holland, Inc., pp. 165–188.

Niki, H. (1974a). Differential activity of prefrontal units during right and left delayed response trials. *Brain Research, 70*, 346–349.

Niki, H. (1974b). Prefrontal unit activity during delayed alternation in the monkey. I: Relation to direction of response. *Brain Research, 68*, 185–196.

Niki, H. (1974c). Prefrontal unit activity during delayed alternation in the monkey. II: Relation to absolute versus relative direction of response. *Brain Research, 68*, 197–204.

Oades, R. D. (1985). The role of noradrenaline in tuning and dopamine in switching between signals in the CNS. *Neuroscience and Biobehavioral Reviews, 9*, 261–282.

Oades, R. D., & Halliday, G. M. (1987). Ventral tegmental (A10) system: Neurobiology. 1. Anatomy and connectivity. *Brain Research Reviews, 12*, 117–165.

Oades, R. D., Rea, M., & Taghzouti, K. (1984). Modulation of selective processes in learning by neocortical and limbic dopamine: Studies of behavioral strategies. In B. E. Will, P. Schmitt, & J. C. Dalrymple-Alford (eds.), *Brain plasticity, learning, and memory*. New York: Plenum Press, pp. 241–251.

Oades, R. D., Taghzouti, K., Rivet, J.-M., Simon, H., & Le Moal, M. (1986). Locomotor activity in relation to dopamine and noradrenaline in the nucleus accumbens, septal and frontal areas: A 6-hydroxydopamine study. *Neuropsychobiology, 16*, 37–43.

O'Kusky, J., & Colonnier, M. (1982). Postnatal changes in the number of neurons and synapses in the visual cortex (A17) of the macaque monkey. *Journal of Comparative Neurology, 210*, 291–296.

Olds, J. (1958). Self-stimulation of the brain. *Science, 127*, 315–324.

Olds, J. (1977). *Drives and reinforcements: Behavioral studies of hypothalamic functions*. New York: Raven Press.

Olds, J., & Miller, P. M. (1954). Positive reinforcement produced by electrical stimulation of the septal area and other regions of rat brain. *Journal of Comparative Physiology and Psychology, 47*, 419–427.

Olds, M. E., & Fobes, J. L. (1981). The central basis of motivation: Intracranial self-stimulation studies. *Annual Review of Psychology, 32*, 523–574.

Olton, D. S., Becker, J. T., & Handelmann, G. E. (1979). Hippocampus, space, and memory. *Behavioral and Brain Sciences, 2*, 313–365.

Ortony, A., & Turner, T. J. (1990). What's basic about basic emotions? *Psychological Review, 97*, 315–331.

Panksepp, J. (1982). Toward a general psychobiology of emotions. *The Behavioral and Brain Science, 5*, 407–468.

Panksepp, J. (1986). The anatomy of emotions. In E. Plutchik & H. Kellerman (eds.), *Emotion: Theory, research, and experience. Volume 3: Biological foundations of emotion*. New York: Academic Press, pp. 91–124.

Panksepp, J., Siviy, S. M., & Normansell, L. A. (1985). Brain opioids and social emotions. In M. Reite & T. Field (eds.), *The psychobiology of attachment and separation*. New York: Academic Press, pp. 3–49.

Papez, J. W. (1937). A proposed mechanism of emotion. *Archives of Neurology and Psychiatry, 79*, 217–224.

Phillips, A. G., & Fibiger, H. C. (1978). The role of dopamine in maintaining intracranial self-stimulation in the ventral tegmentum, nucleus accumbens, medial and sulcal prefrontal cortices. *Canadian Journal of Psychology, 32*, 58–66.

Phillipson, O. T., & Griffiths, A. C. (1985). The topographic order of inputs to nucleus accumbens in the rat. *Neuroscience, 16*, 275–296.

Pipp, S., & Harmon, R. J. (1987). Attachment as regulation: A commentary. *Child Development, 58*, 648–652.

Pizzolato, G., Soncrant, T. T., & Rapoport, S. I. (1985). Time-course and regional distribution of the metablic effects of bromocriptine in the rat brian. *Brain Research, 341*, 303–312.

Plomin, R. (1986). *Development, genetics, and psychology*. New Jersey: Erlbaum.

Ploog, D. (1986). Biological foundations of the vocal expressions of emotions. In E. Plutchick & H. Kellerman (eds.), *Emotion: Theory, research, and experience. Volume 3: Biological foundations of emotion*. New York: Academic Press, pp. 173–197.

Plutchik, R. (1980). *Emotion: A psychoevolutionary synthesis*. New York: Harper & Row.

Plutchik, E., & Kellerman, H. (1986). *Emotion: Theory, research, and experience. Volume 3: Biological foundations of emotion*. New York: Academic Press.

Porrino, L. J. (1987). Cerebral metabolic changes associated with activation of reward systems. In J. Engel & L. Oreland (eds.), *Brain reward systems and abuse*. New York: Raven Press, pp. 51–60.

Porrino, L. J., Crane, A. M., & Goldman-Rakic, P. S. (1981). Direct and indirect pathways from the amygdala to the frontal lobe in rhesus monkeys. *Journal of Comparative Neurology, 198*, 121–136.

Porrino, L. J., & Goldman-Rakic, P. S. (1982). Brain stem innervation of prefrontal and anterior cingulate cortex in the rhesus monkey revealed by retrograde transport of HRP. *Journal of Comparative Neurology, 205*, 63–76.

Posner, M. I., Petersen, S. E., Fox, P. T., & Raichle, M. E. (1988). Localization of cognitive operations in the human brain. *Science, 240*, 1627–1631.

Post, R. M. (1980). Biochemical theories of mania. In R. H. Belmaker & H. M. van Praag (eds.), *Mania: An evolving concept*. New York: Spectrum, pp. 217–267.

Post, R. M., & Uhde, T. W. (1982). Biological relationships between mania and melacholia. *L'Encephale, 8*, 213–228.

Pysh, J. J., & Weiss, M. (1979). Exercise during development induces an increase in Purkinje cell dendritic tree size. *Science, 206*, 230–232.

Rakic, P., Bourgeois, J.-P., Eckenhoff, M. F., Zecevic, M., & Goldman-Rakic, P. S. (1986). Concurrent overproduction of synapses in diverse regions of primate cerebral cortex. *Science, 232*, 232–234.

Reader, T. A., Ferron, A., Descarries, L., & Jasper, H. H. (1979). Modulatory role for biogenic amines in the cerebral cortex. *Brain Research, 160*, 217–229.

Reibaud, M., Blanc, G., Studler, J. M., Glowinski, J., Tassin, J. P. (1984). Non-DA prefronto-cortical efferents modulate D1 receptors in the nucleus accumbens. *Brain Research, 305*, 43–50.

Reite, M., & Field, T. (1985). *The psychobiology of attachment and separation*. New York: Academic Press.

Risch, S. J., & Janowsky, D. S. (1984). Cholinergic-adrenergic balance in affective illness. In R. M. Post & J. C. Ballenger (eds.), *Neurobiology of Mood Disorders*. Baltimore: Williams & Wilkins, pp. 652–663.

Roberts, D. C. S., Corcoran, M. E., & Fibiger, H. C. (1977). On the role of the ascending catecholaminergic systems in intravenous self-administration of cocaine. *Pharmacology, Biochemistry, and Behavior, 6*, 615–620.

Roberts, D. C. S., Koob, G. F., Klonoff, P., & Fibiger, H. C. (1980). Extinction and recovery of cocaine self-administration following 6-hydroxydopamine lesions of the nucleus accumbens. *Pharmacology, Biochemistry, and Behavior, 12*, 781–787.

Roberts, D. C. S., & Zito, K. A. (1987). Interpretation of lesion effects on stimulant self-administration. In M. A. Bozarth (ed.), *Methods of assessing the reinforcing properties of abused drugs.* New York: Springer-Verlag, pp. 119–132.

Robertson, A. (1989). Multiple reward systems and the prefrontal cortex. *Neuroscience and Biobehavioral Reviews, 13,* 163–170.

Robbins, T. W. (1975). The potentiation of conditioned reinforcement by psychomotor stimulant drugs: A test of Hill's hypothesis. *Psychopharmacology, 45,* 103–114.

Roitblat, S. (1987). *Introduction to comparative cognition.* New York: Freeman Press.

Rolls, E. T. (1986). Neural systems involved in emotion in primates. In E. Plutchik & H. Kellerman (eds.), *Emotion: Theory, research, and experience. Volume 3: Biological foundations of emotion.* New York: Academic Press, pp. 125–143.

Rolls, E. T. (1989). Information processing in the taste system of primates. *Journal of Experimental Biology, 146,* 141–164.

Rolls, E. T. (in press). Spatial memory, episodic memory, and neuronal network functions in the hippocampus. To appear in L. Squire (ed.), *The biology of memory, Symposia Hoechst.* Frankfurt, Hoechst, AG.

Rosenkilde, C. E. (1979). Functional heterogeneity of the prefrontal cortex in the monkey: A review. *Behavioral and Neural Biology, 25,* 301–345.

Rosenzweig, M. R., & Bennett, E. L. (1978). Experiential influences on brain anatomy and brain chemistry in rodents. In G. Gottlieb (ed.), *Studies on the development of behavior and the nervous system: Volume 4. Early influences.* New York: Academic Press, pp. 289–330.

Russchen, F. T., Amaral, D. G., & Price, J. L. (1985). The afferent connections of the substantia innominata in the monkey. *Journal of Comparative Neurology, 242,* 1–27.

Sackett, G. P., Bowman, R. E., Meyer, J. S., Tripp, R. S., & Grady, S. S. (1973). Adrenocortical and behavioral reactions by differentially raised rhesus monkeys. *Physiological Psychology, 1,* 209–212.

Sanides, F. (1970). Functional architecture of motor and sensory cortices in primates in the light of a new concept of neocortex evolution. In C. Noback & W. Montagna (eds.), *The primate brain: Advances in primatology, Vol. 2.* New York: Appleton-Century-Crofts, pp. 137–208.

Sawaguchi, T., & Goldman-Rakic, P. S. (1991). D1 dopamine receptors in prefrontal cortex: Involvement in working memory. *Science, 251,* 947–950.

Sawaguchi, T., Matsumura, M., & Kubota, K. (1988). Dopamine enhances the neuronal activity related to a spatial short-term memory task in the primate prefrontal cortex. *Neurocience Research, 5,* 465–473.

Sawaguchi, T., Matsumura, M., & Kubota, K. (1990a). Catecholamine effects on neuronal activity related to a delayed response task in monkey prefrontal cortex. *Journal of Neurophysiology, 63,* 1385–1400.

Sawaguchi, T., Matusumura, M., & Kubota, K. (1990b). Effects of dopamine antagonists on neuronal activity related to a delayed response task in monkey prefrontal cortex. *Journal of Neurophysiology, 63,* 1401–1412.

Schneirla, T. (1959). An evolutionary and developmental theory of biphasic processes underlying approach and withdrawal. In M. Jones (ed.), *Nebraska Symposium on Motivation.* Lincoln: University of Nebraska Press, pp. 27–58.

Schultz, W. (1986). Responses of midbrain dopamine neurons to trigger stumuli in the monkey. *Journal of Neurophysiology, 56,* 1439–1461.

Secunda, S. K., Swann, A., Katz, M. M., Koslow, S. H., Croghan, J., & Chang, S. (1987). Diagnosis and treatment of mixed mania. *American Journal of Psychiatry, 144,* 96–98.

Seeger, T. F., Porrino, L. J., Esposito, R. U., Crane, A. M., Sullivan, T. L., & Pert, A. (1984). Amphetamine effects on intracranial self-stimulation as assessed by the quantitative 2-deoxyglucose method. *Society for Neuroscience Abstracts, 10,* 307.

Shopsin, B. (1989). *Manic illness.* New York: Raven Press.

Simon, H., Scatton, B., & Le Moal, M. (1980). Dopaminergic A10 neurons are involved in cognitive functions. *Nature*, 288, 150–151.

Sirevaag, A. M., Black, J. E., Shafron, D., & Greenough, W. T. (1988). Direct evidence that complex experience increases capillary branching and surface area in visual cortex of young rats. *Developmental Brain Research*, 43, 299–304.

Sirevaag, A. M., & Greenough, W. T. (1985). Differential rearing effects on rat visual cortex synapses. II. Synaptic morphometry. *Developmental Brain Research*, 19, 215–226.

Sitiram, N., Gillin, C., & Bunney, W. E. (1984). Cholinergic and catecholaminergic receptor sensitivity in affective illness: Strategy and theory. In R. M. Post & J. C. Ballenger (eds.), *Neurobiology of mood disorders*. Baltimore: Williams & Wilkins, pp. 629–651.

Silverston, T. (1985). Dopamine in manic depressive illness. *Journal of Affective Disorders*, 8, 225–231.

Soubrie, P. (1986). Reconciling the role of central serotonin neurons in human and animal behavior. *The Behavioral and Brain Sciences*, 9, 319–364.

Spyraki, C., & Fibiger, H. C. (1981). Behavioural evidence for supersensitivity of postsynaptic dopamine receptors in the mesolimbic system after chronic administration of desipramine. *European Journal of Pharmacology*, 74, 195–206.

Sroufe, L. A. (1979). The coherence of individual development. *American Psychologist*, 34, 834–841.

Stein, L. (1962). Effects and interactions of imipramine, chloropromazine, reserpine and amphetamine on self-stimulation: Possible neurophysiological basis of depression. In J. Wortis (ed.), *Recent advances in biological psychiatry*. New York: Plenum Press, pp. 288–308.

Stein, L. (1983). The chemistry of positive reward. In M. Zuckerman (ed.), *The biological basis of sensation seeking, impulsivity, and anxiety*. New Jersey: Erblaum.

Stewart, J., de Wit, H., & Eikelboom, R. (1984). Role of unconditioned and conditioned drug effects in the self-administration of opiates and stimulants. *Psychological Review*, 91, 251–268.

Stone, T. W. (1976). Responses of neurones in the cerebral cortex and caudate nucleus to amantadine, amphetamine and dopamine. *British Journal of Pharmacology*, 56, 101–110.

Stone, T. W., & Bailay, E. V. (1975). Responses of central neurones to amantadine: Comparison with dopamine and amphetamine. *Brain Research*, 85, 126–129.

Sved, A. F., Baker, H. A., & Reis, D. J. (1984). Dopamine synthesis in inbred mouse strains which differ in numbers of dopamine neurons. *Brain Research*, 303, 261–266.

Sved, A. F., Baker, H. A., & Reis, D. J. (1985). Number of dopamine neurons predicts prolactin levels in two inbred mouse strains. *Experientia*, 41, 644–646.

Tassin, J. P., Simon, J., Glowinski, J., & Brockaert, J. (1982). Modulation of the sensitivity of dopamine receptors in the prefrontal cortex and the nucleus accumbens. In E. Ricollu (ed.), *Brain peptides and hormones*. New York: Raven Press, pp. 17–30.

Tellegen, A. (1985). Structures of mood and personality and their relevance to assessing anxiety, with an emphasis on self-report. In A. H. Tuma & J. D. Maser (eds.), *Anxiety and the anxiety disorders*. New Jersey: Erlbaum, pp. 681–706.

Tellegen, A. (1988). The analysis of consistency in personality assessment. *Journal of Personality*, 56, 621–663.

Tellegen, A., Lykken, D. T., Bouchard, T. J., Wilcox, K. J., Segal, N. L., & Rich, S. (1988). Personality similarity in twins reared apart and together. *Journal of Personality and Social Psychology*, 54, 1031–1039.

Tellegen, A., & Waller, N. G. (in press). Exploring personality through test construction: Development of the multidimensional personality questionnaire. To appear in S. R.

Briggs & J. M. Cheek (eds.), *Personality measures: Development and evaluation (vol. 1)*. Greenwich, CN: JAI Press.

Thierry, A.-M., Deniau, J. M., & Feger, J. (1979). Effects of stimulation of the frontal cortex on identified output VMT cells in the rat. *Neuroscience Letters, 15*, 103–107.

Thierry, A.-M., Tassin, J. P., & Glowinski, J. (1984). Biochemical and electrophysiological studies of the mesocortical dopamine system. In L. Descarries, T. Reader, & H. Jasper (eds.), *Monoamine innervation of cerebral cortex*. New York: Alan R Liss, Inc., pp. 233–261.

Thorpe, S. J., Rolls, E. T., & Maddison, S. (1983). Neuronal activity in the orbitofrontal cortex of the behaving monkey. *Experimental Brain Research, 49*, 93–115.

Tinbergen, N. (1951). *The study of instinct*. London: Oxford University Press.

Tronick, E. Z., Winn, S., & Morelli, G. A. (1985). Multiple caretaking in the context of human evolution: Why don't the Efe know the western prescription for child care? In M. Reite & T. Field (eds.), *The psychobiology of attachment and separation*. New York: Academic Press, pp. 293–322.

Turkewitz, G., & Kenny, P. A. (1982). Limitations on input as a basis for neural organization and perceptual development: A preliminary theoretical statement. *Developmental Psychology, 15*, 357–368.

Turner, A. M., & Greenough, W. T. (1983). Synapses per neuron and synaptic dimensions in occipital cortex of rats reared in complex, social, or isolation housing. *Acta Stereologica, 2 (Suppl. 1)*, 239–244.

Turner, A. M., & Greenough, W. T. (1985). Differential rearing effects on rat visual cortex synapses. I. Synaptic and neuronal density and synapses per neuron. *Brain Research, 329*, 195–203.

Turner, B. H., Mishkin, M., & Knapp, M. (1980). Organization of the amygdalopetal projections from modality-specific cortical association areas in the monkey. *Journal of Comparative Neurology, 191*, 515–543.

Uylings, H. B. M., Kuypers, K., & Veltman, W. A. M. (1978). Environmental influences on neocortex in later life. In M. A. Corner, R. E. Baker, N. E. van de Poll, D. F. Swabb, & H. B. M. Uylings (eds.), *Maturation of the nervous system: Progress in brain research, Volume 48*. Amsterdam: Elsevier, pp. 261–274.

Valzelli, L. (1981). *Psychobiology of aggression and violence*. New York: Raven Press.

Van Hoesen, G. W., Pandya, D. N., & Butters, N. (1975). Some connections of the entorhinal (area 28) and perirhinal (area 35) cortices of the rhesus monkey. II. Frontal lobe afferents. *Brain Research, 95*, 25–38.

Volkmar, F. R., & Greenough, W. T. (1972). Rearing complexity affects branching of dendrites in the visual cortex of the rat. *Science, 176*, 1445–1447.

Von Noorden, G. K., & Dowling, J. E. (1970). Experimental amblyopia in monkeys. II. Behavioral studies of strabismic amblyopia. *Archives of Ophthalmology, (Chicago), 84*, 215–220.

Watanabe, T., & Niki, H. (1985). Hippocampal unit activity and delayed response in the monkey. *Brain Research, 325*, 241–254.

Waters, E. (1981). Traits, behavioral systems, and relationships: Three models of infant-mother attachment. In G. Barlow, K. Immelman, M. Main, & L. Petrinovitch (eds.), *The development of behavior*, Cambridge: Cambridge University Press.

Watkins, J. C., & Evans, R. H. (1981). Excitatory amino acid neurotransmitters. *Annual Review of Pharmacology and Toxicology, 21*, 165–204.

Watson, D., & Tellegen, A. (1985). Towards a consensual structure of mood. *Psychological Bulletin, 92*, 426–457.

West, R. W., & Greenough, W. T. (1972). Effect of environmental complexity on cortical synapses of rats: Preliminary results. *Behavioral Biology, 7*, 279–284.

Whitlock, D. G., & Nauta, W. J. H. (1956). Subcortical projections from the temporal neocortex in *Macaca mulatta*. *Journal of Comparative Neurology, 106*, 183–212.

Wiesel, T. N., & Hubel, D. H. (1963). Single-cell responses in striate cortex of kittens deprived of vision in one eye. Journal of Neurophysiology, 26, 1003–1017.

Wilson, W. J., & Soltysik, S. S. (1985). Pharmacological manipulations of the nucleus accumbens: Effects on classically conditioned responses and locomotor activity in the cat. Acta Neurobiologiae Experimentalis, 45, 91–105.

Wise, R. A. (1978). Catecholamine theories of reward: A critical review. Brain Research, 152, 215–247.

Wise, R. A. (1982). Neuroleptics and operant behavior: The anhedonia hypothesis. The Behavioral and Brain Sciences, 5, 39–53.

Yakovlev, P. I. (1948). Motility, behavior, and the brain. Journal of Nervous and Mental Diseases, 107, 313–335.

Yakovlev, P. I. (1959). Pathoarchitectonic studies of cerebral malformation. 3. Arrhinencephalies (holotelencephalies). Journal of Neuropathology and Experimental Neurology, 18, 22–25.

Yokel, R. A., & Wise, R. A. (1975). Increased lever pressing for amphetamine after pimozide in rats: Implications for a dopamine theory of reward. Science, 187, 547–549.

Yokel, R. A., & Wise, R. A. (1976). Attenuation of intravenous amphetamine reinforcement by central dopamine blockade in rats. Psychopharmacology, 48, 311–318.

Zevon, M. A., & Tellegen, A. (1982). The structure of mood change: an idiographic/ nomothetic analysis. Journal of Personality and Social Psychology, 43, 111–122.

Zuckerman, M. (1983). Biological bases of sensation seeking, impulsivity, and anxiety. New Jersey: Erlbaum.

III Influence of Maternal Depression on Infant Affect Regulation

JEFFREY F. COHN & SUSAN B. CAMPBELL

Maternal depression is a major risk factor in a wide range of developmental domains. Within the first year to two, socio-emotional development appears most affected. Infants and toddlers of depressed mothers are at increased risk for developing an insecure attachment (Cummings & Cicchetti, 1990; Radke-Yarrow, Cummings, Kuczynski, & Chapman, 1985), problems in the regulation of affect (Gaensbauer, Harmon, Cytryn, & McKnew, 1984; Zahn-Waxler, Cummings, McKnew, & Radke-Yarrow, 1984), and lack of persistence in meeting age-appropriate cognitive challenges (Redding, Harmon, & Morgan, 1990). By 12 to 18 months, maternal depression is related to mild impairments in general cognitive ability (Lyons-Ruth, Zoll, Connell, & Grunebaum, 1986; Sameroff, Seifer, & Zax, 1982). Later in development, maternal depression is associated with increased risk of poor academic performance (Baldwin, Cole, & Baldwin, 1982), and both behavior problems and affective disorder (Beardslee, Bemporad, Keller, & Klerman, 1983; Caplan, Cogill, Alexandrin, Robson, Katz, & Kumar, 1989; Cytryn, McKnew, Zahn-Waxler, Radke-Yarrow, Gaensbauer, Harmon, & Lamour, 1984; Downey & Coyne, 1990; Zahn-Waxler, Iannotti, Cummings, & Denham, 1990).

The mechanisms responsible for the increased risks associated with maternal depression are not well understood. Especially in bipolar depression, an underlying genetic diathesis may be a contributing factor (Numberger & Gershon, 1984). However, the range and extent of suboptimal outcomes associated with having a depressed parent cannot be attributed simply to genetic factors either in isolation or in conjunction with particular child-rearing environments (Beardslee et al., 1983; Cytryn et al., 1984). Thus, it is important to understand how parental depression is experienced by infants and young children and how that experience might contribute to increased chances of suboptimal socio-emotional and intellectual development.

Preparation of this manuscript was supported in part by NIMH Grant 40867 to the authors.

Even normal adults come to feel depressed after interacting with a depressed person (Coyne, 1976). In infants and young children, who are dependent upon their primary caregivers, the cumulative effects of depressed behavior on their development are likely to be substantial. A guiding question is this: Does depressed maternal behavior and consequent interactional disturbance mediate the effects of maternal depression on infants and young children? Recent research addresses this question.

Reciprocity in the affective and social exchanges between mothers and infants is a robust finding in studies of non-depressed mothers and infants. In mother-infant interactions, the frequency, duration, and timing of infant expressions are closely related to those of the mother (Cohn & Tronick, 1988, 1987; Cohn & Elmore, 1988; Lester, Hoffman, & Brazelton, 1985; Symons & Moran, 1987). Face-to-face interactions are central to the development of communication skills, topic sharing, and the socialization of emotion expression (Kaye, 1982; Malatesta & Haviland, 1982; Schaffer, 1984), and the mother-infant relationship is believed to be crucial to the quality of infant attachment (Ainsworth, Blehar, Waters, & Wall, 1978; Belsky, Rovine, & Taylor, 1984; Egeland & Farber, 1984; Malatesta, Culver, Tesman, & Shepard, 1989). It is therefore likely that the effect of maternal depression is mediated through its influence on the mother's behavior with her infant. To test this proposition, we need to determine that: 1) infants are responsive to depressed behavior; 2) depressed mothers behave in a depressed way with their infants; and 3) infant adaptation to a depressed caregiver is related to socio-emotional outcomes.

Affective disturbances, especially the 'postpartum blues' (Hopkins, Marcus, & Campbell, 1987) are common in the postpartum period, and it is possible that natural selection has made infants relatively immune to disturbances of this sort. Just as a "stimulus barrier" (i.e., habituation) appears to protect babies from over-stimulation, other self-regulatory or relational mechanisms may shield them from experiencing depressed maternal behavior. Infants exert powerful effects of their own on caregivers, and it is possible that an infant can draw out even a mother who is depressed. Depressed mothers may not behave in a depressed way with their baby. This may be particularly true in middle-class, intact, well-functioning families. The demands of parenting also change with development. It is possible that depressed mothers are able to cope well with a young infant, but less so with one who is more demanding of social interaction or autonomy.

Depression also is not a unitary disorder, so the effects on infants are bound to be complex and related to variation in maternal functioning. Affective expression may be sad, depressed, flat, angry, or irritable. The normal timing of affective expressions may also be altered. They may be either slowed down and delayed (as in psycho-motor retardation) or speeded up and frenetic (i.e., hypo-mania). These emotional states may be relatively stable and trait-like (e.g., as in dysthymia); or they may be labile, alternating, for instance, between sad and angry. Affective expression that is sad and withdrawn may have very different effects than depressed affect that is angry or irritable. Individual differences among depressed mothers may be highly salient to infant affective behavior and development. The effects of depression may also depend on how long the episode lasts, whether it recurs, and on the presence of any lingering dysthymia or irritation. Indeed, risk status appears greatest when depression is current (Caplan et al., 1989) or chronic and severe (Sameroff, Seifer, & Zax, 1982; Seifer & Barocas, 1991) or occurs in the context of dysthymia (Frankel, Maslin-Cole, & Harmon, 1991) or other risk factors (Downey & Coyne, 1990; Rutter, Yule, Quinton, Rowlands, Yule, & Berger, 1974; Rutter & Garmezy, 1983).

In this chapter we will review studies showing that infants respond in specific and characteristic ways to depressed maternal affect, and that these effects carry over to situations in which mothers no longer behave in a depressed way. Some of these data come from laboratory manipulations in which mothers distort their typical behavior and act depressed or unresponsive. The assumption in this work is that clinically depressed mothers behave in the way that is modeled in these laboratory simulations. Is this assumption valid? Do depressed mothers interact in a "depressed" way with their infants? And especially important to socioemotional development, do the effects of depressed interactions alter the pattern of infant responsiveness and carryover to new situations?

We will show that current, moderate to severe depression negatively influences mothers and infants, that infant coping remains impaired even after mothers are no longer acting depressed, but that these effects in infants are not irreversible. We will also emphasize the importance of attending to individual differences in patterns of mother-infant adaptation.

Infants have specific and appropriate responses to depressed maternal behavior

To learn whether infants have specific and appropriate responses to depressed maternal behavior, it is necessary to modify the mother's normal behavior and evaluate infant response. Experimental studies of this sort cannot answer questions about the cumulative effects of depressed maternal behavior, but they can discover whether infants are responsive to depressed behavior when first experienced.

As noted above, depressed behavior may take many forms. Clinical reports frequently refer to affective expression that is flat, sad, and withdrawn, or that is angry, hostile, and intrusive. Two studies have tested the hypothesis that sad or withdrawn affective expression leads to negative affect in infants. Cohn and Tronick (1983) instructed mothers of 3-month-old infants to simulate depression or behave normally while interacting with their infant. Infants responded dramatically to this manipulation. They briefly smiled at the mother and when she failed to respond, they quickly turned away. This pattern repeated several times as the infants became increasingly withdrawn and upset.

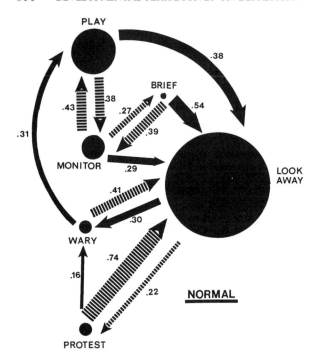

Figure 1. State transition diagram for normal and simulated depressed conditions. The relative proportion of infant time spent in each state is indicated by the size of the circle representing that state. Arrows represent transition probabilities among states. The thickness of arrows represents the relative size of the conditional probabilities of event sequence transition. Striped arrows indicate those transition probabilities for which conditional and unconditional probabilities significantly differ, $p < .05$.
Reprinted with permission from Cohn & Tronick (1983).

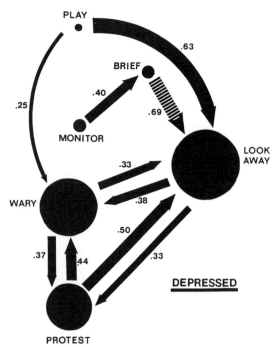

Figure 1, from Cohn and Tronick (1983), shows the difference in infants' behavior between the simulated depressed and normal interactions. The size of the circles represents the proportion of time that infants spent in each affective state. The arrows represent the probability of transitions among states.

In the simulated depressed condition, the proportion of positive affect (denoted by *play*) was far less than in the normal interaction. Extreme reductions in the mother's positive affect resulted in extreme reductions in the positive affect of the baby. When babies became positive, they did so only briefly (*brief positive*). Note, too, that the organization as well as the distribution of infant's behavior was affected. Not only were infants more negative and less positive, but they also organized their behavior differently. They no longer cycled between neutral- (denoted by *monitor*) and positive affective expression. Instead, they cycled between negative affective states and *look away*. Even after mothers again resumed non-depressed behavior, infants remained more negative and withdrawn. Thus, in this experimental manipulation, sad, flat affect reduced both concurrent and subsequent infant positive affective response.

The carry-over effect of depressed interaction found by Cohn and Tronick (1983) has been found to generalize to interactions in which the mother has had chronic depressive symptoms. Field (1984) instructed mothers with high levels of depressive symptoms and non-depressed control mothers to simulate depressed behavior with their infant. Replicating the original findings, infants of non-depressed mothers responded to simulated depression with increased negative affect and remained more negative and less responsive even after their mother resumed non-depressed behavior. Infants of mothers with high levels of depressive symptoms, however, showed little change between the normal and simulated depressed interaction. Field interpreted this finding as suggesting that infants of mothers who were actually depressed saw little change between their mother's normal behavior and a situation in which she was instructed to act sad and withdrawn. Affective expressions other than sad or constricted affect have yet to be studied experimentally.

In the simulated depression experiments, maternal affect and responsiveness were dampened. However, it is possible that depression might differentially affect one or the other aspect of the mother's behavior. For instance, clinically depressed mothers might successfully "simulate" positive affect, but have greater difficulty in coordinating the timing of their expressions. Ekman (1984) has emphasized the role of false smiles in adult interactions, but little attention has been paid to the temporal organization of disingenuous affective expression in interactions with infants and young children.

To test whether the timing as well as the quality of maternal affect influences infant behavior, Cohn and Elmore (1988) modified Tronick's (Tronick, Als, Adamson, Wise, & Brazelton, 1978) still-face procedure. In the original study, Tronick et al. asked mothers to hold a still-face and remain unresponsive while seated *en face* with their baby. In the modification by Cohn and

Elmore, mothers of 3-month-old babies were instructed to become still-faced for 5 seconds contingent on their infant becoming positive. This perturbation of the usual relation between mothers' and infants' affect provided a test of how closely infants monitor the temporal relationship between their own and their mother's affect.

Consistent with earlier research (Cohn & Tronick, 1987; Kaye & Fogel, 1980), mothers were almost always in a positive state when their infant became positive. But when mothers briefly became still-faced contingent on infants' positive expression, the infants became less likely to cycle between positive and neutral expression and more likely to turn away.

This study demonstrated that babies are sensitive to the reciprocity of their mother's affective behavior. However, the mismatches (cf. Tronick & Cohn, 1989) between mothers' and infants' affect in this manipulation were relatively long (5 seconds) and were defined primarily in terms of facial expression of affect. Timing violations of shorter duration and in other modalities might have less effect. The durations of maternal vocalizations are much briefer than those of maternal facial expressions, and infants may be more sensitive to their mother's latency to respond vocally.

Interactions between depressed mothers and infants are less positive and more negative than those of non-depressed mother-infant pairs

Given the strong experimental evidence that infants are sensitive to depressed maternal affective expression, at least of the type studied to date, it is important to learn whether depressed mothers behave in a "depressed" way with their infants. Do depressed mothers show distortions of affective expression and timing in their interactions? Are interactions between depressed mothers and infants less positive and more negative than those of non-depressed mother-infant pairs? The answers to these questions depend in part on how depression is defined.

Diagnostic and related issues. Most research on infants (Bettes, 1988; Cohn, Matias, Tronick, Lyons-Ruth, & Connell, 1986; Cohn & Tronick, 1989; Field, 1984; Field, Healy, Goldstein, Perry, Schanberg, Zimmerman, & Kuhn, 1988) has used self-report measures of mothers' depressive symptoms rather than a standard clinical interview to diagnose depression. Commonly used self-report instruments are the Center for Epidemiologic Studies Depression Scale (CES–D: Radloff, 1977) and the Beck Depression Inventory (BDI: Beck, Ward, Mendelson, et al., 1961). These are Likert-type scales that include items about mood and cognitive and vegetative symptoms associated with depression. High scores suggest greater severity and are considered diagnostic for screening purposes. Self-report measures in the postpartum period, however, over-diagnose depression and fail to identify some women who meet formal diagnostic criteria (Campbell & Cohn, 1991; Gotlib, Whiffen, Mount, Milne, & Cordy, 1989; O'Hara, Neunaber, & Zekoski, 1984). Elevated levels of depressive symptoms may index a range of psychiatric disorders, and not just depression (Garrison & Earls, 1986).

Table 1. Correspondence between RDC and CES–D Score to Determine Depression's Prevalence

	CES–D Score			
	Depressed		Not Depressed	
	N	%	N	%
RDC				
Depressed	55	59.8	37	40.2
Not Depressed	77	8.4	838	91.6

Note. Cut-score on the CES–D was 16.
Kappa = .43. Adapted from Campbell & Cohn (in press).

Table 1 shows the correspondence between a diagnostic interview and the CES–D in a middle-class primiparous sample of about 1000 women (Campbell & Cohn, in press). Prevalence according to RDC (Spitzer, Endicott, & Robins, 1978) is 9%; prevalence according to the CES–D is about half again as much. The CES–D serves well as a screening instrument; but were depressed subjects identified with the CES–D, almost half would fail to meet diagnostic criteria. Thus, studies that do not use diagnostic criteria can be only suggestive of effects related to depression as opposed to more general distress.

More generally, little is known about the prevalence, duration, and course of depression in postpartum women. Most epidemiologic studies concentrate on community samples without particular reference to the transition to parenthood (e.g., Myers & Weissman, 1980), and diagnostic differences across studies make what data exist difficult to evaluate. With the exception of recent work by Gotlib (Gotlib et al., 1989) and by O'Hara (O'Hara et al., 1984, 1990), few studies have used standard diagnostic criteria to define depression in postpartum women. Only one study has used standard diagnostic criteria to study the course of depression beyond the postpartum period (Campbell, Cohn, Flanagan, Popper, & Meyers 1992).

Depression is an episodic disorder of variable duration. In unselected community and clinical groups, individual episodes may last any where from several weeks to a half year or more (Akiskal, 1982; Clayton, 1983). Campbell et al. (1992) document a similar course in postpartum women. Rate of relapse is high: approximately 50% within 2 years of recovery (Belsher & Costello, 1988; NIMH/NIH Consensus Conference [1985], cited in McLean & Hakstian, 1990). Thus, it is difficult to know how many infants may have a depressed mother, how long her depression might last, or whether it is likely to re-occur. Few women might have chronic depressions, but those few may have the most significant effects on their infants.

Depression is also frequently confounded with other risk factors, such as poverty, family disruption, and child abuse and neglect. Some epidemiologic evidence suggests that depression in the absence of multiple risk factors may be of less consequence to infant or child behavior and development (Robins, 1974; Rutter et al., 1974; for review, see Rutter & Garmezy, 1983), although appropriate studies remain to be done. Thus, findings from studies that recruit subjects unsystematically, assess depression through self-report instruments, or confound depression with other risk factors cannot support strong inferences about the influence of depression. It is important, therefore, to make careful distinctions with respect to presence or absence of other risk factors.

High levels of depressive symptoms in the context of other risk factors. Using the BDI to assess depression in women of low SES, Field conducted a series of cross-sectional studies that suggest depressed mothers and their infants show fewer positive- and more negative facial expressions and vocalize less than non-depressed mothers and infants (Field, 1984). Depressed mother-infant pairs were more likely to share negative affect, whereas non-depressed dyads were more likely to share positive affect (Field, Healy, Goldstein, & Guthertz, 1990). Infants of depressed mothers were also more likely to respond with increased negative and less positive affective expressions during interactions with a non-depressed female stranger (Field, Healy, & Goldstein et al., 1988). These studies by Field suggest that negative affect is more common in interactions between depressed versus non-depressed mothers and infants in multi-problem families.

Individual differences. Depression is a heterogeneous disorder. In an exploratory study, we studied individual differences in the expression of negative affect in mothers with chronic depressive symptomatology (Cohn et al., 1986; Cohn & Tronick, 1989). Subjects were thirteen mothers and their 6- to 7-month-old infants. They were all part of a longitudinal study conducted by Lyons-Ruth (Lyons-Ruth et al., 1987). The mothers had moderate to severe levels of depressive symptoms, as assessed with the CES–D, and high rates of factors associated with risk of childhood behavior disorder, such as child neglect, substance abuse, and low SES (Rutter & Garmezy, 1983).

The behavior of these mothers was strikingly unlike that of mothers in normative studies. Mothers in well functioning families typically display positive affect about half the time and do not show expressions of angry or rough behavior. By contrast, the mothers in this clinical group were withdrawn or interacted in an aggressive, intrusive way with few positive affective expressions. Anger/poke, which refers to angry or intrusive behavior, occurred about 25% of the time (Table 2). Disengagement, such as leaning back and away from the baby and being unresponsive, occurred about 40% of the time. With few exceptions, the mothers in this study all showed at least some negative affect. Negative behavior is rare in normative studies. The infants' behavior was also less positive.

Table 2. Percentage of Time in Negative and Positive States.

	Depressed	Normative
Mothers		
Anger/Poke	23	0
Play	21	42
Infants		
Avert/Protest	64	22
Play	6	15

Note. Depression data are adapted from Cohn & Tronick (1989).
Normative, comparison data are adapted from Cohn & Tronick (1987).

The number of subjects was small, but variations among mothers in type of negative affect shown was pronounced (Figure 2). At the extreme of disengagement, two mothers (M-Disengaged) showed a pattern similar to some clinical descriptions of depressed mothers (Weissman & Paykel, 1974) and what Cohn and Tronick (1983) and also Field (1984) had modeled in the simulated depression studies. These mothers were disengaged more than 75% of the time. They slouched back in their chairs, often turned away, and spoke in an expressionless voice. They were responsive only to active infant distress.

At the other extreme was the largest group (M-Intrusive): six mothers with high proportions of angry or intrusive behaviors, such as rough handling, poking at their babies, and speaking in an angry tone. Two others (M-Mixed) also showed *anger/poke*, although less so, together with some *play* and much *elicit* (attempts to get the baby's attention). A small group of three mothers (M-Positive) showed high rates of positive expression, comparable to those found among non-depressed mothers (Cohn & Tronick, 1987; Kaye & Fogel, 1980).

Maternal disengagement and intrusiveness had quite different effects on infants. Infants of disengaged mothers had the highest proportions of *protest*, which suggests that the most distressing behavior for infants may be the pattern of maternal disengagement (Figure 3). Infants of intrusive mothers had the highest proportions of *look away*, which is consistent with previous work indicating that increases in maternal intensity are unsuccessful in re-establishing mutual interaction when infants are looking away (Cohn & Tronick, 1987; Kaye & Fogel, 1980). The infants of the most positive mothers had the highest proportions of *play*. These individual differences were unrelated to any particular combination of risk factors. Within this clinical group, depressive symptoms and other risk factors did not predict maladaptive

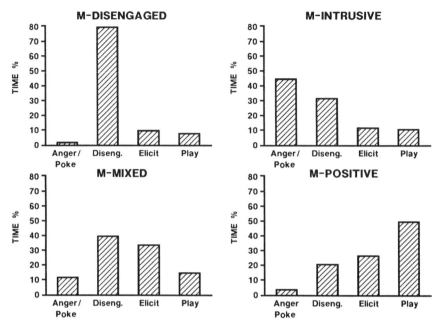

Figure 2. Individual differences among mothers in the percentage of time spent in behavioral states during face-to-face interaction with their babies. Reprinted with permission from Cohn & Tronick (1989).

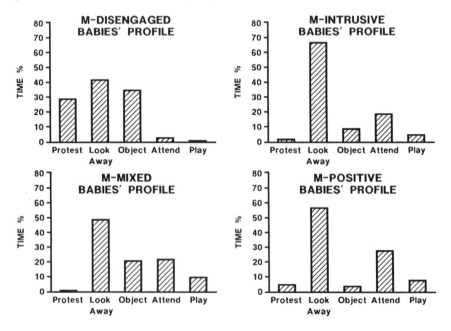

Figure 3. Individual differences among babies in the percentage of time spent in behavioral states during face-to-face interaction with their mothers. Reprinted with permission from Cohn & Tronick (1989).

interaction patterns in a simple one-to-one fashion. Infants' affective behavior was specific to the affective quality and reciprocity of mothers' behavior. **High levels of depressive symptoms in the absence of multiple risk factors.** Some studies indicate that depression has an impact on mothers and infants in low-SES, multi-problem families. Even subclinical levels of depression may influence mother's interactive behavior significantly. But what about depression when it occurs in the absence of other risk factors? Do mothers behave in a less positive, more negative way?

Using the BDI to assess depression in middle-class mothers, Bettes (1988) studied the timing and acoustic contours of mothers' vocalizations to 3-month-old infants. The mothers she studied had subclinical to mild depression according to the BDI. Depressed mothers were slower to respond to their infant's vocalizations, and were less likely to use the expanded intonation contours that are typical of infant-directed speech. Depressed mothers also used vocal utterances and pauses of more variable duration. Predictable utterance and pause durations and exaggerated contours are believed to promote dyadic interaction. Although differences in vocal behavior between depressed and non-depressed mothers in this study were striking, Bettes reported no differences in infant behavior. One reason may be the low levels of depression; or that measurements of infant behavior were limited to vocal utterances and pauses and measures of mothers' behavior were limited to the vocal expression. It is possible that maternal facial expression, in particular, did not vary between depressed and non-depressed groups. Alternatively, the influence of depression on infant behavior in the absence of multiple risk factors may be less pervasive.

Depression assessed according to diagnostic criteria

The studies reviewed in the preceding section all used self-report symptom ratings to assess depression; depression often co-occurred with other risk factors; with few exceptions assessments were not longitudinal; and because subjects were recruited informally or through service providers, little was known about how representative subjects were of other mothers and infants.

To pursue these and related issues, we (Campbell & Cohn, 1991; Campbell et al., 1992; Cohn et al., 1990, 1992) are studying the prevalence and course of depression in the postpartum period, its influence on the developing relationship between mothers and infants, and the infant's capacity to regulate affect in response to age-appropriate stressors. We first will present findings based on telephone screening of approximately 1000 postpartum mothers at 6 postpartum weeks. We then will present initial findings based on intensive longitudinal study of our initial subjects (n with complete data to date ranges from 50 to 65 at each age).

Subject recruitment and study design. We recruit mothers from delivery records at Magee Womens' Hospital, the major obstetrics hospital in Pittsburgh. Mothers are then interviewed over the phone at 6 weeks postpartum to determine whether they meet diagnostic criteria for depression. To be included in the screening population, mothers and infants must meet criteria intended to minimize the occurrence of other risk factors. Diagnostic screening interviews are scored according to modified Research Diagnostic Criteria. We also obtain from each mother a self-report measure of depression (CES–D). Scores above 16 are considered to reflect severe symptoms (Myers & Weissman, 1980).

Women meeting screening criteria for depression and non-depressed controls are interviewed in their homes at 2 months. For diagnoses, we administer the SADS–L (Endicott & Spitzer, 1978) as modified by O'Hara (O'Hara et al., 1984) for postpartum women. Women are asked about mood and the major symptoms of depression (sleep disturbance, appetite changes, fatigue, loss of interest or anhedonia, concentration difficulties, guilt, agitation or retardation, and thoughts of suicidal ideation).

Mood and symptoms are rated on 6-point scales, from 1 (not present or present to a normal degree) to 6 (serious and incapacitating). Only ratings of 3 and above are considered clinically significant. Further, since this is a postpartum sample in which changes, especially in sleep, fatigue, and appetite are expected (Campbell & Cohn, in press; O'Hara et al., 1984), sleep disruptions that are accounted for by the baby waking up are not counted as a symptom. Similarly, increases in appetite are considered a normal reaction to the birth of a baby and are coded as clinically significant only in extreme cases, especially in the first few postpartum months, and for breast-feeding women. Loss of interest in sex is not included as a symptom, but women who reported loss of interest in the baby are considered to evidence loss of interest. The duration of mood and symptoms is also recorded.

Sad mood and anhedonia and at least three symptoms must be present together for at least two weeks to meet criteria for a diagnosis of depression. Further, women must endorse the SADS questions about help seeking and/or functional impairment to receive a diagnosis. Women with three symptoms rated as clinically significant are considered to meet criteria for minor depression; those with four symptoms are considered as probable major depression; and women with five or more symptoms are considered to meet criteria for definite major depression. So far, 86% of the depressed women have met criteria for probable or definite major depression.

In some of the analyses we distinguish between two groups of depressed mothers — those with current and acute depression and those whose depression was already remitting by 2 months postpartum. Twenty-seven mothers met modified RDC and also had CES–D scores above 16. These women were both clinically depressed, as determined by psychiatric interview and diagnosis, and reported subjective feelings of acute distress. Ten women met RDC only. Their depressions in many cases had remitted by the time of the 2-month assessment. Thirty-one mothers were non-depressed control subjects. We excluded women who had clinically significant CES–D scores (i.e., 16) but who did not also meet criteria for depression. Thus, we distinguish two groups of depressed mothers: those meeting Research Diagnostic Criteria at some time during the first two postpartum months and also experiencing high levels of self-reported distress, and those mothers who meet RDC only. By defining these subgroups, we were able to determine whether psychiatric criteria alone, or psychiatric criteria together with high levels of self-reported distress, was crucial for mediating mothers' and infants' behavior.

Behavioral observations are conducted in the families' home at 2, 4, and 6 months and in the laboratory (Strange Situation assessment) at 12 months. Observations include structured and spontaneous mother-infant interactions and infant response to the mother remaining unresponsive (still-face). We also conduct a telephone assessment of depression at 9 months.

During the structured and still-face interactions, mothers and infants behavior is videotaped and later coded on a 1-s time base by staff blind to mothers' diagnosis. (See Cohn et al., 1990 for details). Home visitors, who are not blind to diagnosis, complete rating scales descriptive of mothers' and infants' behavior during the 2- to 3-hour interview and observation period. The scales are derived from previous research on maternal sensitivity (Ainsworth, Blehar, Waters, & Wall, 1978), maternal affect and engagement (Lyons-Ruth, Connell, Zoll, & Stahl, 1987; Vaughn, Taraldson, Crichton, & Egeland, 1980), and infant responsiveness (Vaughn et al., 1980). In all, 12 maternal, infant, and dyadic behaviors were rated. These ratings were then subjected to a principal components analysis with varimax rotation. Two factors, affect and sensitivity accounted for about 60% of the variance in mothers' behavior at each age. An affect factor also accounts for about 60% of the variance in infant behavior at each age. (See Cohn et al., 1990 for details).

To summarize, we assess depression, mother-infant interaction, infant response to age-appropriate stressors (still-face at 2 through 6 months and Strange Situation at 12 months), and other features of mothers' and infants' adjustment longitudinally over the course of the first year. (Assessments through 30 months are in progress, but are not described here.)

Demographic comparisons between depressed and non-depressed mothers. In the screening sample (Campbell & Cohn, 1991) we find minor but significant differences in SES between postpartum depressed and non-depressed subjects. SES in both groups is middle class, but is slightly lower quantitatively on the Hollingshead scale in depressed women. Minor pregnancy and delivery complications, also tend to be slightly more common in the depressed mothers. Thus, even in an otherwise low-risk population, depression still tends to occur together with other risk factors. As Downey and Coyne emphasize (1990), findings such as these suggest caution in making inferences specific to depression.

Reports of pregnancy experiences. Depressed mothers in the longitudinal sample (Campbell et al., in press) reported higher rates of psychological distress during pregnancy. Postpartum depressed mothers more often hadn't planned their pregnancy. Not surprisingly, they also reported a much higher prevalence of negative thoughts about their pregnancy. These group

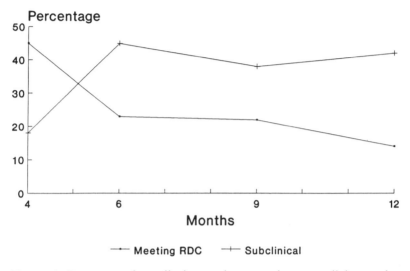

Course of Depression in Primiparous Mothers Meeting RDC at 2 Months

Figure 4. Percentage of initially depressed women who were still depressed or showed subclinical symptoms of depression through 12 months.

differences suggest that the antecedents of postpartum depression may be found within the pregnancy period.

Course of depression. Depression remitted in about 80% of depressed mothers by 6 months, although depressed mood or related symptoms continued in about half of all remitted cases. Figure 4 shows the percentage of mothers who were still depressed through 12 months. Also shown is the percentage who, while no longer meeting criteria for depression, continued to experience subclinical levels of depressed mood or symptoms.

Stability of mothers' and infants' behavior

To assess the stability of mothers' and infants' affect over time, we computed stability coefficients for both the face-to-face interactions and the home ratings. In both sets of analyses, we found evidence of moderate stability. The test-retest correlation between a 2- and 4-month composite for positive affect (high and low positive) was approximately .5; from 4- to 6 months, this correlation increased to about .7. From 4 to 6 months negative affect in mothers became more stable. This was due to increasing negativity in some depressed mothers. Infant behavior was less stable but also showed an increase in stability for negative affect. Figure 5 shows the stability coefficients for mothers' and infants' affect in face-to-face interaction between 4 and 6 months.

Stability Coefficients:
Four to Six Months

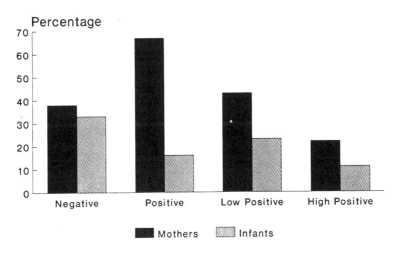

coeffs > .25, p < .05

Figure 5. Stability coefficients for percentage of time mothers and babies spent in affective states.

These stability coefficients are much larger than those reported in another context by Bakeman and Brown (1980). One reason may be the wide range of mothers we studied. It may also be the case that mothers' and infants' behavior during even brief interactions is far more stable than has previously been assumed (Kaye, 1982).

The same pattern was found in the home ratings. Mothers' behavior showed moderate stability, increasing over time. Infant stability coefficients were low but significant from 4 to 6 months. Thus, mothers provided a consistent affective environment to which their infant responded, and we see evidence that a possible cumulative effect was to bring about increasing stability in infant behavior.

Reciprocity of affect. A consistent finding in previous studies is that mothers and infants reciprocate affect. We have conducted two analyses of mother-infant reciprocity. First, we have correlated the distributions of mother and infant negative and positive affect during face-to-face interactions. This analysis tells us whether mother-infant pairs are matching affective level over time. The second analysis is a time-series regression to assess synchrony and mutual influence. A consistent finding at each age is that mothers and infants matched each other's level of positive and negative affect. We find a moderate correlation between mothers' and infants' affect at each age.

Moment-to-moment synchrony, or coherence, increases from 2 to 4 months, but is unrelated to diagnostic status. In our analyses so far, we have found no differences in synchrony related to depression (Cohn et al., 1990). Mutual influence appears equal in each group. Mothers and infants respond contingently to each other's affective displays.

Generalizability of affect expression during face-to-face interactions. Significant correlations between behavior in the two settings were found in the larger sample at 2 and at 4 months, although not at 6 months. Thus, the two assessments, structured interaction and naturalistic observation, showed moderate stability and also low to moderate concurrent validity.

Depressed mothers and infants are more negative and less positive than non-depressed mothers. RDC/CES–D mothers, those both meeting psychiatric criteria and having high levels of subjective distress, more clearly differed from both RDC only and control subjects (Figure 6). RDC/CES–D mothers had a narrower range of positive affect (lower percentages of high positive/exaggerated expressions). The amount of negative affect at 2 months in RDC/CES–D mothers, while not significant signalled an important developmental trend. With development, prevalence of negative rather than positive affect more consistently discriminated depressed from non-depressed mothers.

The infant data parallel those for the mothers. Infants of depressed mothers had lower proportions of low positive, or interest, and more negative affect. These differences were due to the infants of RDC/CES–D mothers (Figure 7).

In the subjects we have studied to date, we have not found strong differences in face-to-face interaction among any of the groups at 4 or 6 months, with the exception of the increase in the number of depressed mothers who show negative affect.

In the home ratings, we again found that RDC/CES–D dyads accounted for depression effects at 2 months. We also found evidence of continued impairments in this group at 4 months. Maternal sensitivity, which primarily reflected negative affect, differentiated these groups at 2 and 4 months. Thus, in both the structured face-to-face interaction and in the home ratings we found an increase in maternal negative affect over time in RDC/CES–D mothers.

Infants' response to age appropriate stressors. Both the still-face and attachment assessments stress the infant's resources to cope with challenges around salient developmental issues. A central developmental issue for infants 2 through 6 months is the sharing of positive affect and the regulation of face-to-face exchanges. When mothers fail to match infant affect, the infant's task is to initiate a change in her behavior. Positive elicits in response to the still-face demonstrate the infant's ability in this regard. At 12 months the attachment relationship is a central developmental issue. The infant must regulate negative affect through an adaptive working model of the attachment relationship and use of the mother when distressed. Thus, both assessments tap the infant's expectations about the mother's responsiveness and the infant's ability to cope when stressed. Maternal depression is believed to decrease the likelihood of both positive elicits during the still-face (Field, 1984) and attachment security (Cicchetti & Aber, 1986; Cummings & Cicchetti, 1990). We wanted to tested these hypotheses and also learn whether positive

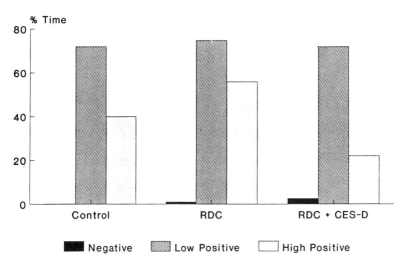

Figure 6. Percentage of mothers' time spent in affective states at 2 months.

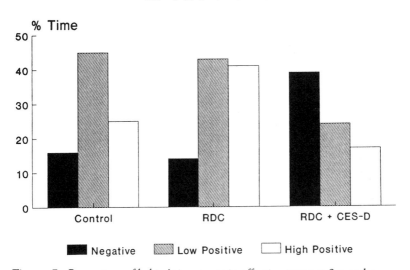

Figure 7. Percentage of babies' time spent in affective states at 2 months.

elicits predict attachment security. An early pilot study (Tronick, Ricks, & Cohn, 1982) suggested this might be true.

Consistent with the findings of Field (1984), infants of RDC/CES–D mothers had lower frequencies of positive elicits at 4 months, although not at 2 or 6 months. Differences between groups at those ages were in the expected direction, and may achieve statistical significance once our sample is complete. Diagnostic status at 2 months did not contribute to the prediction of attachment; however, we have found a trend suggesting that chronicity of depression is associated with increased insecurity. Of six mothers who were still depressed at 6 months, five had infants who were classified as avoidant or resistant.

Experience with alternative caregivers may have moderated a depression effect. Non-maternal care was common by six months: about 20 hours per week on average. In infants of mothers who were depressed at 2 months, increased time in non-maternal care was associated with an increased probability of secure attachment at 12 months. Using a logistic regression, positive elicits at 6 months and the interaction of 2-month depression status with hours in non-maternal care predicted 68% of the 12-month attachment classifications (odds ratio = 6.84). Ambivalent classifications could not be predicted. When they were omitted from the logistic regression, 72% of avoidant and secure classifications were correctly predicted (odds ratio = 8.55) (Cohn et al., 1992).

Discussion

Infants of non-depressed mothers respond dramatically to simulated depressed affect and to distortions in the timing of their mother's behavior in relation to their own. In response to simulated depression, infants become wary, they try to positively elicit their mother to change, and, when unsuccessful, they become increasing negative and unresponsive (Cohn & Tronick, 1983). This increased negative affect and lack of responsiveness then carries over into situations in which the mother is no longer acting depressed. These data suggest that were the mothers to behave continually with depressed affect, infant's affect would come to resemble the mother's. Indeed, in the studies by Field (1984), this seemed to be the case. Infants of mothers with high levels of depressive symptoms were more negative and less responsive than infants of non-depressed mothers, and their behavior varied little between simulated depressed and 'normal' interactions.

Depressed affect may include anger and irritation. Depressed mothers may also be highly intrusive. The experimental study of "simulated" depression has so far been restricted to sad and flat affective expression. Cohn et al. (1986) speculated that restricted maternal affect and lack of responsiveness led to increased infant distress, whereas maternal anger and intrusiveness led to increased avoidance. In the absence of further experimental studies, we do not know whether variation in the type of negative affect mothers show will lead to qualitative differences in infant response. However, studies do indicate that earlier maternal intrusiveness is related to the development of avoidant attachment (Belsky et al., 1984; Egeland & Farber, 1984; Malatesta et al., 1989).

Infants have dramatic reactions to violations of the expected temporal relationship between their own and their mothers' positive affect. Cohn and Elmore (1988) found that when mothers sobered in response to their infant's becoming affectively positive, the infant's response was to sober and look away. Inappropriate timing of affective displays is a likely concomitant of maternal depression. Bettes (1988), for instance, found that in mothers with mild to moderate levels of depressive symptoms, vocal utterances were more variable and turns were of longer duration than in non-depressed mothers. The primary focus to date has been on the affective aspects of depression. Temporal aspects may be equally important to infant behavior and development.

With few exceptions, research about the influence of maternal depression during the first year has tended to ignore diagnostic criteria and to confound depression with other risk factors. Results from these studies suggest that depressed mothers and their babies are more negative and less positive than non-depressed mother-infant pairs. In the study by Cohn (Cohn et al., 1986; Cohn & Tronick, 1989), negative affect was characteristic of almost all of the depressed mothers, although there were substantial individual differences in how negative affect was expressed. In families that have fewer risk factors the influence of depression appears moderated. Bettes (1988), for instance, found consistent effects in mothers' vocal behavior but no differences in infant behavior related to depression. In our ongoing investigation of depression in postpartum mothers, we find more moderate effects on maternal behavior in mothers who are depressed in the absence of other risk factors. In the absence of multiple and severe risk factors, depression appears to have reduced impact on mothers and infants.

A necessary question to ask is whether our current findings must be qualified by the postpartum status of the mothers in our study. More specifically, is depression in the postpartum period different from or more heterogeneous than depressions occurring at other times? Stated differently, it is possible that postpartum depression is distinct from other depressions, and that some or all of the depressed women we studied were experiencing postpartum rather than "true" depression. Neither the RDC nor DSM make a distinction between depression in the postpartum and other times; nor have prospective studies found differences between depression in the postpartum period and at other times (Gotlib, Whiffen, Wallace, & Mount, 1991). None the less, it is possible that had we been able to differentiate among postpartum depressions, we might have found stronger effects of depression.

Our data contraindicate this interpretation. First, we followed the RDC in defining depression, and were careful to take into account the normal changes of parturition in applying the criteria for clinically significant symptoms. Eighty-six percent of the women we studied met criteria for probable or definite major depression, and all either experienced functional impairment or sought help for their depression. Second, depression is an episodic disorder, and approximately half the depressed mothers in our study had experienced at least one or more previous episodes of depression. Among those for whom the present depressive episode was their first, there is no way of knowing what proportion will go on to experience additional episodes. However, the age of the women in our study is well within the period in which first episodes occur (Boyd & Weissman, 1981). Third, if postpartum depression is more heterogeneous than depressions at other times, one might expect an increased prevalence relative to community samples. We did not find this to be the case. Others have found no difference in prevalence rates between postpartum women and demographically matched non-postpartum women (Gotlib et al., 1991; O'Hara, Zekoski, Phillips, & Wright, 1990). We did find a high remission rate for depression. However, that finding is consistent with what is known about depressions occurring at other times. Depression is an episodic disorder of variable duration. Thus, we find no evidence to indicate that inferences about depression in the postpartum period must be qualified by the uniqueness of depression at this time. On the other hand, the experience of being depressed and having a new baby is, of course, specific to this period (Campbell et al., 1992).

Also consistent with what is known about depression at other times in the life cycle, depression was associated with small but significant increases in rates of other risk factors. These include marital distress during pregnancy, higher prevalence of minor delivery complications, and increased infant difficultness (Campbell et al., 1992; Sameroff, Seifer, & Zax, 1982; cf. Zuckerman, Bauchner, Parker, & Cabral, 1990). Downey and Coyne (1990) have emphasized that depression often co-occurs with marital distress, which may independently influence child outcomes. Because experimental designs are of limited feasibility, it may be difficult to disentangle reliably the unique effects of maternal depression from those of other risk factors. Studies that include non-depressed psychiatric and also medical control groups (e.g., Gotlib, 1990) may be informative in this regard. Our work suggests that the influence of depression is attenuated in the absence of other severe risk factors.

An important factor mediating infant effects may be infant's age. Over the age range from 2 through 6 months, incidence of negative affect in depressed mothers increased steadily. Reasons for this increase are unclear. Older infants may require more active social engagement, which a mother who is depressed finds difficult to manage. Older infants are also more demanding of autonomy. The phenomenology of depression may also change over time. When the increasing demands of parenting an older child are concurrent with the emotional strain of enduring depression, adverse child outcomes may become more likely.

A mother's subjective feelings of distress were more important than her diagnostic status alone. Mothers' self-reported level of subjective distress was a central factor in mediating mothers' and infants' affect through six months. A mother's experience of her own distress was more important than her having met diagnostic criteria within the first 8 weeks postpartum. On most measures, women who met RDC without having high levels of subjective distress were indistinguishable from non-depressed controls. Mothers who met criteria and had higher subjective distress, clearly differed on almost all measures at two months, and continued to be more negative through six months. Negativity in fact increased over this time period. Thus, in mothers with high levels of initial symptoms, the continuing effect of depression may be more evident in negative rather than positive affect expression. Alternatively, it may be stability in low levels of positive affect that proves more influential. We are not yet ready to distinguish between these alternatives.

We did not find a relationship between a brief depressive episode within the first 8 weeks and infant attachment at one year. However, preliminary data suggest that longer lasting depressive episodes were associated with an increased rate of insecure attachment. Infants of mothers who remained depressed through 6 months were more likely to be classified as insecurely attached at 12 months than infants of mothers whose depression remitted. This finding is preliminary and so must be interpreted with caution, but it does suggest that chronicity and currency of depression are more important than prior diagnosis. A chronicity effect would also be consistent with the view of Cicchetti and colleagues (Cicchetti & Aber, 1986; Cummings & Cicchetti, 1990). They have theorized that insecure attachment is more likely in infants who have experienced maternal depression during their second year, as would be likely in the case of chronic or frequently occuring maternal depression.

Other data are consistent with the hypothesis that chronicity and currency of depression are of more consequence than is past diagnostic status. Consider Radke-Yarrow et al.'s (1985) study of depression history and toddler attachment. (Depression was defined according to life-time history. In some women, episodes predated the child's birth. The percentage of current depressions was not reported.) Radke-Yarrow and colleagues reported an increased prevalence of insecure attachment in the depressed group. A close reading of their findings, however, shows that the relationship between attachment and depression was due entirely to the inclusion of bipolar subjects in the depressed group. Diagnosis of unipolar depression (Major or Minor Depression) alone was unrelated to attachment. This can be seen by reanalyzing the tabular data in the published report (Table 3).

Bipolar depression is a chronic disorder characterized by cycles of mania and depression and is not always well controlled. Unipolar depression, on the other hand, is characterized by depression only and it may or may not be chronic. In unipolar depression impairment is much less severe, on average. It is not possible to say from this study whether chronicity, currency, or an index

Table 3. Toddler Attachment by Mothers' Diagnosis

Diagnosis	Percent Insecure	p
Not Depressed	9/31 (29%)	—
Bipolar + Unipolar	30/55 (55%)	.025
Bipolar only	11/14 (79%)	.005
Unipolar only	19/41 (46%)	N.S.

Note. Adapted from Yarrow-Radke et al. (1985).

of severity over time, was more important, but it is clear that a diagnosis of major depression was unrelated to insecure attachment.

Strongly related to attachment in the Radke-Yarrow et al. study were contemporaneous observations of mothers' affect with her child. Reduced positive affect and involvement were associated with insecurity. Similar findings have been reported at 12 months by Lyons-Ruth (et al., 1987) and at about 20 months by Teti, Gelfand, Messinger, & Isabella (1991). Sameroff, Seifer, and Zax (1982) found that chronicity and severity of depression were of more consequence to a range of developmental outcomes than diagnostic status alone. Future studies should differentiate past from current and chronic episodes of depression and should examine more carefully the relative contribution of diagnostic variables and affective behavior over time.

Mother-infant interactions are regulated through a process of bidirectional influence (Cohn & Tronick, 1988; Lester, Hoffman, & Brazelton, 1985). The contributions of each partner, however, may not be equal. When we consider the very sizable stability of maternal positive affect over time, and the increasing stability of infant negative affect, it is clear that maternal affect is potentially more influential in determining infant response. The mother's affect and sensitivity are a consistent environment within which the infant develops. Spitz (1965) emphasized the cumulative nature of affective exchanges in shaping infant personality. Mothers with chronic or recurrent episodes of depressed mood may represent a high-risk environment for young children.

In this regard, it may not only be a question of whether a mother has at one time been diagnosable, but rather that she experience currently significant negative or reduced positive mood. As Tronick and Cohn (Cohn & Tronick, 1989; Tronick, 1987) have argued, infants don't experience diagnoses; they don't directly experience many of the symptoms of depression, such as mothers' sleep disruption or changes in appetite. But they do have daily interchanges mediated by affect and timing. And infants are exquisitely sensitive to these components, and by their dependence on caregivers, extremely vulnerable to distorted affect or timing. A mother with persistent irritable or sad mood, who is intrusive and rough in her handling, will increase the chances of impaired infant affect regulation, including avoidant attachment.

In a previous report (Cohn et al., 1990), we found that mothers' work status had a positive effect on mother-infant interaction at 2 months in the depressed group. A similar but more profound effect emerged here. In infants of depressed mothers, hours of non-maternal care were positively related to secure attachment. Time with alternative caregivers may have provided babies of postpartum depressed mothers with emotionally corrective experiences at a time when their mothers were either depressed or in the process of recovering. Alternatively, it may be that work outside of the home independently contributes to a mothers' ability to relate to her baby. The isolation of rearing a young baby, when coupled with depression, may be a particularly difficult stressor for the mother-infant relationship. Opportunities for social support and more varied responsibilities may contribute to a sense of greater effectance than would otherwise be the case in depressed mothers. Teti and Gelfand (1990) found that the effect of depression on mother-infant interaction was mediated through a mother's sense of effectance. Fathers also may be more supportive of the mother and more involved with their babies when the mother is working outside of the home. Further research on this topic is needed. In particular, it is important that we consider circumstances in which non-maternal care may lead to increased security. Past research has focused on the relationship between non-maternal care and avoidance (Belsky, 1988; Clarke-Stewart, 1989), without considering possible beneficial effects of non-maternal care on attachment security.

Research on the influence of maternal depression on infant adaptation has important implications for clinical practice. Mothers with brief depressions who recover relatively soon should be reassured. Anticipatory guidance in these cases should emphasize that the baby may take some time to show normal responsiveness, but that no long term impairment is expected. Mothers with more chronic depressions, or who have histories of dysthymia or other chronic mood disorders, on the other hand, should be encouraged to consider treatment. Help with the baby and opportunities that enhance feelings of effectance may be essential to the well-being of mother and baby. The role of maternal employment and non-maternal care is not clear, but care from a sensitive alternative caregiver for infants of severely depressed mothers may be a protective factor.

Mothers with similar risk factors may behave dissimilarly with their babies. Past diagnosis of depression or any combination of other risk factors may be predictive only weakly of mothers' and infants' behavior. It may be more important to focus on maternal affect and patterns of mother-infant adaptation than on group differences related to past diagnostic status.

Mother-infant interaction assessment can provide the clinician with valuable information about how symptomatology is related to caregiving behavior and infants' response. Although treatment efforts commonly focus on the individual patient, a broader focus may be warranted when the patient is a woman with a young child. Depressive symptoms, especially in the presence of other risk factors, may have dramatic effects on infant affective behavior and development. Medication or other treatments may successfully treat some aspects of symptomatology. We do not know whether successful treatment also remedies the kinds of maternal behavior of salience to infants. Maladaptive patterns of interaction may continue even after clinically significant symptoms remit. Insecure attachment is a potential outcome. Thus, clinicians should be alert to the possibility of directing intervention efforts to the mother-infant dyad, as well as to the mother herself. Increased attention to patterns of mother-infant adaptation would guide clinicians in this direction.

REFERENCES

Akiskal, H.S. (1982). Factors associated with incomplete recovery in primary depressive illness. *Journal of Clinical Psychiatry, 43*, 266–271.

Ainsworth, M.D., Blehar, M.C., Waters, E., & Wall, S. (1978). *Patterns of attachment: A psychological study of the Strange Situation*. Hillsdale, NJ: LEA.

Bakeman, R. & Brown, J. (1980). Early interaction: Consequences for social and mental development at three years. *Child Development, 51*, 437–447.

Baldwin, A.L., Cole, R.E., & Baldwin, C.P. (1982). Parental pathology, family interaction, and the competence of the child in school. *Monographs of the Society for Research in Child Development, 47*, Serial No. 187, entire issue.

Beardslee, W.R., Bemporad, J., Keller, M.B., & Klerman, G.L. (1983). Children of parents with major depressive disorder: A review. *American Journal of Psychiatry, 54*, 1254–1268.

Beck, A.T., Ward, C.H., Mendelson, M., Mock, J.E., & Erbaugh, J.H. (1961). An inventory for measuring depression. *Archives of General Psychiatry, 4*, 561–571.

Belsher, G. & Costello, C. (1988). Relapse after recovery from unipolar depression: A critical review. *Psychological Bulletin, 104*, 84–96.

Belsky, J. (1988). "Effects" of infant daycare revisited. *Early Education Quarterly, 3*, 235–272.

Belsky, J., Rovine, M., & Taylor, D.G. (1984). The Pennsylvania Infant and Family Development Project: 3. The origins of individual differences in infant-mother attachment: Maternal and infant contributions. *Child Development, 55*, 718–728.

Bettes, B. (1988). Maternal depression and motherese: Temporal and intonational contours. *Child Development, 59*, 1089–1096.

Boyd, J. & Weissman, M. (1981). Epidemiology of affective disorders. *Archives of General Psychiatry, 38*, 1039–1046.

Campbell, S.B. & Cohn, J.F. (1991). Prevalence and correlates of postpartum depression in first-time mothers. *Abnormal Psychology, 1000*, 594–599.

Campbell, S.B., Cohn, J.F., Meyers, T., Popper, S., & Flanagan, C. (1992). The course and correlates of postpartum depression during the transition to parenthood. *Development and Psychopathology, 4*, 29–49.

Campbell, S.B., Cohn, J.F., Ross, S., Elmore, M., & Popper, S. (April, 1990). Postpartum adaptation and postpartum depression in primiparous women. International Conference on Infant Studies, Montreal.

Caplan, H.L., Cogill, S.R., Alexandria, H., Robson, K., Katz, R., & Kumar, R. (1989). Maternal depression and the emotional development of the child. *British Journal of Psychiatry, 154*, 818–822.

Cicchetti, D. (1990). An historical perspective on the discipline of developmental psychopathology. In J. Rolf, A. Masten, D. Cicchetti, Neuchterlein, K., & S. Weintraub (eds.), Risk and protective factors in the development of psychopathology. NY: Cambridge University.

Cicchetti, D. & Aber, J.L. (1986). Early precursors of later depression: An organizational perspective. In L. Lipsett & C. Rovee-Collier (eds.), Advances in Infancy, Volume 4. Norwood, NJ: Ablex.

Clarke-Stewart, A. (1989). Infant daycare: Maligned or malignant. American Psychologist, 44, 266–273.

Clayton, P.J. (1983). The prevalence and course of the affective disorders. In J.M. Davis & J.W. Maas (eds.), The affective disorders (pp. 193–202). Washington, DC: American Psychiatric Association.

Cohn, J.F., Campbell, S.B., Matias, R., & Hopkins, J. (1990). Face-to-face interactions of postpartum depressed mother-infant pairs at 2 months. Developmental Psychology, 26, 15–23.

Cohn, J.F., Campbell, S.B., & Ross, S. (1991). Infant response in the still-face paradigm at 6 months predicts avoidant and secure attachment at 12 months. Development and Psychopathology, 3, 367–376.

Cohn, J.F. & Elmore, M. (1988). Effect of contingent changes in mothers' affective expression on the organization of behavior in 3-month-old infants. Infant Behavior and Development, 11, 493–505.

Cohn, J.F., Matias, R., Tronick, E.Z., Lyons-Ruth, K. & Connell, D. (1986). Face-to-face interactions, spontaneous and structured, of mothers with depressive symptoms. In T. Field & E.Z. Tronick (eds.), Maternal Depression and Child Disturbance, New Directions for Child Development, No. 34, 31–46. San Francisco: Jossey-Bass.

Cohn, J.F. & Tronick, E.Z. (1983). Three-month-old infants' reaction to simulated maternal depression. Child Development, 54, 185–193.

Cohn, J.F. & Tronick, E.Z. (1987). Mother-infant interaction: The sequence of dyadic states at 3, 6, and 9 months. Developmental Psychology, 23, 68–77.

Cohn, J.F. & Tronick, E.Z. (1988). Mother-infant interaction: Influence is bidirectional and unrelated to periodic cycles in either partner's behavior. Developmental Psychology, 24, 386–392.

Cohn, J.F. & Tronick, E.Z. (1989). Specificity of infants' response to mothers' affective behavior. Journal of the American Academy of Child and Adolescent Psychiatry, 28, 242–248.

Coyne, J. (1976). Depression and the response of others. Journal of Abnormal Psychology, 85, 186–193.

Cummings, E.M. & Cicchetti, D. (1990). Toward a transactional model of relations between attachment and depression. In M.T. Greenberg, D. Cicchetti, & E.M. Cummings (eds.), Attachment in the preschool years: Theory, research, and intervention. Chicago: University of Chicago.

Cytryn, L., McKnew, D.H., Zahn-Waxler, C., Radke-Yarrow, M., Gaensbauer, T.J., Harmon, R.J., & Lamour, M. (1984). A developmental view of affective disturbances in children of affectively ill parents. American Journal of Psychiatry, 141, 219–222.

Downey, G. & Coyne, J.C. (1990). Children of depressed parents: An integrative review. Psychological Bulletin, 108, 50–76.

Egeland, B. & Farber, E.A. (1984). Infant-mother attachment: Factors related to its development and changes over time. Child Development, 55, 753–771.

Ekman, P. (1984). Expression and the nature of emotion. In K.R. Scherer & P. Ekman (eds.), Approaches to emotion (pp. 319–344), Hillsdale, NJ: Erlbaum.

Endicott, J. & Spitzer, R.L. (1978). A diagnostic interview: The Schedule for Affective Disorders and Schizophrenia. Archives of General Psychiatry, 35, 837–844.

Field, T. (1984). Early interactions between infants and their postpartum depressed mothers. *Infant Behavior and Development, 7*, 527–532.

Field, T., Healy, B., Goldstein, S., & Guthertz, M. (1990). Behavior-state matching and synchrony in mother-infant interactions of nondepressed versus depressed dyads. *Developmental Psychology, 26*, 7–14.

Field, T., Healy, B., Goldstein, S., Perry, S., Debra, B., Schanberg, S., Zimmerman, E.A., & Kuhn, C. (1988). Infants of "depressed" mothers show depressed behavior even with nondepressed adults. *Child Development, 59*, 1569–1579.

Frankel, K., Maslin-Cole, C., & Harmon, R.J. (April, 1991). *Depressed mothers and their preschoolers: What they say is not what they do.* Presented at the Society for Research in Child Development, Seattle.

Gaensbauer, T.J., Harmon, R.J., Cytryn, L., & McKnew, D.H. (1984). Social and affective development in infants with a manic-depressive parent. *American Journal of Psychiatry, 141*, 223–229.

Garrison, W.T. & Earls, F.J. (1986). Epidemiologic perspectives on maternal depression and the young child. In T. Field & E.Z. Tronick (eds.), *Maternal Depression and Child Development*, New Directions for Child Development, No. 34, 13–30. San Francisco: Jossey-Bass.

Gotlib, I.H. (1990). Unpublished data. University of Western Ontario.

Gotlib, I.H., Whiffen, V.E., Mount, J.H., Milne, K., & Cordy, N.I. (1989). Prevalence rates and demographic characteristics associated with depression in pregnancy and the postpartum. *Journal of Consulting and Clinical Psychology, 57*, 269–274.

Gotlib, I.H., Whiffen, V.E., Wallace, P.M., & Mount, J.H. (1991). Prospective investigation of postpartum depression: Factors involved in onset and recovery. *Abnormal Psychology, 100*, 122–132.

Hopkins, J., Marcus, M., & Campbell, S.B. (1987). Postpartum depression: A critical review. *Psychological Bulletin, 95*, 498–515.

Kaye, K. (1982). *The mental and social life of babies.* Chicago: University of Chicago.

Kaye, K. & Fogel, A. (1980). The temporal structure of face-to-face communication between mothers and infants. *Developmental Psychology, 16*, 454–464.

Lester, B., Hoffman, J., & Brazelton, T.B. (1985). The rhythmic structure of mother-infant interaction in term and preterm infants. *Child Development, 56*, 15–27.

Lyons-Ruth, K., Zoll, D., Connell, D., & Grunebaum, H.U. (1986). The depressed mother and her one-year-old infant: Environment, interaction, attachment and infant development. In T. Field & E.Z. Tronick (eds.), *Maternal Depression and Child Disturbance*, New Directions for Child Development, No. 34, 61–82.

Lyons-Ruth, K., Connell, D.B., Zoll, D., & Stahl, J. (1987). Infants at social risk: Relations among infant maltreatment, maternal behavior, and infant attachment behavior. *Developmental Psychology, 23*, 223–232.

Malatesta, C.Z., Culver, C., Rich-Tesman, J., & Shepard, B. (1989). The development of emotion expression during the first two years of life. *Monographs of the Society for Research in Child Development, 54*, (1–2, Serial No. 219).

Malatesta, C.Z., & Haviland, J.M. (1982). Learning display rules: The socialization of emotion expression in infancy. *Child Development, 53*, 991–1033.

McLean, P.D. & Hakstian, A.R. (1990). Relative endurance of unipolar depression treatment effects: Longitudinal follow-up. *Journal of Consulting and Clinical Psychology, 58*, 482–488.

Myers, J.K. & Weissman, M.M. (1980). Use of a self-report symptom scale to detect depression in a community sample. *American Journal of Psychiatry, 137*, 1081–1084.

Nurnberger, J. & Gershon, E.S. (1984). Genetics of affective disorders. In R. Post & P. Ballenger (eds.), *Neurobiology of mood disorders.* Baltimore: Williams & Wilkins.

O'Hara, M.W., Neunaber, D.J., & Zekoski, E.M. (1984). Prospective study of postpartum depression: Prevalence, course, predictive factors. *Journal of Abnormal Psychology, 93*, 158–171.

O'Hara, M.W., Zekoski, E.M., Phillips, & Wright, E.J. (1990). A controlled, prospective study of postpartum mood disorders: Comparison of childbearing and non-childbearing women. *Journal of Abnormal Psychology, 99*, 3–15.

Radke-Yarrow, M., Cummings, M., Kuczynski, L., & Chapman, M. (1985). Patterns of attachment in two- and three-year-olds in normal families and in families with parental depression. *Child Development, 56*, 884–893.

Radloff, L.S. (1977). The CES–D Scale: A self-report depression scale for research in the general population. *Applied Psychological Measurement, 3*, 385–401.

Redding, Harmon, & Morgan (1990). Relationships between maternal depression and infants' mastery behaviors. *Infant Behavior and Development, 13*, 391–395.

Robins, L. (1974). *Deviant children grown up.* NY: Krieger.

Rutter, M., Yule, B., Quinton, D., Rowland, O., Yule, W., & Berger, M. (1974). Attainment and adjustment in two geographical areas: III. *British Journal of Psychiatry, 123*, 520–533.

Rutter, M. & Garmezy, N. (1983). Developmental psychopathology. In *Handbook of Child Psychology: Vol. 2*, ed. M.N. Haith, J.J. Campos, & P.H. Mussen (series ed.) NY: Wiley, pp. 775–911.

Sameroff, A., Seifer, R., & Zax, M. (1982). Early development of children at risk for emotional disorder. *Monographs of the Society for Research in Child Development, 47*, (7, No. 199).

Schaffer, H.R. (1984). *The child's entry into a social world.* London: Academic.

Seifer, R. & Barocas, R. (April, 1991). *A comparison of maternal diagnosis, severity of illness, and symptom dimensions as predictors of 4-year child status.* Presented at the Society for Research in Child Development, Seattle.

Spitz, R. (1965). *The first year of life.* NY: International Universities Press.

Spitzer, R.S., Endicott, J., & Robins, E. (1978). Research Diagnostic Criteria: Rationale and reliability. *Archives of General Psychiatry, 36*, 773–782.

Symons, D.K. & Moran, G. (1987). The behavioral dynamics of mutual responsiveness in early face-to-face mother-infant interactions. *Child Development, 58*, 1488–1495.

Teti, D.M. & Gelfand, D.M. (April, 1990). *Maternal depression, parenting, and maternal self-efficacy: A longitudinal study of mothers and infants.* In T. Field (Chair), Maternal depression: Effects on infants. A symposium presented at the International Society for Infant Studies, Montreal, Quebec.

Teti, D.M., Gelfand, D.M., Messinger, D., & Isabella, R. (April, 1991). *Security of infant attachment and maternal functioning among depressed and nondepressed mothers and infants.* Presented at the Society for Research in Child Development, Seattle.

Tronick, E.Z. & Cohn, J.F. (1989). Infant-mother face-to-face interaction: Age and gender differences in coordination and miscoordination. *Child Development, 59*, 85–92.

Tronick, E., Als, H., Adamson, L., Wise, S., & Brazelton, T.B. (1978). The infant's response to entrapment between contradictory messages. *Journal of the American Academy of Child and Adolescent Psychiatry, 17*, 1–13.

Tronick, E.Z., Ricks, M., & Cohn, J.F. (1982). Maternal and infant affective exchange: Patterns of adaptation. In T.M. Field & A. Fogel (eds.), *Emotion and early interaction.* Hillsdale, NJ: LEA.

Tronick, E.Z., (April, 1987). In B.S. Zuckerman (Chair), Maternal depression and child disturbance: Research and clinical implications. *Biennial Meeting of the Society for Research in Child Development.*

Vaughn, B.E., Taraldson, B., Crichton, L., & Egeland, B. (1980). Relationship between neonatal behavioral organization and infant behavior during the first year of life. *Infant Behavior and Development, 3*, 47–66.

Weissman, M.M. & Paykel, E.S. (1974). *The depressed woman: A study in social relationships*. Chicago: University of Chicago.

Zahn-Waxler, C., Cummings, E.M., McKnew, D.H., & Radke-Yarrow, M. (1984). Altruism, aggression, and social interactions in young children with a manic-depressive parent. *Child Development, 55*, 112–122.

Zahn-Waxler, C., Iannotti, R.J., Cummings, E.M., & Denham, S. (1990). Antecedents of problem behaviors in children of depressed mothers. *Development and Psychopathology, 2*, 271–291.

Zuckerman, B., Bauchner, H., Parker, S., & Cabral, H. (1990). Maternal depressive symptoms during pregnancy and newborn irritability. *Developmental and Behavioral Pediatrics, 11*, 190–194.

IV Maternal Depressive Symptoms, Disorganized Infant-Mother Attachment Relationships and Hostile-Aggressive Behavior in the Preschool Classroom: A Prospective Longitudinal View from Infancy to Age Five

KARLEN LYONS-RUTH

Introduction

One central emphasis of a developmental approach to psychopathology is a focus on the junctures where normal and deviant developmental pathways begin to diverge, that is, where forerunners to later disorder can first be identified. This emphasis on early points of divergence has led developmental researchers to begin a series of prospective longitudinal studies in order to observe the processes associated with the presence of risk factors from the beginning of life. This chapter reports on one such prospective longitudinal study of infants at risk due to the combined effects of poverty and maternal depressive symptoms.

This work grew out of the need to offer a more developmentally-grounded and process-oriented view of the often-reported association between low SES and increased rates of childhood psychopathology (e.g. Rutter, Yule, Quinton, Rowlands, Yule, & Berger, 1974). Low-income per se is not a psychological construct and its relation to negative outcomes for children can only be understood through an understanding of how socioeconomic status sets a social context which increases the likelihood of maladaptive developmental processes. The data to be reviewed here summarize our findings regarding

Work reported in this chapter was funded by NIMH grant #35122 and grants from the A.L. Mailman Family Foundation, the Milton Fund of Harvard University, and an anonymous foundation. Preparation of this chapter was completed while the author was a fellow at the Henry A. Murray Research Center, Radcliffe College.

some of the poverty-related risk factors identified during infancy which were associated with maladaptive social interactions during the first five years of life.

Previous studies explaining how poverty places children at risk have selected families for study on the basis of poverty-related demographic variables such as single parenthood or early parenthood which are associated with poorer child outcomes among low-SES families. Family processes within these subgroups have then been studied. We employed the reverse strategy. Reasoning that, at the most proximal level, risk resides in a distortion of the regulatory process between parents and infant rather than in demographic factors per se, we asked pediatric and social service workers to identify the infants in their caseloads who were at greatest risk due to caretaking inadequacies. We then looked at a variety of research measures of the family situation which might differentiate low-income families experiencing caretaking difficulties from their socioeconomically similar low-income controls.

One of the structured assessments that best discriminated the group of low-income mothers displaying caregiving problems from their low-income controls was the level of depressive symptoms reported by the mother at entry into the study. As we proceeded with the study, it became apparent that maternal depressive symptoms remained a critical variable associated with child outcomes both in infancy and kindergarten.

We were also interested in whether the organization of infant attachment behaviors toward the mother in the first and second years would be sensitive to the family's caretaking difficulties and perhaps mediate some of the variance in child adaptation during the preschool years. This is the first study to report prospective longitudinal data on the interrelationships between maternal depressive symptoms, disorganized attachment relationships in infancy and later child adjustment in kindergarten.

In relation to the larger literature on the effects associated with parental depression among school-aged children, the findings from the current study begin to extend downward to infancy many of the relationships reported in the literature on older children of depressed parents (see Coyne, Downey, & Boergers, this volume; Hammen, this volume). Thus, longitudinal findings from the current study begin to bridge the gap between current research findings related to infancy and the later child outcomes of interest to students of childhood psychopathology.

Developmental Models of Psychopathology

In contrast to the studies of school-aged children of depressed parents, which have emerged from earlier research on adult psychopathology, studies of risk populations in infancy have grown out of previous research with normal populations. Therefore, the theoretical model guiding our work and other work in developmental psychopathology differs in emphasis at several points from earlier theory and research in the study of adult psychopathology

(Cicchetti, 1990a; Garmezy, Masten, & Tellegen, 1984; Sroufe & Rutter, 1984; Rutter & Garmezy, 1983). Earlier medically-grounded models have implicitly assumed discontinuity, often biologically based, between processes operating in the creation of "health" and "illness". One alternative model of the interrelations between normal and pathological development which is more contextual, developmental and process-oriented has been articulated by Bowlby (1988).

In Bowlby's view, normal and abnormal development are inextricably related. His model rests on the assumption that the flexible regulation of affect and behavior associated with social adaptation is a developmental achievement. This achievement rests on the mastery of a series of related social competencies beginning in early infancy, with later competencies developing from and integrating earlier competencies. The availability of more complex forms of cognition with development propels this successive reregulation of social competencies toward more integrated, flexible and adaptive forms (e.g. Fischer & Pipp, 1984). Such a hierarchical model of development also implies considerable continuity in social-developmental adaptation over time.

A second important tenet of current theory in developmental psychopathology is that flexible regulation of affect, and the social competencies underlying affect regulation, are learned in relationships (Sameroff & Emde, 1989). While these developmentally-acquired skills are not the only factors determining later emotional dysregulation or psychopathology, they are assumed to make an important contribution. The extent of this contribution has not yet been established and needs to be explored in process-oriented, prospective longitudinal studies if the relational skills involved in eventual social adaptation are to be understood.

Two further aspects of this developmental and relational perspective deserve mention. The first tenet is that symptomatic behavior in childhood often reflects not simply a current disturbance but also a failure to acquire underlying broad-based social competencies (Sroufe, 1989; Cicchetti, 1990b). In this view maladaptation needs to be assessed not simply in terms of symptomatic behavior but also in terms of the normative social-regulatory competencies that may have been interfered with in earlier development.

A related, but more recent, emphasis (Sroufe, 1989; Bowlby, 1988) is that a particular deviation from more normative pathways also needs to be understood in terms of its own distinct organizational features, or goal-corrected direction, as well as in terms of the failure to acquire normative competencies. Thus, one must also explore the extent to which alternative organizational principles, or overriding goals, may have replaced the central organizing principles seen under more normal social conditions. For example, Aber and Allen (1987) in attempting to account for the deficits in mastery behavior and cognitive performance observed among maltreated preschoolers, have advanced a "secure readiness to learn" hypothesis. According to this hypothesis, when comforting access to an attachment figure is consistently in jeopardy, the attachment-exploration balance becomes disrupted, and normal motivation to explore may become superceded by constant preoccupation with the state of the relationship. This preoccupation both interferes with the acquisition of normative competencies and substitutes a different organizing focus for segments of the child's behavior that might otherwise be directed toward exploration and learning.

Thus, in contrast to a more purely taxonomic approach to describing syndromes of disorder, a developmental approach views individual adaptive efforts as related to one another over time and as related to an age-graded series of predictable adaptational demands articulated by the culture. These adaptive efforts are seen as taking place along a fluid interface between adaptation and maladaptation. Processes which have the potential to shift the individual's pathway in relation to age-related adaptational demands then become the focus of investigation. These views are particularly relevant to students of infancy, a period when neurobiological maturation and developmental change is rapid and where the inseparability of the developing organism from its regulating social-relational context is particularly evident (Sameroff & Emde, 1989).

The Attachment System as Social Regulator

A second distinctive theoretical emphasis emerging from developmental work on infancy is a view of the organized structure of interactions comprising the child-caregiver attachment relationship, which regulates the infant and child's felt security and the balance between exploration and comfort-seeking.

An early and central contribution of this work on attachment relationships has been the insight that the organization of relationships cannot be understood by the assessment of single behaviors or indicators. Instead, multiple facets of behavior and affect are organized toward the achievement of felt security. The resulting pattern of organization is what must be understood and described.

These organized relational patterns are accompanied by organized representational models of present and past relationships (Main, Kaplan & Cassidy, 1985). Furthermore, these relational representations can be assessed prior to the establishment of a particular relationship, such as prior to the birth of the infant or prior to establishing particular peer relationships, and have been shown to predict aspects of relationships that are established months or years later (e.g. Arend, Gove & Sroufe, 1979; LaFreniere & Sroufe, 1985; Oppenheim, Sagi, & Lamb, 1988; Ward, Carlson, Altman, Levine, Greenberg & Kessler, 1990; Waters, Wippman & Sroufe, 1979). These insights first emerged from work on early attachment relationships between parent and infant, as articulated by Ainsworth, Blehar, Waters and Wall (1978) and, more recently, from work by Main and colleagues (Main, Kaplan & Cassidy, 1985; Main & Solomon, 1990; Main & Hesse, 1990.)

A large research literature on attachment relationships now supports the view that the pattern of regulation of attachment-related affect and behavior is relatively stable over time for both parent and child, at least in low-risk populations. Furthermore, work by Ainsworth et al. (1978) and Main et al. (1985) has described four distinct organized patterns of behavior governing the regulation of attachment-related affects in infancy. The pattern labeled *Secure* has been related to a history of warm and responsive interaction with the parent during the first year (Belsky, Rovine, & Taylor, 1984; Ainsworth et al., 1978) and with more positive social behaviors at later ages. For example, infants with secure attachment relationships have been found to display less anger and non-compliance with their parents in toddlerhood (Londerville & Main, 1981; Matas, Arend, & Sroufe, 1987) and greater cooperation and sociability with peers in nursery school (for review, see Lyons-Ruth, 1991). From studies done so far, it is not clear whether the significant prediction from these infant behaviors to later social adaptation stems from continuity in infant behavioral regulation over time, from continuity in parental behavior associated with these infant patterns, from more complex interaction effects, and/or from as yet unidentified correlates or "third variables". The potential of this theoretical framework for illuminating the study of developmental psychopathology is only beginning to be explored, with the work presented in this chapter as one contribution.

Maternal Depressive Symptoms as Indices of Relational Dysregulation

Studies of school-aged children of depressed parents have used DSM–III–R diagnostic criteria for maternal major depression, and use of diagnostic criteria have recently been considered necessary to adequate research design (e.g. Downey & Coyne, 1990). However, the most recent well-designed studies comparing both DSM–III–R diagnosis and maternal symptom levels in relation to child outcomes have found symptom levels to be the more critical variable mediating child effects.

In the study by Hammen and colleagues that most closely examined the interrelationships among maternal affective diagnosis, maternal stress, maternal depressive symptoms and child psychiatric diagnosis, several conclusions emerged. First, risk to children was attributable not just to maternal psychopathology but also to concurrent chronic stress in families (Hammen, Gordon, Burge, Adrian, Jaenicke & Hiroto, 1987). Furthermore, current depressive symptoms and chronic stress continued to be significant predictors of negative aspects of mother-child interaction and of child affective diagnosis with maternal lifetime history of major depression controlled. In addition, lifetime history failed to contribute significant additional variance after the former two variables were controlled (Gordon, Burge, Hammen, Adrian, Jaenicke & Hiroto, 1989; Hammmen, Adrian, Gordon, Burge, Jaenicke & Hiroto, 1987). As the authors note, chronic stress and current symptoms of depression may be elevated in women without affective disorders as well as absent in psychiatrically ill women in remission. In final structural equations models of maternal and child variables influencing child outcomes, maternal diagnosis played no role in prediction (Hammen, Burge & Stansbury, 1990). The maternal assessment showing the most consistent relation to the entire set of child outcomes, including child psychiatric disorder, was the extent of maternal depressive symptoms. Depressive symptoms predicted significant incremental variance in most of the child outcomes after controlling for the contributions of maternal diagnosis and chronic stress. Further evidence of the importance of depressive symptoms for child outcomes, even in the context of a maternal diagnosis of major depression, can be found in Cohn, Campbell & Matias (1990).

Prior to the current study, a few previous studies have related maternal depressive diagnosis or depressive symptoms during the preschool years to early child behavior problems (Ghodsian, Zajicek & Wolkind, 1984; Richman, Stevenson & Graham, 1982; Fergusson, Hons, Horwood, Gretton & Shannon, 1985; Brody & Forehand, 1986). These data have been equivocal, however, due to the reliance on mothers' ratings of child problems. In the one study using both mothers and teachers as informants (Fergusson et al., 1985), the relationship between maternal depressive symptoms and child behavior problems failed to occur in the teachers' ratings, leaving it unclear whether child problems were evident only in the home during early childhood or whether depressed mothers were overrating their children's problems (see also Friedlander, Weiss, & Traylor, 1986; Richters & Pellegrini, 1989, in relation to this debate).

Despite the methodological issues related to maternal report data, similarities are notable across two prospective longitudinal studies which have reported data on chronicity of maternal depressive episodes in relation to child outcome variables. Both studies have reported later effects of previous maternal depression during the first year and half of the child's life on child functioning at age four or five, even in the absence of maternal depression at the time of the later assessment. Cogill, Caplan, Alexandra, Robson, and Kumar (1986), studying 94 consecutive obstetric patients representing all social classes, reported that during the child's first 12 months of life, 23.4% of mothers were diagnosed as depressed by a psychiatrist using a semi-structured interview. At four years of age, children of these mothers showed significant 10 point decrements on the McCarthy scales of children's abilities, particularly those scales assessing perceptual and motor performance. At age four, only 8.5% of mothers were depressed on clinical interview (depressive symptoms per se were not assessed) and depression at age four was not significantly related to McCarthy scores. These effects of early maternal depression on later child ability occurred primarily among women of lower social status or those with marital conflict or whose husbands also earned psychiatric diagnoses.

A second study was conducted by Wolkind and colleagues of 108 women selected randomly from all births in an inner-city London borough. Maternal depression was assessed by Present State Exam. In Wolkind's low-income sample, as will be reported for the current sample, there was strong continuity in maternal depression over time (4–42 months child age), with 74.8% of mothers having the same depression status at 42 months as at 4 months (Wolkind, Zajicek-Coleman & Ghodsian, 1980). Using maternal reports of child behavior problems at 42 months, Ghodsian et al. (1984) found that both 42 months' depression alone and chronic depression related significantly to maternal reports of child behavior problems at 42 months. Maternal depression at 14 months child age also had a significant effect on later behavior problems, even when the depression did not continue. The effects of previous (14 months) depression were dependent on the presence of a younger sibling by 14 months child age, but no other demographic or social factors could be found which mediated the relationship between early maternal depression and later problems.

In Richman, Stevenson & Graham's (1982) longitudinal study from age three to age eight of 94 three-year-olds with behavior problems and their matched controls, maternal depressive symptoms at age three were significantly related to both neurotic and antisocial disorders at age eight. Maternal depressive symptoms at age three were more strongly related to child disorder at age eight than were marital distress or maternal criticism at age three. By age eight, the larger emotional environment comprising all of these factors was most significant.

The Harvard Family Support Project: Maternal Depressive Symptoms, Family Support Services and Infant-Mother Attachment

The findings discussed in this chapter are part of an ongoing, prospective longitudinal study of a cohort of infants from low-income families, including 41 infants considered at risk for later disorder due to observed caregiving difficulties and 35 infants from the same communities who were closely matched to the at-risk group on demographic indicators. Demographic and risk characteristics of the sample are shown in Table 1.

Mothers and infants in the two high-risk groups were referred to the study by calls from staff members of health, educational, and social service agencies serving low-income families because of staff concerns about the quality of the caregiving environment for the infant. To be eligible for family support services, infants were required to be aged birth to 9 months at study entry. Referral calls were followed up by staff screening to verify risk status and by extensive recruitment efforts with the families.

Two nonintervention groups were also assessed. The second group, a group of 10 families labeled the high-risk untreated group, was identified through the same clinical referral process used to identify the high-risk infants, but this group was assessed at 18 months prior to the provision of short-term intervention services.

The third group, a group of 35 families labeled the community group, was a

Table 1. Demographic and Risk Characteristics of the Sample

	High-risk treated	High-risk untreated	Community untreated
N	31	10	35
Demographic characteristics			
High school graduate	58.1%	60.0%	53.0%
Mean weekly income (per person)	$45.99	$43.95	$46.98
Non-Caucasian mother	16.1%	40.0%	14.3%
Mean maternal age (yrs.)	25.6	21.8	24.8
Male infant	51.6%	80.0%	57.1%
First-born infant	38.7%	80.0%	40.0%
Risk characteristics			
High depressive symptoms	64.5%	60.0%	22.9%
Ever psychiatrically hospitalized	31.3%	30.0%	0.0%
Maltreating	32.3%	0.0%	0.0%

Note. All community group mothers and infants were individually matched to a high-risk mother and infant on the six demographic characteristics shown. Group x Risk $X^2(2,N=76)$, all $p<.001$. Group x Demographic $F(2,73)$ or $X^2(2,N=76)$, all p n.s. From "Infants at Social Risk" by K. Lyons-Ruth, D. B. Connell, H. U. Grunebaum, and S. Botein, 1990, *Child Development, 61*, p. 85. Copyright 1990 by the Society for Research in Child Development, Inc. Reprinted by permission.

matched comparison group of mothers and infants from the same neighborhoods who had never sought or received social services directed at parenting skills, had never been identified as maltreating, and had never undergone extensive psychiatric treatment. The community-group mothers were individually matched to high-risk mothers on the demographic variables shown in Table 1. Although, as a group, the community sample was lower in risk, 22.9% of community mothers reported high levels of depressive symptoms on interview. Additional details are available in Lyons-Ruth, Connell, Grunebaum, and Botein, 1990.

Oral interviews on the Center for Epidemiological Studies Depression Scale (Radloff, 1977) were conducted with each mother at study entry and at 18 months infant age. A cutoff score of 16 or above has been established for the CESD as indicating possible clinical disorder. In comparison to concurrent diagnoses with the SADS diagnostic interview, the cutoff point of 16 differentiates well between depressed and non-depressed people, with a false-positive rate of 6.1% and a false-negative rate of 36.4% (Myers & Weissman, 1980).

Myers and Weissman (1980) also point out, however, that because only a small proportion of people are depressed, the 6.1% of people in a total population sample who are "false-positive" constitute almost half of the group classified as "depressed" (CESD ≥16) on the CES–D.

Diagnostic Interview Schedule (DIS) interviews (Robins, Helzer, Croughan, & Ratcliff, 1981), excluding the sections detailing psychotic symptoms, were administered to all mothers between 12 and 18 months infant age. DIS interviews were not included as formal research measures. Interviews were conducted by clinically trained staff.

Ten demographic variables were coded from maternal interviews: mother's race, whether mother was a high school graduate, per person weekly income (including government assistance and food stamps), mother's age at birth of the target child, child's sex and birth order, mother's age at the birth of her first child, whether mother was a single parent, whether the family was supported by government assistance, and the number of siblings under age 6. A cumulative demographic risk score was computed from these variables.

A maternal childhood history interview was conducted at the mother's home at study entry. Childhood history information was gathered in two parts. First, the mother was asked to trace all changes in adult caregivers from her birth to age sixteen. Additional questions were asked about the incidence of psychiatric hospitalization, drug or alcohol abuse, or time in prison of adults within the mother's family of origin. The occupational levels of both of the mother's parents were rated on the nine-point Occupational Scale from the Hollingshead Four-Factor Index of Social Status (Hollingshead, 1975).

The second part of the childhood history interview consisted of thirty-five structured items probing five domains of early life experience hypothesized to relate to the mother's social adjustment and mothering capacities, including family warmth, conflict, and structure, and peer and school experiences. Internal consistency for the five qualitative childhood history scales, assessed by Cronbach's Alpha ranged from .56 to .74. Further details are available in Lyons-Ruth, Zoll, Connell, and Grunebaum, 1989.

Naturalistic mother-infant interaction was videotaped at home for forty minutes when the infants were twelve and eighteen months of age. Maternal behavior was coded in ten four-minute intervals on twelve five-point rating scales and one timed variable. Coders were blind to other information on the families, and all ratings were reliable. Methodological details are available in Lyons-Ruth, Connell, Zoll, and Stahl (1987).

The Bayley Scales of Infant Development, Mental and Motor Scales (Bayley, 1969), were administered to each infant in laboratory visits at 12 and 18 months of age. To provide an estimate of maternal intelligence, the Similarities subscale of the Wechsler Adult Intelligence Scale (WAIS), 1955 edition, was also administered as part of the twelve-month laboratory visit (Wechsler, 1955).

Within two weeks of home videotaping, mothers and infants were videotaped in the Ainsworth Strange Situation. In this procedure, the infant is videotaped in a playroom during a series of eight structured three-minute episodes involving the baby, the mother, and a female stranger. During the observation, the mother leaves and rejoins the infant twice, first leaving the infant with the female stranger, then leaving the infant alone. The procedure is designed to be mildly stressful in order to increase the intensity of activation of the infant's attachment behavior. All videotapes were coded as described by Ainsworth, Blehar, Waters, and Wall (1978) and Main and Solomon (1990). Coders were blind to all other data on the families and all coding was reliable. Further methodological details are available in Lyons-Ruth, Connell, Grunebaum, and Botein (1990).

Depressive Symptoms and DSM–III Diagnosis

As shown in Table 1, sixty-three percent of mothers perceived as having caregiving difficulties reported high levels of depressive symptoms (CESD score ≥16) on the CES depression questionnaire while only 23% of low-risk mothers did. Thus, a high level of maternal depressive symptoms was the most prevalent single correlate of caregiving inadequacy among this low-income sample and maternal depressive symptoms on the CES–D were surprisingly stable over time among these low-income mothers. Six-months stability (12–18 months) for the low-risk community mothers was 85% for depressive classification, with $r=.74$ for continuous scores. Eleven-month stability for high-risk mothers (7–18 months) was similar, 84% for classification, $r=.67$ for continuous scores. Three-and-a-half year stability (from 18 months to age 5) for the sample ($N=64$) was similarly high, 75% for classification, $r=.68$ for continuous scores.

It is also pertinent to ask how the CES–D data relate to affective disorders as defined by DSM–III (the existing diagnostic system at the time of study). Table 2 displays the DIS diagnoses for the matched groups of high-risk and community mothers. Lifetime rates of diagnosis as revealed by the DIS were similar to the rates of current depressive symptoms, and the DSM–III affective disorders were clearly the diagnoses that differentiated best between high-risk and community groups, with a 41.2% difference in incidence of major depression and a 20.6% difference in incidence of dysthymic disorder. The presence of any lifetime DSM–III affective diagnosis was a significant predictor of maternal caregiving problems (high-risk status) as perceived by community service providers, $X^2(1,N=68)=13.25, p<.001, Phi=.44$.

As shown in Table 3, agreement between a "depressed" classification on the CES–D and a lifetime DSM–III diagnosis was 64.5% at 18 months and 72.1% at age 5. "False positives" on the CES–D were low at 13.9% at 18 months and 8.2% at 5 years, indicating that most women with high CES–D scores earned lifetime DIS diagnoses of major depression (22.2%), dysthymic disorder (27.7%) or both (19.4%). Equivalent percentages at age 5 were 22.2%, 37.0%, and 25.9%. The "false negative" rate for the CES–D was higher, at

Table 2. Diagnostic Interview Schedule Diagnoses for SES-Matched
High Risk and Community Mothers

DIS diagnosis	High-risk mothers	Community mothers
N	34	34
Affective diagnoses		
Major depression	47.1%	5.9%
Dysthymic disorder	47.1%	26.5%
"Double depression"	20.6%	5.9%
Bipolar disorder	2.9%	0.0%
Any affective diagnosis	73.6%**	26.5%
Other diagnoses		
Alcohol abuse	14.7%	2.9%
Other substance abuse	17.6%	2.9%
Cyclothymic disorder	20.6%	11.8%
Panic disorder	23.5%	14.7%
Phobic disorder	50.0%	41.2%
Obsessive compulsive disorder	41.2%	41.2%

Note. High-risk and community mothers individually matched on mother's ethnicity and education, per-person family income, and infant sex and birth order. Mothers without individual matches not included in table.
** High-risk vs. Community, $X^2(1,N=68)=13.25$, $p<.001$, $Phi=.44$.

21.5% at 18 months and 19.7% at 5 years. This indicates that a number of mothers with lifetime diagnoses were not currently reporting depressive symptoms at the two CES–D assessment points.

It is notable that the high rate of continuity of depressive symptoms from 18 months to 5 years in this sample cannot be attributed solely to the fact that a substantial subgroup of mothers with depressive symptoms also had experienced a major depressive episode in their lifetimes. Continuity of depressive symptoms was also high among mothers experiencing dysthymic disorder only and among those with no lifetime diagnosis, as shown in Table 4. In summary, the group of mothers classified as "depressed" on the CES–D at 18 months had a high incidence of lifetime DSM–III affective diagnoses, their depressive symptoms had generally been stable for 6 to 12 months prior to the 18 months' assessment and most continued to exhibit depressive symptoms three and a half years later.

Table 3. Agreement Between Lifetime Unipolar Affective Diagnosis on the DIS Assessment at 18 Months and Depression Classified by CESD Scores

| | | Proportion depressed by CESD score | |
| | | Child age 18 months | Child age 5 years |
	N	78	61
Overall agreement (DIS/CESD)			
Agreement (DIS/CESD)		.65 (51)	.72 (44)
False positive-CESD		.14 (11)	.08 (5)
False negative-CESD		.22 (16)	.20 (12)
Subgroup agreement (DIS/CESD)			
No diagnosis on DIS		.30 (37)	.18 (27)
Dysthymic disorder only		.50 (20)	.59 (17)
+ Double depression group		.61 (28)	.67 (24)
Major depression only		.62 (13)	.60 (10)
+ Double depression group		.71 (21)	.71 (17)
Double depression		.87 (8)	.86 (7)

Note. Cell n's in parenthesis. One subject with bipolar disorder is not included. She also met criteria for double depression but was not depressed by CESD score.

Maternal Depressive Symptoms, Maternal Behavior, Infant Security of Attachment and Infant Mental Development

The primary social outcome measure in infancy was the patterning of attachment behaviors toward the mother at 18 months. This measure was chosen both because of the theoretical centrality of a secure attachment relationship in providing optimal regulation of felt security in infancy and because of the large research literature now correlating secure attachment behaviors in infancy with positive social behaviors at subsequent ages. The attachment assessment results in the categorization of the overall pattern of infant behavior into one of four categories.

Secure attachment behavior is generally characterized by the infant's indicating some protest or distress when left by the parent and by refusing comforting contact from the unfamiliar research assistant in the room. When the parent returns, the infant usually greets the parent positively or, if distressed, actively seeks physical contact with the parent for comforting. Infants with secure attachment relationships are easily soothed by contact with the parent and return to further play and exploration.

Table 4. CESD Classifications of Maternal Depression at Child Age 5 Years: Agreement with 18-month CESD and DIS Assessments

	Proportion depressed by CESD score at 5 years
Overall agreement	
Depressed by CESD at 18 months	.75 (61)
Subgroups	
Depressed by CESD at 18 months and lifetime DIS unipolar dx	.83 (18)
Depressed by CESD at 18 months but no lifetime DIS unipolar dx	.71 (7)
Not depressed by CESD at 18 months but lifetime DIS unipolar dx	.44 (16)
Not depressed by CESD at 18 months and no lifetime DIS unipolar dx	.00 (20)

Note. Cell n's in parenthesis. One subject with bipolar disorder excluded. DIS diagnoses included major depression and dysthymic disorder.

Three additional patterns of insecure infant behavior have also been described. Insecure-*Avoidant* infants show an absence of protest or distress at separation and continued active engagement with toys, combined with an avoidance of eye contact or physical contact with the mother when she returns. Insecure-*Ambivalent* infants combine protest and distress at separation, often of extreme proportions, with physical contact-seeking combined with direct or displaced angry behavior toward mother when she returns. *Ambivalent* infants also often fail to be comforted by contact with the parent and one subgroup of ambivalent infants shows extreme passivity combined with continued distress (for further detail see Ainsworth et al., 1978).

A third and more recently discovered form of insecure attachment behavior has been termed Insecure-*Disorganized* (Main & Solomon, 1990). This form of behavior tends to combine elements of more than one of the above patterns, as well as other signs of conflict, apprehension or helplessness. In the current study, infants most often combined distress during the parent's absence with avoidance of the parent on the parent's return and strong resistance to contact if the parent approached. Angry behavior both toward the toys and toward the parent was frequent. In several cases, the female research assistant was favored over the parent for comforting. In previous work, Disorganized infant attachment behavior has been associated with maternal alcohol use (O'Connor, Sigman, & Brill, 1987), maternal history of loss, particularly unresolved losses (Main, Kaplan, & Cassidy, 1985), and child maltreatment (Carlson, Cicchetti, Barnett, & Braunwald, 1989).

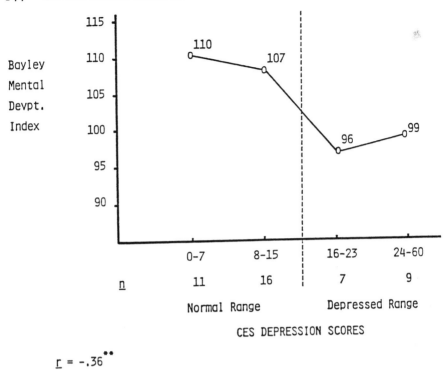

Figure 1. Infant mental development at 18 months of age as a function of maternal depressive symptoms.

In order to evaluate the effects associated with maternal depressive symptoms independently of any effects associated with intervention, our first set of analyses examined the subgroup of 45 infants who had received no intervention services. Two additional infants were excluded from the non-depressed group because their mothers had histories of hospitalization for non-depressive disorders. None of the unserved infants were protective service cases. Only two of the depressed mothers in this sub-sample had ever experienced psychiatric hospitalization.

Figures 1 and 2 present the social and cognitive infant outcome data plotted by maternal depression scores obtained at first contact with the family. Several aspects of the data are notable. First, among low-income mothers with few depressive symptoms, infant scores for both mental development and infant security of attachment are close to the norms for non-poverty samples available in current literature. Bayley mental development scores have a standardized mean of 100 in representative samples; the proportion of infants classified securely attached in the Ainsworth attachment assessment usually varies between 60% and 70% in middle-class samples (see Ijzendoorn & Kroonenberg, 1988, for meta-analysis of worldwide samples).

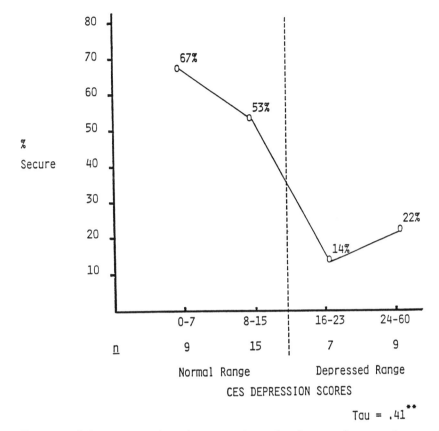

Figure 2. Infant security of attachment at 18 months of age as a function of maternal depressive symptoms.

Second, the infant data provide striking convergent evidence for the validity of the cut-off point established in previous studies of the CES–depression scale. This cut-off point, established to indicate possible clinical disorder, had been previously set for the CES–D scale in relation to its ability to discriminate patients with a clinical diagnosis of major depression. These infant data provide further convergent evidence of the validity of the cutoff score, in that the cut-off point is identifying maternal depressive symptoms severe enough to be associated with serious disregulation of the parent-infant relationship.

Our observations of the same mothers and infants at home at both 12 and 18 months revealed that elevated depressive symptoms were associated with an increased incidence of maternal hostile-intrusive behaviors toward the infant (Lyons-Ruth, Zoll, Connell & Grunebaum, 1986; Lyons-Ruth et al, 1990). The hostile-intrusive cluster included contributions (.50) from variables indexing covert hostility, interference with the infant's goal-directed

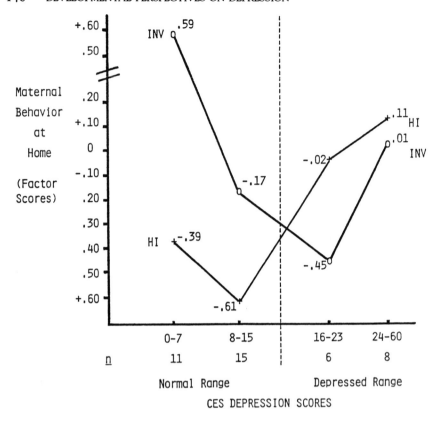

Figure 3. Maternal interaction at home as a function of maternal depressive symptoms.

behavior, overt anger, and a lack of tenderness in physical comforting and caretaking behavior. Thus, these research assessments, coded by students unaware of any other data on the families, confirm the initial association found in the data between depressive symptoms and caregiving problems observed clincially by pediatric and social service providers. Associations between depressive symptoms and negative parental behaviors have also been reported in a number of studies in relation to older children (e.g. Hammen (this volume); Richman, Stevenson, & Graham, 1982; Weissman & Paykel, 1984). In other studies of infant attachment security, similar maternal behaviors, such as maternal rejection, intrusiveness, and discomfort in holding and touching the infant, have been associated with insecure infant-mother attachment relationships (Ainsworth et al., 1978; Belsky et al., 1984; Main & Weston, 1981). These data are shown in Figure 3.

Maternal involvement varied in more complex ways in relation to the level of depressive symptoms. The mother's engagement with her infant dropped off as depressive symptoms moved into the range associated with clinical disorder and then rebounded as mothers with the highest levels of symptoms became very intrusive and controlling with their infants.

Maternal Childhood History, Current Family Circumstances and Depressive Symptoms

A number of aspects of past and present family context were associated both with maternal depressive symptoms and with negative maternal behavior. Table 5 shows the aspects of mother's childhood history and present family context which were related to the mother's current depressive symptoms.

Aspects of the mother's childhood history were also significantly related to her current mothering behavior, with two distinct clusters of associations emerging in the data. The first cluster of associations was a family cohesiveness cluster. Mothers who had experienced more supervision, fewer moves of family residence and no losses due to parental death or divorce were more likely to provide involved, attentive caregiving to their own infants, while mothers from less cohesive households were more distant and less likely to interact with their infants at home. By 18 months, 20% of the variance in the mother's current involvement with her infant at home could be accounted for by these childhood family cohesiveness variables, $R=.44$.

The second cluster of childhood history variables indexed the affective quality of family and peer relationships. The mother's current hostile-intrusive behavior toward her infant was related to her own history of hostile family relationships, as characterized by family conflict, severe punishment, lack of warmth, and psychopathology in her own mother, as well as poor quality peer relationships. Hostile relationships in the mother's childhood accounted for 27% of the variance in her own hostile-intrusiveness toward her 18-month old infant, $R=.52$, with psychopathology of her own mother accounting for 12% of the variance and the quality of childhood peer relationships accounting for 15%.

These two clusters of relationships were evident both among the group of mothers experiencing the most difficult backgrounds, defined as including maternal psychopathology, out-of-home placement, or repeated severe punishment, and among the group of mothers with more benign childhoods, who had experienced none of these. Socioeconomic status in childhood also did not account for any of these associations.

One particularly notable finding that deserves further exploration was the independent effect of positive peer relationships in decreasing later hostile-intrusive parenting behaviors. This direct effect occurred among mothers with the most negative early family relationships, as well as among mothers with less conflicted family relationships. Peer relationships are rarely explored in studies of the prediction available from childhood experiences and deserve

Table 5. The Association Between Maternal Depressive Symptoms and Current and Past Family Characteristics

| | Depressive symptoms | |
	Severity	"Depressed" classification (CESD≥16)
Current family characteristics		
Family on assistance	$F(1,54)=5.73$*	$X^2(1,N=56)=7.65$**
Infant not first born	$F(1,54)=2.94^x$	
Mother's age at birth of child	NS	
Male companion in home	NS	
Maltreatment documented	NS	
Family occupational level	NS	
Mother non-Caucasian	NS	
Mother no high school diploma	NS	
Per person weekly income	NS	
Sex of infant	NS	
Childhood history information		
Parental warmth	$r=-.43$***	$F(1,54)=14.11$***
Positive peer relationships	$r=-.39$**	$F(1,54)=2.99^x$
Lack of family conflict	$r=-.37$**	$F(1,54)=12.34$***
Psychopathology of family members	$r=.32$**	$F(1,54)=4.91$*
Maternal psychopathology	$F(1,54)=4.67$*	$X^2(1,N=56)=3.66$**
Paternal psychopathology		
Positive school experience	$r=-.20^x$	
Structure and supervision		
Parents' occupational level	$r=-.28$*	
Number of moves	$r=.24$*	
Parental death/separation		
Child in foster care	$F(1,54)=4.59$*	

Note. $N=56$. From "The Depressed Mother and Her One-Year Old Infant" by K. Lyons-Ruth, D. Zoll, D. Connell, and H. Grunebaum, 1986, *New Directions for Child Development*, 34, p. 61. Copyright 1986 by Jossey-Bass. Reprinted by permission.
$^x p<.10$ *$p<.05$ **$p<.01$ ***$p<.001$

further attention from researchers. Further discussion of these findings is available in Lyons-Ruth, Zoll, Connell, and Grunebaum (1989).

Aspects of the mother's current demographic status and family situation were much less strongly related to her current mothering behavior in this uniformly low-income sample. Ten aspects of the mother's current situation were evaluated, including mothers age, race and education, child's sex and birth order, weekly per person family income, mother's age at first child, single parenthood, AFDC status, and number of children under age 6. Of these, only two, number of children in the home under age six and mother's age at the birth of her first child, were significantly correlated with maternal behavior toward her infant at home.

Several hypotheses could be developed about the interrelationships between maternal depressive symptoms and these past and present aspects of family context in the prediction of negative maternal behavior. Two possible models of the relationships among these domains are implicit in much of the literature on depression.

In a strong theory or threshold model of the effects of depression, depression is viewed as an alternation in mood state that then has ramifications for many areas of life functioning. In this view, the depressive state is a critical mediator of symptomatic behavior, including hostile-intrusiveness or withdrawn mothering. Many biological and social factors may contribute to whether the mother becomes depressed, but according to this model the importance of these factors lies in whether or not the threshold for depression is reached. The depressive state itself is then the most important variable predicting other correlated aspects of life functioning.

A weaker theory might be called the correlate model. In this view, depression is one possible correlate of a range of past or present family stresses associated with negative maternal behavior. The family stresses are viewed as primary, however, and as mediating hostile-intrusive or withdrawn mothering, whether or not the mother also responds to these stresses by developing depressive symptoms.

To evaluate whether a threshold model or a correlate model provided a better description of the relationships between maternal depressive symptoms and maternal behavior, a series of hierarchical multiple regression analyses were performed on the two maternal behavior factors, entering significant childhood history variables, current situation variables, and maternal depression scores in forward and backward orders to assess the shared and non-shared variance in maternal behavior associated with each predictor. To avoid implying causality, a formal causal modeling approach was not used and all associations are diagrammed as potentially bidirectional. Figures 4 and 5 diagram the variance in maternal behavior that can be accounted for by direct and indirect effects of childhood history, current circumstances and maternal depressive symptoms.

As shown in Figure 4, maternal depressive symptoms played no role in the prediction of maternal involvement in this sample, probably due to the

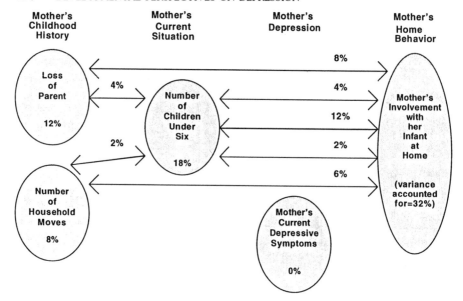

Regression Results: F(3,45)=7.06, p<.001, Multiple R=.57

Figure 4. Variance in maternal involvement accounted for by other variables.

curvilinear nature of the relationship, as was shown in Figure 3. In contrast, the lack of stable relationships in childhood contributed both directly to the prediction of lower maternal involvement (14% of variance) and was also associated with the likelihood of the mother's bearing closely spaced children, which in turn independently predicted the level of maternal involvement (18% of variance).

In relation to maternal hostile-intrusive behavior, the significant relationship between maternal depression and maternal behavior was entirely accounted for by aspects of the mother's childhood history, as can be seen in Figure 5. The psychopathology of the mother's own mother in childhood and the quality of the mother's childhood peer relationships accounted for all of the variance in mothering related to maternal depressive symptoms, as well as an additional significant portion of variance not related to depressive symptoms. Teenage parenthood was the only current circumstance that significantly predicted hostile-intrusiveness, and teen parenthood was unrelated to the extent of maternal depressive symptoms, although it was related to earlier family relationships.

Thus, a particular version of the correlate model, which we labeled the Relational model, emerged from these data. According to this model, early relationships exert direct effects on later parenting, independent of current stresses or current depressive symptoms. Depressed mothers appear to be one

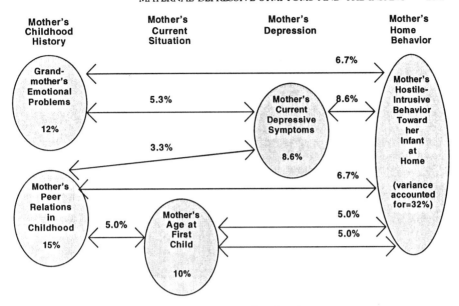

Regression Results: $\underline{F}(4,45)=5.41$, $\underline{p}<.001$; Multiple R=.57

Figure 5. Variance in maternal hostile-intrusiveness accounted for by other variables.

subgroup of the larger group of mothers who have experienced conflicted early family relationships, and depressive symptoms appear to be better understood as one correlate of these intergenerational patterns of conflict rather than as a primary independent factor influencing maternal behavior.

This should be considered an exploratory analysis, given the modest sample size and the number of variables involved. However, a similar (and unanticipated) direct effect of childhood relationships on later parenting has been reported by Belsky, Hertzog and Rovine (1986) in a middle class sample (depressive symptoms were not assessed), so the direct effects of early relationships on later parenting behavior appear to generalize beyond low-income groups. A simple effect of reporting bias, that is, that depressed mothers see their childhoods negatively, cannot explain the pattern of results reported here since the prediction from childhood history also occurred independently of depressive symptoms. Other research using family informants or siblings of depressed patients has further ruled out the tenability of such a biased-reporting explanation (Crook, Raskin & Eliot, 1981; Parker, Tupling & Brown, 1979; Robins, Schoenberg, Holmes, Ratcliff, Benham & Works, 1985). The strength of these crossgenerational relationships is also consistent with recent data from attachment research on the important role of mental representations of earlier attachment relationships in mediating current parenting behavior (see Main, Kaplan & Cassidy, 1985).

Early Family Support Services and Developmental Outcomes

High-risk families with infants under 9 months of age were offered a weekly one-hour home-visiting service, designed both to support adequate parenting and to address a range of family social service needs. Services were provided until 18 months infant age, with an average of 13 months duration and 47 home visits/family. Families receiving weekly services were randomly assigned to professional or paraprofessional visitors. Since both groups showed equivalent progress on all assessment measures, however, those two subgroups were combined in all subsequent analyses (Lyons-Ruth, Zoll, Connell, & Odom, 1987). The four central goals of the home visiting service were similar for the two service levels (paraprofessional/professional) as follows: (1) Providing an accepting and trustworthy relationship; (2) Increasing the family's competence in accessing resources to meet basic needs, including social, financial, legal, health and educational services; (3) Modeling and reinforcing more interactive, positive and developmentally appropriate exchanges between mother and infant, including the use of Levenstein's (Madden, O'Hara, & Levenstein, 1984) toy demonstration model (paraprofessional service), with emphasis on the mother's dual role as teacher and source of emotional security for her infant; (4) Decreasing social isolation from other mothers through encouraging weekly participation in parenting groups (professional service) or monthly participation in a drop-in social hour (paraprofessional service). A more qualitative description of services provided and clinical issues encountered in working with these high-risk families can be found in Lyons-Ruth, Botein & Grunebaum (1984).

Several potential routes of impact of services on the mother-infant relationship were envisioned. One possible route was that the provision of a supportive confidant for the mother would decrease maternal depressive symptoms (e.g. Brown & Harris, 1975), thereby decreasing symptom-associated negative mothering behaviors. A second possible route was that maternal social isolation would be decreased through the group-related activities, as well as through the service linkages established, thereby decreasing maternal depressive symptoms and/or negative maternal behaviors (e.g. Kotelchuk, 1982). Finally, a direct route of impact was envisioned in which the provision of new models of relationship, including the model of the home visitor's responses to the mother, as well as the home visitor's modeling about parent-infant interaction, would have a direct impact on maternal behavior, with other changes in social isolation or depressive symptoms less central to the process of change.

Our data regarding the effects of the home visiting services are most consistent with the latter route of influence. As noted earlier, maternal depressive symptoms were remarkably stable over time in both the served and unserved groups, with few mothers changing depression status over the course of the service provision. Maternal social contacts in the five days preceding the assessment also did not show a clear relationship to service provision, although there was a strong but non-significant trend for depressed mothers

Table 6. Pearson Correlations Between Time in Intervention and Maternal Behavior at 12 and 18 Months

| | 12 months | | 18 months | |
	Raw	Partial	Raw	Partial
Maternal behavior	r	r^a	r	r^a
d.f.	27	22	30	25
Involvement factor	.36*	.49**	– .18	–.09
Sensitivity	.24	.31	– .28	–.24
Warmth	.33*	.45*	– .18	–.13
Disengagement	– .40*	–.51**	.11	–.02
Verbal communication	.41*	.56**	– .19	–.11
Quantity of comforting touch	.33*	.51**	.04	.05
Quality of comforting touch	.17	.21	– .17	–.19
Quantity of caretaking touch	.20	.18	– .01	.01
Anger	– .28	–.30	– .13	–.06

Note. From "Infants at Social Risk" by K. Lyons-Ruth, D. B. Connell, H. U. Grunebaum, and S. Botein, 1990, *Child Development, 61*, p. 85. Copyright 1990 by the Society for Research in Child Development, Inc. Reprinted by permission.

[a]Adjusted for maternal depression, psychiatric hospitalization and maltreatment status at service entry.

*p<.05 **p<.01

receiving services to have more social contacts than depressed mothers who did not receive services.

Despite the absence of effects on these potential mediating variables, mothers' positive interactions with their infants at home at 12 months of age were significantly correlated with the amount of time they had received home-visiting services, as shown in Table 6. After controlling for any initial variation in risk status, mothers who had received a longer term of home visiting by 12 months infant age were significantly more involved with their infants at home, as indicated by higher levels of verbal communication, less withdrawal, greater warmth in interaction, and more frequent physical comforting of the infant. By 18 months of age, all mothers had received at least 9 months of home-visiting services, and variations in service time from 9 to 18 months no longer correlated with differences in maternal behavior.

Infant developmental outcomes were also significantly associated with the provision of home-visiting services. As can be seen in Table 7, infants of depressed mothers who received services achieved significantly higher mental development scores than both groups of infants of depressed mothers who did

Table 7. Bayley Mental Development Index at 18 Months by Treatment Group and Depressive Symptoms

Depression status		High-risk treated infants	High-risk untreated infants	Community untreated infants
	N	31	10	35
Full sample	mean	103.10 (31)	97.10 (10)	106.51 (35)
	S.D.	13.38	11.32	13.47
Non-depressed	mean	101.45 (11)	103.75 (4)	110.11 (27)
	S.D.	16.78	13.50	12.10
Depressed	mean	104.00 (20)	92.67 (6)	94.38 (8)
	S.D.	11.49	7.89	10.91

Note. Cell *n*'s in parenthesis. From "Infants at Social Risk" by K. Lyons-Ruth, D. B. Connell, H. U. Grunebaum, and S. Botein, 1990, *Child Development, 61,* p. 85. Copyright 1990 by the Society for Research in Child Development, Inc. Reprinted by permission.

not receive services, Duncan multiple range test *p*<.05, with treated infants outperforming untreated infants by 11 and 10 points respectively, or two-thirds of a standard deviation in the normative Bayley sample. As also shown in Table 7, infants of low-income mothers not reporting high depressive symptoms, whether treated or untreated, were attaining mean scores consistent with national norms.

In relation to the security of the infants' attachment relationships, a similar difference between served and unserved infants of depressed mothers was noted, as shown in Table 8, Mann Whitney *U*=70.0, *p*<.05. Unserved infants of depressed mothers exhibited particularly high rates of attachment behavior that was both avoidant or resistant *and* disorganized. The rate of such inse-cure-disorganized behavior was more than twice that shown by infants of depressed mothers who received home-visiting services, 54% vs. 22%.

Given the presence of a subgroup of maltreated infants in the group receiving services, it was also of interest to examine treatment by depression effects among infants without maltreatment histories. When maltreating mothers were eliminated from the comparisons, the difference in infant attachment status related to service provision became more pronounced. As can be seen in Table 9, compared to unserved infants of depressed mothers, served infants of depressed mothers displayed twice the rate of fully secure attachments and only one-sixth the rate of the least secure attachments, 9% vs. 54%, Mann-Whitney *U*=3.05, *p*<.01.

Given the non-random assignment of subjects to the service group, extensive control analyses were performed to assess whether any demographic or risk differences between groups could account for the pattern of effects associated

Table 8. Infant Attachment Classifications at 18 Months by Treatment Group and Depressive Symptoms

Depression status	High-risk treated infants	High-risk untreated infants	Community untreated infants
N	28[a]	10	32[a]
Non-depressed mothers			
Forced B classification			
Secure-not disorganized	.30 (3)	.00	.48 (12)
Secure-disorganized	.20 (2)	.00	.08 (2)
Forced A or C classification			
Insecure	.10 (1)	.50 (2)	.20 (5)
Insecure-disorganized	.40 (4)	.50 (2)	.24 (6)
Depressed mothers			
Forced B classification			
Secure-not disorganized	.33 (6)	.17 (1)	.14 (1)
Secure-disorganized	.28 (5)	.17 (1)	.00
Forced A or C classification			
Insecure	.17 (3)	.00	.43 (3)
Insecure-disorganized	.22 (4)	.67 (4)	.43 (3)

Note. Cell *n*'s in parenthesis. From "Infants at Social Risk" by K. Lyons-Ruth, D. B. Connell, H. U. Grunebaum, and S. Botein, 1990, *Child Development, 61*, p. 85. Copyright 1990 by the Society for Research in Child Development, Inc. Reprinted by permission.
[a]Four tapes originally classified as secure, three from the treated group and one from the community group, could not be recoded for the Disorganized category and are not included.

with service provision. None of the 10 demographic variables shown in Table 5 (plus maternal IQ scores) nor their interaction effects nor their cumulative effects could account for the results of service provision on infant outcome. The treatment effects were consistent over all demographic subgroups in the study (see Lyons-Ruth et al., 1990, for details of these analyses).

Longitudinal Continuity in Adaptation:
Behavior Problems at Age Five

When the children were four to five years old (49 to 71 months), 64 children and their families, or 82.1% of the original sample, participated in a follow up study. The percentage of subjects lost to follow-up was similar for depressed and non-depressed groups (17.6% vs. 18.2%). There were no

Table 9. Security of Attachent Among Treated and Untreated Infants of Depressed Mothers

Infant attachment classification		Depressed mother subgroups (maltreating group excluded)		
		High-risk treated infants	High-risk untreated infants	Community untreated infants
	N	11[a]	6[b]	7
Forced B classification				
Secure		.36 (4)	.17 (1)	.14 (1)
Secure-disorganized		.45 (5)	.17 (1)	.00
Forced A or C classification				
Insecure		.09 (1)	.00	.43 (3)
Insecure-disorganized		.09 (1)	.67 (4)	.43 (3)

[a]Three mothers had a history of hospitalization; those infants were classified secure, secure-disorganized and insecure-disorganized.

[b]One mother had a history of hospitalization; her infant was classified Insecure-disorganized.

significant associations between maternal depressive symptoms at age five and the six major demographic factors in this closely matched sample, as shown in Table 10.

Teacher ratings of children's problem behavior at school were obtained using the Preschool Behavior Questionnaire (PBQ), developed by Behar and Stringfield (1974) after Rutter's (1967) Children's Behavior Questionnaire. The top 10% of scores on each of the four PBQ problem scales indicates problems serious enough to warrant evaluation for services. Fifty-one teachers rated the children.

Because we were concerned about possible differences across teachers in their baselines for rating problem behavior, we also asked teachers to rate the three same-sexed classmates nearest in age. These three scores were averaged to yield a mean classmate score. Since significant correlations did occur between teachers' ratings of subjects and classmates, classmate control scores were included as covariates in all analyses of teacher data.

Mothers' behavior problem ratings for their children were obtained using the Simmons Behavior Checklist (SBCL), a maternal report scale developed and validated for the preschool age range (Reinherz & Gracey, 1983; Reinherz, Gordon, Morris, & Anastas, 1983). Mothers were also reassessed on the CES Depression Scale and children were assessed for verbal and performance IQ and social-cognitive skills. Methodological details are available in Alpern and Lyons-Ruth (submitted for publication). Only the teacher data will be discussed here.

Table 10. Demographic Characteristics of Depressed and Non-Depressed Groups

Demographic characteristics	Maternal CES–D depression classification		
	Not depressed (CESD<16)	Depressed (CESD≥16)	F or x^2 p value
N^a	34	28	
Maternal characteristics			
% White	91.2%	82.2%	ns
% High school graduate	67.7%	50.0%	ns
Mean per person weekly income	$50.00	$43.00	ns
Mean maternal age at child's birth	25.6 yrs.	24.3 yrs	ns
Infant characteristics			
% Male	61.8%	57.1%	ns
% First-born	47.1%	46.4%	ns
Risk characteristics			
Protective service cases	11.8%	21.4%	ns
Mean CES–D scores	6.98	25.54	.001

[a]Includes the 62 subjects with both maternal and teacher data.

Behavior Problem Scores of Low-Income Classmates

The behavior problem scores of classmate control children revealed that even within very low-income classrooms the proportion of children with deviant scores on total problems and on hostile behavior was not far over the 10% observed in the nationally representative validation sample for the PBQ. However, there was a tendency for low-income children generally to show elevated rates of anxious and hyperactive behavior (see also Fergusson et al., 1985). By contrast, the elevated rates of hostile behavior were specific to the children of mothers with high levels of depressive symptoms, even in low-income classrooms.

Current Depressive Symptoms and Child Behavior Problems

As in earlier analyses, behavior problem scores over the cut-off point for serious behavior disturbance were first examined for the children who had received no intervention services and whose mothers had no maltreatment histories and no psychiatric hospitalizations unrelated to depression. Again,

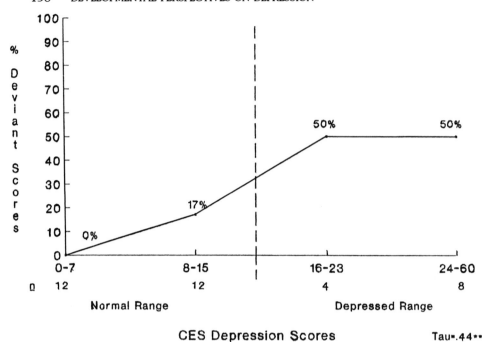

CES Depression Scores   Tau=.44**

Figure 6. Hostile-aggressive behavior in kindergarten as a function of concurrent maternal depressive symptoms.

level of current depressive symptoms was significantly related to child outcomes, particularly to hostile behavior toward peers, and the convergent validity of the CES–D cutoff scores was again supported by the child problem data, as seen in Figure 6. Results were similar, though slightly weaker, for the full sample, and further analyses were based on the entire sample.

Neither protective service status nor any of the set of demographic variables assessed in the study could account for the relationship between maternal depressive symptoms and child hostile behavior problems. There were no protective service cases represented in the untreated group data shown in Figure 6 and, in the full sample at age 5, protective service status was unrelated to both maternal depressive symptoms and child behavior problem scores.

Continuity in Social Adaptation from Infancy to Age Five

In addition to the continuity found in maternal depressive symptoms, a major hypothesis of the longitudinal study was that there would be continuity in infant social adaptation from infancy to kindergarten, manifested in a significant contribution of attachment history to later relationships with peers in the classroom. Our hypotheses were less definitive regarding the degree to which the infant's attachment classification would contribute unique variance to prediction or whether early maternal symptoms and behaviors would account equally well for the attachment-related variance in child outcome. Attachment theory would predict, however, that the form of relational regulation internalized by the infant would tend to maintain itself over time, independent of additional stability contributed by continuities in maternal behavior or family ecology.

Assessments of maternal and child social-emotional functioning in infancy were significantly predictive of later hostile behavior scores in the deviant range. Security of attachment in infancy showed the most consistently strong predictive relationships with later problem behavior, predicting both total problems and hostile-aggressive behavior. Further analysis revealed that infants classified as disorganized in infancy were at greatest risk for later hostile-aggressive behavior, with 44.4% of children who were classified as disorganized/disoriented in their attachment relationships in infancy showing highly hostile-aggressive behavior in the kindergarten classroom, compared to only 8.7% of children classified in infancy as securely attached and 25% of children classified in infancy as avoidant. Thus, even in low-income families, children classified as secure in their attachment relationship in infancy did not show elevated rates of hostile-aggressive behavior at age five, while infants classified as disorganized/ disoriented did show elevated rates compared to children with other attachment histories. Additional details are available in Lyons-Ruth, Alpern, and Repacholi, (in press).

Maternal psychosocial problems and maternal hostile-intrusive behavior were also significant predictors of later child hostile behavior. The maternal psychosocial problems variable primarily represented variance due to depressive symptoms. This variable was coded positive if mothers had high levels of depressive symptoms during the child's infancy or had histories of psychiatric hospitalization or child maltreatment. Most of the variance in child outcome was accounted for by the presence of serious depressive symptoms. With the 10 maltreating mothers removed, the association between maternal psychosocial problems and child outcome remained the same. Among the 52 non-maltreating mothers, 16 had high levels of depressive symptoms, 3 had depressive symptoms plus a history of hospitalization and 3 mothers had psychiatric hospitalization histories without depressive symptoms. To evaluate whether the variance accounted for by the three significant infancy predictors was redundant or whether buffering or potentiating effects of one risk factor on another risk factor might be present, a series of multiple discriminant function analyses were performed. These analyses revealed that both security of attachment and maternal psychosocial problems made significant independent and additive contributions to the prediction of child hostile behavior, each continuing to account for significant variance after the other was entered. No buffering or potentiating interaction patterns among the variables were significant.

Consistent with an additive effect, in the absence of both disorganized attachment behavior and maternal psychosocial problems only 5.3% of

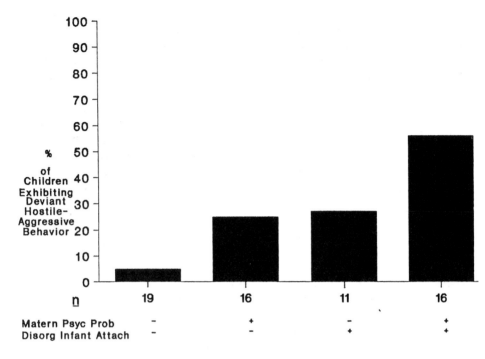

Figure 7. Additive effect of disorganized infant attachment classification and maternal psychosocial problems on later child hostile-aggressive behavior.

children showed deviant levels of hostile-aggressive behavior at school. If only maternal problems were present, this rose to 25.0%; if only disorganized attachment was present, the rate was similar at 27.3%. If the infant displayed disorganized attachment behavior *and* the mother had a psychosocial problem, the rate of aggressive behavior in preschool doubled to 56.3%, or a majority of the group.

Integrative Summary: Symptoms, Diagnosis and Relational Models

The current study was not designed as a study of affective disorders but as a study of the processes that link low socioeconomic status with adverse infant and child outcomes. However, one critical link in the process that emerged in these findings was the chronically high level of depressive symptoms that characterized mothers of infants and children with seriously maladaptive social behaviors. These high levels of depressive symptoms were also associated with high rates of lifetime DSM–III affective disorders, although for a subgroup of low-income women severe and chronic depressive symptoms occurred in the absence of a lifetime affective disorder. Data from other studies also indicate that rates of serious depressive symptoms may be elevated in the context of chronic stressors without a corresponding increase in rates of major depressive episodes (Breslau & Davis, 1986; Robins, Helzer, Weissman, Orvaschel, Grunberg, Burke & Regier, 1984).

What are the implications of these findings for research on affective disorders using structured diagnostic instruments? The psychiatric diagnostic manual includes three major affective diagnostic categories: bipolar disorder, major depression and dysthymic disorder. Most research using structured interviews has concentrated on assessing major depression only and most terms such as "clinical depression" or "depressive disorder" implicitly refer to criteria for major depression, with less attention to the other clinically recognized diagnostic category of dysthymic disorder.

Parents meeting criteria for dysthymic disorder are more rarely studied, yet the pattern of child effects emerging in recent studies suggests that child risk is more strongly associated with chronic dysphoria in a parent than with episodic major depressive episodes per se. Even in the context of major depressive disorder, evidence indicates that about 40% of those diagnosed with major depression also suffer from "double depression", or a combination of major depressive episodes and more longstanding dysthymic disorder (Keller & Shapiro, 1982; Taylor, Harding, & Dickstein, 1988). Given the importance of chronic depressive symptoms emerging in recent studies, dysthymic disorder and "double depression" may warrant more intensive study.

Whether or not the patterns of depressive symptoms exhibited by women experiencing chronic adversity conform to a diagnostic category currently included in the DSM–III–R, however, they appear to play an important role in the family contexts associated with child disorder. Current DSM–III–R categories probably underrepresent psychological syndromes associated with low-income status and chronic stress in general. For example, post-traumatic syndromes related to chronic sexual or physical abuse are still not well-understood or well-described in the standard diagnostic manual, although improved criteria are likely to be included in DSM–IV. Likewise, the "burnt out" chronic hopelessness of many poor women, whose histories of trauma are only beginning to be explored, do not always map onto current diagnostic categories very well. However, the level of experienced pain and impaired functioning in relationships accompanying these chronic dysthymic conditions are becoming evident. Thus, the current diagnostic manual should not be reified to the exclusion of gaining a better understanding of the debilitating syndromes of distress and hopelessness associated with chronic adversity and child maladaptation (see also McLoyd, 1990, for review of literature on economic stress and psychological distress among black families).

Understanding the impact of depressive symptoms and chronic adversity is also important in middle-class environments where adversity in the form of chronic child or adult illnesses also produces chronically elevated parental depressive symptoms. These symptoms, in turn, are associated with elevated rates of child psychiatric disorders (Hammen, Adrian et al., 1987; Breslau & Davis, 1986). Breslau and Davis (1986) note that "the notion that depressive symptoms are a worthy object of study *in their own right* (italics theirs), even if they are of little utility as indicators of [major depressive disorder], appears to us to be intuitively sound . . . (p. 313)." Given the rates of infant and child disorder now found to be associated with chronic maternal depressive symptoms, this conclusion appears even more pressing.

This high rate of affective symptoms and disorder among inadequately parenting mothers was not anticipated. Depressive symptoms were not an obvious aspect of many mothers' initial presentations to care providers or study staff. Instead, nurses and social workers observed neglect, apathy or anger in the mother's response to her infant. For the small proportion of mothers in the study with histories of psychiatric hospitalization, previous hospitalizations were often not known by service providers at the time of referral to the study. However, most of the highly symptomatic women in the study had no prior psychiatric contacts and were resistant to seeking conventional psychiatric care.

Depressive symptoms were important for two reasons. First, serious and chronic depressive symptoms were much more frequent than other significant indicators of parenting risk, such as a history of child maltreatment or prior psychiatric hospitalization. In the current study, 23% of community control mothers and 64% of mothers exhibiting parenting difficulties had high depressive symptom levels. These rates are consistent with other studies. Brown and Harris (1975) reported a 31% incidence of depression assessed by psychiatric interview among working class women with a child under six and Richman et al (1982), using symptom scales, reported a 30% rate among working-class mothers with three-year-olds who were matched demographically to families of three-year-olds with behavior problems. Orr and James (1984) found that 35% of a sample of 240 urban mothers seen for pediatric healthcare met CES–D criteria for depression. In that sample, low income, minority status and female head-of-household status substantially increased the risk for maternal depression to 50% for women living alone and who were either low income or Black.

Depressive symptoms were also important because high levels of depressive symptoms emerged as an important indicator that parental coping abilities had been undermined. Depressive symptom scales used as the only criteria for defining a depressed group do have important limitations, however. These emerge most strikingly in regard to assessing disorder among socially and economically well-buffered groups, such as university students, where high levels of depressive symptoms have been found to be transient in a number of cases (Coyne & Gotlib, 1983; Hammen, 1980). However, in the current study, depressive symptoms of women assessed by the CES–D showed little resemblance to the "mild and transient distress" referred to by Coyne and Gotlib (1983). In contrast, depressive symptoms among adult women in stressful economic circumstances are often quite stable, as reported here and elsewhere (Wolkind et al., 1983; Richman et al., 1982). High symptoms in the context of chronic stressors seem to have a different meaning and course, which may be better captured by longitudinal administrations of depressive symptom scales than by a single administration alone. These chronically elevated symptom levels appear to be important correlates of disrupted parenting capacities.

The predictive associations observed in the present study among maternal depressive symptoms, disorganized attachment behavior in infancy and deviant levels of child hostile-aggression at age five extend downward to infancy an emerging literature on the stability and family contexts associated with high rates of oppositional and conduct disorders in childhood. Data from the longitudinal study of three-to-eight-year-old children by Richman, Stevenson and Graham (1982) support several aspects of the current data, including the high rate of maternal depressive symptoms among lower SES mothers, the relationship of maternal depressive symptoms to later conduct disorder in children, and the absence of strong sex differences in symptomatology during the preschool period (see also Radke-Yarrow, Richters, & Wilson, 1988).

In a second large cohort ($N=527$) of children followed from ages five to nine (Reinherz, Gordon, Morris & Anastas, 1983), teacher-rated PBQ scores for hostility and hyperactivity at age 5 were strong predictors of receipt of later guidance services for emotional or behavioral disorders in grades 1–3. So children in the current study rated as deviant by their teachers at age five are likely to continue to show serious problems in subsequent years. Other studies have indicated significant continuity in antisocial behavior or conduct disorders from early school age through adulthood (Loeber, 1982; Olweus, 1979; Robins, 1978).

Data from the current study suggest that a majority of the family contexts from which the small subgroup of antisocial children will be drawn may be identifiable in the first two years of life. The finding that maternal psychosocial problems in infancy, particularly maternal depressive symptoms, were important predictors of later child hostile-aggression also extends downward the recent literatures on both child conduct disorders and children of depressed parents, since both of these literatures identify maternal depression as a frequent concurrent correlate of child conduct disorder during the school years (Behar & Stewart, 1982; Downey & Coyne, 1990; Hammen, this volume; Stewart, deBlois & Cummings, 1980). The current longitudinal data further indicate that the chronicity of parental depressive symptoms may be important in the genesis of conduct disorders and that parental depressive symptoms may be present from early in the life of a conduct disordered child.

Despite the tendency to see current emotional state as the primary "causal" factor influencing the depressed woman's interactions with family members, this association can also be viewed from other perspectives. For example, the frequent co-occurence of marital distress with maternal depression and child disorder has prompted Downey and Coyne (1990) to suggest that marital conflict may account for the association between maternal major depression (or depressive symptoms) and child disorder. Data from the current study and the associated literature on the development of attachment relationships suggests another way of viewing these associations. Our data suggest that conflictual, dysregulated relationships in childhood may play a more primary role in the structuring of later relationships and account for both the dysregulated affect manifested in symptom formation at an individual level and in the dysregulated interactions manifested in interpersonal conflict at a relational level.

From an attachment perspective, relational representations have a general application across different relationships, including relationships to parents, peers, teachers, and later, spouses (see Main, Kaplan, & Cassidy, 1985; Main & Hesse, 1990; Sroufe & Fleeson, 1986). From this viewpoint, distressed marital relationships and distressed parent-child relationships emanate, in part, from a common template or working model of the regulation of affect in relationships. Rather than a causal relationship from marital distress to parenting or peer interactions, both sets of distressed relationships may be reflections of a common relational pattern. Such a relational view does not posit that all aspects of marital or parental functioning are accounted for by working models of attachment, only that an important source of common variance will reside in these relationship models. From this perspective, the parents' working models of attachment relationships should be accounted for first before assessing the residual influences between marital problems and child outcomes (see Belsky, Youngblade, & Pensky, 1989; Quinton, Rutter, & Liddle, 1984, for approaches to this issue outside the framework of attachment theory).

In relation to data from the current study, we had reliable knowledge of the absence of current relationships for many of the single mothers in the study, due to our weekly home-visiting relationships. However, a relational perspective can explain the similarities in infant risk and maternal behavior between mothers with conflicted current relationships with a male and mothers with no current relationship but whose past relationships were conflicted.

Another implication of a relational model is that addressing the depressive symptoms or major depressive illness alone may have only limited impact on the underlying relationship patterns. This model is consistent with evidence regarding the continued negative parenting behaviors of previously depressed women not currently experiencing a major depressive episode (Gordon et al, 1989; Weissman & Paykel, 1974). Conversely, targeting the relationship patterns may not have an immediate impact on the level of dysphoria, as our intervention data suggested.

As Coyne and Downey (1991) have pointed out in relation to the literature on stress and coping, we may be making logical errors in dividing a set of conceptually related phenomena into separately assessed variables and then positing causal relationships between what are essentially different assessments of the same underlying construct. The most striking support for this relational, or common factor, view comes from the four-generational prospective longitudinal data of the Berkeley Guidance Study, initiated in 1928. The degree of intergenerational prediction of problem behavior and marital conflict for these families led Caspi and Elder (1988) to conclude that "attributing adult outcomes to proximal events . . . is spurious because these effects derive from attributes of individuals, already evident in late childhood . . ." (p. 135). (Also see Belsky & Pensky, 1988, for review of intergenerational influences.) Further prospective work on the longitudinal course of relationship patterns is clearly needed.

An important frontier in the study of developmental psychopathology now lies in developing a set of conceptual tools for understanding relational patterns at a more organizational level. We need to move beyond the current practice of using a variety of separate indicators, such as amount of negative affect, rate of interaction, conflict resolution tactics, etc., to index relational processes and move to a more conceptually grounded and integrated view of the central functions of relationships and of the overall patterning of behavior in relation to these functions.

This move to an organizational, or "goal-corrected" view of interpersonal behavior occurred in the area of caregiver-infant interaction in relation to the security-maintaining functions of the caregiving system posited by Bowlby. Mary Ainsworth then described at a reliable behavioral level the several organized patterns of behavior and affect that emerged in infant-parent interaction in relation to this function. These initial insights from the field of attachment research have now generated a second generation of research findings characterizing the patterns of mental representation of older children and adults regarding attachment-related themes (Crowell & Feldman, 1988; Fonagy, Steele, & Steele, 1991; Main et al., 1985; Ward et al., 1990). These new methods of assessment offer a more organizationally-based understanding of relational behavior in relation to attachment issues and offer a conceptual and methodological model which treats interpersonal behavior at a more integrated and qualitative level of organization than that inherent in most previous approaches.

In the next generation of studies we need to explore the extent to which different expressions of relational behavior by the same individual, as manifest, for example, in peer, parental and marital relationships, and also in the self-regulation of affect and self-esteem, should be conceived as independent domains or whether they should be seen as conceptually and empirically related behavioral expressions of internalized mental representations of relationships. Understanding more clearly how these diverse manifestations may be expressions of a central representational model will also help us to conceptualize more clearly how some genetic influences, external circumstances and life choices contain elements independent of these internalized models and have the power to set in motion a process of representational change.

The intervention data reported here indicate that new models of relationship offered by responsive, supportive, and reliable home visitors may represent one such independent agent of change. Provision of these responsive and non-hostile relationship models had significant impact on patterns of affect regulation between mothers and infants which were then carried over into children's relationships with new social partners in kindergarten. Describing the central organizational features of relationships and how and under what circumstances they are transformed constitutes an important current frontier in the study of developmental psychopathology.

REFERENCES

Aber, J.L., Allen, J.P., Carlson, V., & Cicchetti, D. (1989). The effects of maltreatment on development during early childhood: Recent studies and their theoretical, clinical, and policy implications. In D. Cicchetti & V. Carlson (eds.), *Child maltreatment: Theory and research on the causes and consequences of child abuse and neglect* (pp. 570–619). Cambridge: Cambridge University Press.

Aber, J.L., & Allen, J.P. (1987). The effects of maltreatment on young children's socioemotional development: An Attachment theory perspective. *Developmental Psychology, 23,* 406–414.

Ainsworth, M.D.S., Blehar, M., Waters, E., & Wall, S. (1978). *Patterns of attachment.* Hillsdale, NJ: Lawrence Erlbaum Associates.

Alpern, L., & Lyons-Ruth, K. (1990). Preschool children at social risk: Chronic and non-chronic maternal depressive symptoms, child I.Q. and child behavior problems at school and at home. Submitted for publication.

Arend, R., Gove, F., & Sroufe, L.A. (1979). Continuity of individual adaptation from infancy to kindergarten: A predictive study of ego-resiliency and curiosity in preschoolers. *Child Development, 50,* 950–959.

Bayley, N. (1969). *The Bayley scales of infant development.* New York: The Psychological Corporation.

Behar, D., & Stewart, M.A. (1982). Aggressive conduct disorder of children: the clinical history and direct observation. *Acta Psychiatrica Scandinavica, 65,* 210–220.

Behar, L., & Stringfield, S. (1974a). *Manual for the preschool behavior questionnaire.* (Available from Dr. Lenore Behar, 1821 Woodburn Road, Durham, NC 27705.)

Behar, L., & Stringfield, S. (1974b). A behavior rating scale for the preschool child. *Developmental Psychology, 10*(5), 601–610.

Belsky, J., Youngblade, L., & Pensky, E. (1989). Childrearing history, marital quality, and maternal affect: Intergenerational transmission in a low-risk sample. *Development and Psychopathology, 1,* 291–304.

Belsky, J., & Pensky, E. (1988). Developmental history, personality and family relationships: Toward an emergent family system. In R.A. Hinde & J. Stevenson-Hinde (eds.), *Relationships within families* (pp. 193–217). Oxford: Oxford University Press.

Belsky, J., Hertzog, C., & Rovine, M. (1986). Causal analysis of multiple determinants of parenting: Empirical and methodological advances. In M. Lamb, A. Brown, & B. Rogoff (eds.), *Advances in developmental psychology: Vol. 4* (pp. 153–202). Hillsdale, NJ:Erlbaum.

Belsky, J., Rovine, M., & Taylor, D. (1984). The Pennsylvania infant and family development project III: The origins of individual differences in infant-mother attachment: Maternal and infant contributions. *Child Development, 55,* 718–728.

Bowlby, J. (1988). *A secure base*. New York: Basic Books.

Breslau, N., & Davis, G. (1986). Chronic stress and major depression. *Archives of General Psychiatry, 43*, 309–314.

Brody, G. & Forehand, R. (1986). Maternal perceptions of child maladjustment as a function of the combined influence of child behavior and maternal depression. *Journal of Consulting and Clinical Psychology, 54*, 237–240.

Brown, G. & Harris, T. (1975). *Social origins of depression: A study of psychiatric disorders in women*. New York: The Free Press.

Carlson, V., Cicchetti, D., Barnett, D., & Braunwald, K. (1989). Disorganized/disoriented attachment relationships in maltreated infants. *Developmental Psychology, 25*(4), 525–531.

Caspi, A., & Elder, G. (1988). Childhood precursors of the life course: early personality and life disorganization. In E.M. Hetherington, R. Lerner, & M. Perlmutter (eds.), *Child development in life-span perspective* (pp. 115–142). Hillsdale, NJ: Lawrence Erlbaum Associates.

Cicchetti, D. (1990a). An historical perspective on the discipline of developmental psychopathology. In J.Rolf, A. Masten, D. Cicchetti, K. Neuchterlein, & S. Weintraub (eds.), *Risk and protective factors in the development of psychopathology.* (pp 2–28). New York: Cambridge University Press.

Cicchetti, D. (1990b). The organization and coherence of socio-emotional, cognitive, and representational development. In R. Thompson (ed.), *Nebraska symposium on motivation* (pp. 275–382). Lincoln: University of Nebraska Press.

Cicchetti, D. (1984). The emergence of developmental psychopathology. *Child Development, 55*(1), 1–7.

Cogill, S.R., Caplan, H.L., Alexandra, H., Robson, K., & Kumar, R. (1986). Impact of maternal postnatal depression on cognitive development of young children. *British Medical Journal, 292*, 1165–1167.

Cohn, J., Campbell, S., & Matias, R. (1990, April). Face-to-face interactions of depressed and non-depressed mother- infant pairs at 2, 4, and 6 months. Paper presented at the International Conference on Infant Studies, Montreal.

Coyne, J.C., & Downey, G. (1991). Social factors in psychopathology. *Annual review of psychology, 42*, 401–25.

Coyne, J.C., & Gotlib, I.H. (1983). The role of cognition in depression: a critical appraisal. *Psychological Bulletin, 94*, 472–505.

Crook, T., Raskin, A., & Eliot, J. (1981). Parent-child relationships and adult depression. *Child Development, 52*, 950–957.

Crowell, J.A., & Feldman, S.S. (1988). Mothers' internal models of relationships and children's behavioral and developmental status: A study of mother-child interaction. *Child Development, 59*, 1273–85.

Downey, G., & Coyne, J.C. (1990). Children of depressed parents: An integrative review. *Psychological Bulletin, 108*, 50–76.

Fergusson, D.M., Hons, B., Horwood, L.J., Gretton, M.E., & Shannon, F.T. (1985). Family life events, maternal depression and maternal and teacher descriptions of child behavior. *Pediatrics, 75* (1), 30–35.

Fischer, K.W., & Pipp, S.L. (1984). Development of the structures of unconscious thought. In K.S. Bowers & D. Meichenbaum (eds.), *The unconscious reconsidered* (pp. 88–148). New York: John Wiley & Sons.

Fonagy, P., Steele, H., & Steele, M. (1991). Maternal representations of attachment during pregnancy predict the organization of infant-mother attachment at one year of age. *Child Development, 62*, 891–905.

Friedlander, S., Weiss, D.S., & Traylor, J. (1986). Assessing the influence of maternal depression on the validity of the Child Behavior Checklist. *Journal of Abnormal Child Psychology, 14*(1), 123–133.

Garmezy, N., Masten, A.S., & Tellegen, A. (1984). The study of stress and competence in children: A building block for developmental psychopathology. *Child Development*, *51*, 97–111.

Ghodsian, M., Zajicek, E., & Wolkind, S. (1984). A longitudinal study of maternal depression and child behavior problems. *Journal of Child Psychology and Psychiatry, 25*, 91–109.

Gordon, D., Burge, D., Hammen, C., Adrian, C., Jaenicke, C., & Hiroto, D. (1989). Observations of interactions of depressed women with their children. *American Journal of Psychiatry, 146*, 50–55.

Hammen, C.L. (1980). Depression in college students: Beyond the Beck Depression Inventory. *Journal of Consulting and Clinical Psychology, 48*, 126–128.

Hammen, C., Adrian, C., Gordon, D., Burge, D., Jaenicke, C., & Hiroto, D. (1987). Children of depressed mothers: Maternal strain and symptom predictors of dysfunction. *Journal of Abnormal Psychology, 96*, 190–198.

Hammen, C., Burge, D., & Stansbury, K. (1990). Relationship of mother and child variables to child outcomes in a high-risk sample: A causal modeling analysis. *Developmental Psychology, 26*, 24–30.

Hammen, C., Gordon, G., Burge, D., Adrian, C., Jaenicke, C., & Hiroto, G. (1987). Maternal affective disorders, illness, and stress: Risk for children's psychopathology. *American Journal of Psychiatry, 144*, 736–741.

Hirsch, B.J., Moos, R.F., & Reischl, T.M. (1985). Psychosocial adjustment of adolescent children of a depressed, arthritic, or normal parent. *Journal of Abnormal Psychology, 94*, 154–164.

Keller, M., & Shapiro, R. (1982). "Double Depression": Superimposition of acute depressive episodes on chronic depressive disorders. *American Journal of Psychiatry, 139*, 438–442.

Klein, D., Taylor, E., Harding, K., & Dickstein, S. (1988). Double depression and episodic major depression: Demographic, clinical, familial, personality, and socioenvironmental characteristics and short-term outcome. *American Journal of Psychiatry, 145*, 1226–1231.

Kotelchuk, M. (1982). Child abuse and neglect: prediction and misclassification. In R. Starr, Jr. (ed.), *Child abuse prediction: policy implications* (pp. 67–104). Cambridge, MA: Ballinger Publishing Company.

LaFreniere, P., & Sroufe, L.A. (1985). Profiles of peer competence in the preschool: Interrelations between measures, influence of social ecology, and relation to attachment history. *Developmental Psychology, 21*, 56–69.

Loeber, R. (1982). The stability of antisocial and delinquent child behavior: a review. *Child Development, 53*, 1431–46.

Londerville, S., & Main, M. (1981). Security of attachment, compliance, and maternal training methods in the second year of life. *Developmental Psychology, 17*(3), 289–299.

Lyons-Ruth, K. (1991). Rapprochement or approchement: Mahler's theory reconsidered from the vantage point of recent research on early attachment relationships. *Psychoanalytic Psychology, 8*(1), 1–23.

Lyons-Ruth, K., Botein, S., & Grunebaum, H. (1984). Reaching the hard-to-reach: Serving multirisk families with infants in the community. In B. J. Cohler & J. S. Musick (eds.), *Intervention with psychiatrically disabled parents and their young children* (pp. 95–122). (New Directions for Mental Health Services, no. 24). San Francisco: Jossey-Bass, 1984.

Lyons-Ruth, K., Connell, D., & Zoll, D. (1989). Patterns of maternal behavior among infants at risk for abuse: Relations with infant attachment behavior and infant development at 12 months of age. In D. Cicchetti & V. Carlson (eds.), *Child maltreatment: Theory and research on the causes and consequences of child abuse and neglect* (pp. 464–93). New York: Cambridge University Press.

Lyons-Ruth, K., Connell, D.B., Grunebaum, H., & Botein, S. (1990). Infants at social risk: Maternal depression and family support services as mediators of infant development and security of attachment. *Child Development, 61*, 85–98.

Lyons-Ruth, K., Connell, D., Zoll, D., & Stahl, J. (1987). Infants at social risk: Relations among infant maltreatment, maternal behavior, and infant attachment behavior. *Developmental Psychology, 23*, 223–232.

Lyons-Ruth, K., Alpern, L., & Repacholi, B., (in press). Disorganized infant attachment classification and maternal psychosocial problems as predictors of hostile-agressive behavior in the preschool classroom. *Child Development.*

Lyons-Ruth, K., Zoll, D., Connell, D., & Grunebaum, H. (1989). Family deviance and family disruption in childhood: Associations with maternal behavior and infant maltreatment during the first two years of life. *Development and Psychopathology, 1*, 219–236.

Lyons-Ruth, K., Zoll, D., Connell, D., & Grunebaum, H. (1986). The depressed mother and her one-year-old infant: Environmental context, mother-infant interaction and attachment, and infant development. In E. Tronick & T. Field (eds.), *Maternal depression and infant disturbance* (pp. 61–82). San Francisco: Jossey Bass.

Lyons-Ruth, K., Zoll, D., Connell, D., & Odom, R. (1987, April). *Maternal depression as mediator of the effects of home-based intervention services.* Paper presented at the biennial meeting of the Society for Research in Child Development, Baltimore, MD.

Main, M., & Hesse, E. (1990). Parents' unresolved traumatic experiences are related to infant disorganized attachment status: Is frightened and/or frightening parental behavior the linking mechanism? In M. Greenberg, D. Cicchetti, & E.M. Cummings (eds.), *Attachment in the preschool years: Theory, research and intervention* (pp. 161–184). Chicago: University of Chicago Press.

Main, M., Kaplan, N., & Cassidy, J. (1985). Security in infancy, childhood and adulthood: A move to the level of representation. In I. Bretherton & E. Waters (eds.), *Growing points of attachment theory and research. Monographs of the Society for Research in Child Development,* No. 209, *50* (1–2), 66–104.

Main, M., & Solomon, J. (1990). Procedures for identifying infants as disorganized-disoriented during the Ainsworth Strange Situation. In M. Greenberg, D. Cicchetti & E.M. Cummings (eds.), *Attachment in the preschool years: Theory, research and intervention* (pp.121–160). Chicago: University of Chicago Press.

Main, M., & Weston, D. (1981). The quality of the toddler's relationship to mother and father: Related to conflict behavior and the readiness to establish new relationships. *Child Development, 52*, 932–940.

Matas, L., Arend, R.A., & Sroufe, L.A. (1987). Continuity of adaptation in the second year: The relationship between quality of attachment and later competence. *Child Development, 49*, 547–556.

McLoyd, V.C. (1990). The impact of economic hardship on black families and children: Psychological distress, parenting, and socioemotional development. *Child Development, 61*, 311–346.

Myers, J.K., & Weissman, M.M. (1980). Use of a self-report symptom scale to detect depression in a community sample. *American Journal of Psychiatry, 137*, 1081–1084.

Olweus, D. (1979). Stability of aggressive reaction patterns in males: a review. *Psychological Bulletin, 86*, 852–875.

Oppenheim, D., Sagi, A., & Lamb, M. (1988). Infant-adult attachments on the kibbutz and their relation to socioemotional development four years later. *Developmental Psychology, 24*, 427–433.

O'Connor, M., Sigman, M., & Brill, N. (1987). Disorganization of attachment in relation to maternal alcohol consumption. *Journal of Clinical and Consulting Psychology, 55*, 831–836.

Orr, S., & James, S. (1984). Maternal depression in an urban pediatric practice: Implications for health care delivery. *American Journal of Public Health, 74*(4), 363–365.

Parker, G., Tupling, H., & Brown, L. (1979). A parental bonding instrument. *British Journal of Medical Psychology, 52*, 1–10.

Quinton, D., Rutter, M., & Liddle, C. (1984). Institutional rearing, parenting difficulties, and marital support. *Psychological Medicine, 14*, 107–124.

Radke-Yarrow, M., Richters, J., & Wilson, W.E. (1988). Child development in a network of relationships. In R.A. Hinde & J. Stevenson-Hinde (eds.). *Relationships within families* (pp. 48–67). Oxford: Oxford University Press.

Radke-Yarrow, M., Cummings, E.M., Kuczynski, L., & Chapman, M. (1985). Patterns of attachment in two- and three-year-olds in normal families and families with parental depression. *Child Development, 56*, 884–893.

Radloff, L. (1977). The CES-D scale: A self-report depression scale for research in the general population. *Applied Psychological Measurement, 1*(13), 385–401.

Reinherz, H., Gordon, A., Morris, K., & Anastas, T. (1983). Who shall be served? Issues in screening for emotional and behavioral problems in school. *Journal of Primary Prevention, 4*(2), 73–95.

Reinherz, H., & Gracey, C. (1983). *Simmons Behavior Checklist: Technical information.* Boston: Simmons College School of Social Work.

Richman, N., Stevenson, J., & Graham P. (1982). *Preschool to school: A behavioral study.* London: Academic Press.

Richters, J., & Pellegrini, D. (1989). Depressed mothers' judgments about their children: An examination of the depression-distortion hypothesis. *Child Development, 60*, 1068–1075.

Robins, L. (1978). Sturdy predictors of adult antisocial behavior: replication from longitudinal studies. *Psychological Medicine, 8*, 611–622.

Robins, L.N., Helzer, J.E., Croughan, J., & Ratcliff, K.S. (1981). The NIMH Diagnostic Interview Schedule: Its history, characteristics and validity. *Archives of General Psychiatry, 38*, 381–389.

Robins, L.N., Helzer, J.E., Weissman, M.M., Orvaschel, H., Grunberg, E., Burke, Jr., J.D., & Regier, D.A. (1984). Lifetime prevalence of specific psychiatric disorders in three sites. *Archives of General Psychiatry, 41*, 949–958.

Robins, L.N., Schoenberg, S., Holmes, S., Ratcliff, K., Benham, A., & Works, J. (1985). Early home environment and retrospective recall: A test for concordance between siblings with and without psychiatric disorders. *American Journal of Orthopsychiatry, 55*(1), 27–41.

Rutter, M. (1967). A children's behavior questionnaire for completion by teachers: Preliminary findings. *Journal of Child Psychology and Psychiatry, 8*, 1–11.

Rutter, M., & Garmezy, N. (1983). Developmental psychopathology. In E. M. Hetherington (ed.), *Handbook of child psychology, Vol IV, Socialization, personality, and social development* (pp. 775–912). New York: Wiley

Rutter, M., Yule, B., Quinton, D., Rowlands, O., Yule, W., & Berger, M. (1974). Attainment and adjustment in two geographical areas: III. Some factors accounting for area differences. *British Journal of Psychiatry, 126*, 520–533.

Sameroff, A.J., & Emde, R.N. (eds.). (1989). *Relationship disturbances in early childhood: A developmental approach.* New York: Basic Books.

Sroufe, L.A. (1989). Pathways to adaptation and maladaptation: Psychopathology as developmental deviation. In D. Cicchetti (ed.), *The emergence of a discipline: Rochester symposium on developmental psychopathology, Vol. 1* (pp. 13–40). Hillsdale, NJ: Erlbaum.

Sroufe, L., & Fleeson, J. (1986). Attachment and the construction of relationships. In W. Hartup & Z. Rubin (eds.), *Relationships and development* (pp. 36–54). Hillsdale, NJ: LAwrence Erlbaum Associates.

Sroufe, L., & Rutter, M. (1984). The domain of developmental psychopathology. *Child Development, 55*, 17–29.

Stewart, M.A., deBlois, C.S., & Cummings, C. (1980). Psychiatric disorder in the parents of hyperactive boys and those with conduct disorder. *Journal of Child Psychology and Psychiatry, 21*, 283–292.

Van Ijzendoorn, M., & Kroonenberg, P. (1988). Cross-cultural patterns of attachment: A meta-analysis of the strange situation. *Child Development, 59*, 147–56.

Ward, M., Carlson, E., Altman, S., Levine, L. Greenberg, R., & Kessler, D. (1990, April). *Predicting infant-mother attachment from adolescent mothers' working models of relationships.* Paper presented at the biennial meeting of the International Society on Infant Studies, Montreal.

Waters, E., Wippman, J., & Sroufe, L.A. (1979). Attachment, positive affect, and competence in the peer group: Two studies in construct validation. *Child Development, 50*, 821–829.

Wechsler, D. (1955). *Wechsler Adult Intelligence Scale manual.* New York: Psychological Corporation.

Weissman, M., & Paykel, E. (1974). *The depressed woman: A study of social relationships.* Chicago: University of Chicago Press.

Wolkind, S.N., Zajicek-Coleman, & Ghodsian, M. (1980). Continuities in maternal depression. *International Journal of Family Psychiatry, 1*, 167–182.

V Emotional Dysregulation in Disruptive Behavior Disorders

PAMELA M. COLE & CAROLYN ZAHN-WAXLER

In this chapter we present a view of disruptive behavior disorders as **affective** disorders and, from that perspective, discuss the emotional characteristics which are associated with the development of aggressive, antisocial behavior. The formal term, affective disorder, has been reserved traditionally for depression-related disorder; we use it to include broader affect-related dysfunction. We refer to disruptive behavior disorders as involving affective disorder because we think that (a) patterns of emotional dysregulation play an important role in the development and maintenance of disruptive behavior disorders in children, and (b) that the affective disturbances associated with disruptive behavior disorders are not as distinctly or discretely different from depression-related disorders as they sometimes appear to be.

The role of emotion in disruptive behavior disorders has not received as much attention as the roles of socialization, learning or cognitive control. In this chapter we illustrate the affective underpinnings of disruptive behavior disorders, examine the distinctions and overlap between these disorders and traditional affective disorder, and consider the developmental paths, particularly in early childhood, that may lead to the emergence of particular patterns of emotional dysregulation and stable disruptive behavior (see also Cicchetti & Schneider-Rosen, 1986).

In the first sections of the chapter, we provide an overview of the disruptive behavior disorders, the history of the traditional segregation of behavior disorder from affective disorder, and the evidence and arguments for comorbidity of affective and disruptive disorders. Next, we describe the emotional characteristics associated with behavior disorders, and from the standpoint of an emotion regulation perspective, we consider possible developmental

AUTHOR'S NOTE. The authors wish to thank the National Institute of Mental Health, Intramural Program, and the John T. and Catherine D. MacArthur Foundation for their support of this work.

trajectories leading to these disorders. We focus particularly on the role of emotion in early childhood and its implications for the development of defiant and aggressive behavior later in childhood and adolescence.

Overview of the disruptive behavior disorders

Disruptive behavior represents the most common concern and referral problem among child-focused presenting problems, and disruptive behavior disorders are the most common diagnoses among children and adolescents (Anderson, Williams, McGee, & Silva, 1987; Cerreto & Tuma, 1977; Faulstich, Monroe, Carey, Ruggiero, & Gresham, 1986; Offord, Adler, & Boyle, 1986; Rutter, Cox, Tupling, Berger, & Yule, 1975; Schroeder, Gordon, Kanoy, & Routh, 1983; Stewart, DeBlois, Meardon & Cummings, 1980). The three major diagnoses in the DSM–III–R (American Psychiatric Association, 1987) category of disruptive behavior disorders are conduct disorder, oppositional defiant disorder, and attention deficit with hyperactivity disorder. The formal diagnosis of conduct disorder (CD) is restricted currently to antisocial behavior that violates specific rules of conduct (e.g., stealing, physical aggression). Oppositional defiant disorder (ODD) is defined by defiant, disobedient behavior without clear antisocial acts, and attention deficit disorder is associated with disruptiveness that appears to stem from the core features of distractibility and impulsivity.

Conduct and oppositional disorders have in common behavior that is consistently defiant of authority and noncompliant with family, classroom, and societal rules. Although conduct disorder is distinguished from ODD by its violations of the rights and properties of others, it is not fully clear whether these two diagnoses represent different basic entities or different manifestations of the same problem (Achenbach, Conners, Quay, Verhulst, & Howell, 1989; Frick, Lahey, Loeber, Stouthamer-Loeber, Green, Hart, & Christ, 1991; Reeves, Werry, Elkind, & Zametkin, 1987; Rey, Bashir, Schwarz, Richards, Plapp, & Stewart, 1988; Schachar & Wachsmuth, 1990). Some argue that oppositional defiant disorder is a milder version of conduct disorder (Loeber, Lahey, & Thomas, 1991; Werry, Reeves, & Elkind, 1987). What the two diagnoses share in particular are symptoms that involve hostile confrontation with others (Quay, 1986).

Theoretically, attention deficit disorder (ADD) seems more distinct, involving difficulty deploying and modulating attention, and not intentional noncompliance or transgression. We include it in this discussion, however, because ADD frequently co-occurs with the other disruptive behavior disorders (Barkley, 1990; Shapiro & Garfinkel, 1986), and differential diagnosis between conduct disorder and ADD has been persistently difficult (Loney & Milich, 1982; Prinz, Conner, & Wilson, 1981; Quay, 1979; Stewart et al., 1980). There is an assumption and hope that research will help to tease apart syndromes that are based on antisocial versus attentional problems (Hinshaw,

1987). Nonetheless, school age children who appear to be hyperactive without conduct problems still have twice the risk of engaging in criminal activity as nonproblem children (Farrington, Loeber, & Van Kammen, 1990), and so, in practical terms, attention deficit disorder is another form of behavior disorder. A certain degree of comorbidity among different types of disruptive behavior disorders appears to exist (Reeves et al., 1987; Stewart et al., 1980). Some have suggested that these types of disruptive problems be grouped as cases of "disinhibitory psychopathology" (Gorenstein & Newman, 1980).

Disruptive behavior disorders and their major symptoms — aggressivity, impulsivity, noncompliance — tend to be relatively stable over the course of childhood, adolescence and adulthood (Kohlberg, LaCrosse, & Ricks, 1972; Huesmann, Eron, Lefkowitz, & Walder, 1984; MacFarlane, Honzik, & Allen, 1962; Olweus, 1979; Robins, 1966; Rose, Rose, & Feldman, 1989). Retrospective reports of adolescent delinquents and adult antisocial personalities often allude to the presence of problematic behavior prior to or at school entry (e.g., Robins, 1966), although prospective research indicates that not all behavior problem preschoolers develop disruptive disorders (Campbell, Breaux, Ewing, & Szumowski, 1986; Richman, Stevenson, & Graham, 1975). Early onset of disruptive behavior, however, is a predictor of more stable behavior problems (Loeber, 1990; Moffitt, 1990).

Although the stability of early disruptive behavior is usually contrasted with the transience of early "emotional" problems (e.g., worries, fears, moodiness; MacFarlane et al., 1962), it is not known whether the presence of significant disruptive behavior in early childhood might also present risk for later internalizing disorders. Some studies suggest that, in fact, aggressive young girls may not continue to display externalizing behavior over the course of development but may be at increased risk for depression and somatic problems (Achenbach, Howell, Quay, & Conners, 1991; Moskowitz & Schwartzman, 1989; Robins, 1986).

Research with children prior to school entry reinforces the evidence of the early establishment of disruptive patterns for some significant number of behavior problem preschoolers (Campbell et al., 1986; Chamberlin, 1981; Lerner, Inui, Trupin, & Douglas, 1985; Loeber, Tremblay, Gagnon, & Charlebois, 1989; MacFarlane et al., 1962; Richman et al., 1975). We think these years may be particularly important in understanding the development of disruptive behavior disorders because it is during these years that the source of influence of emotional and behavioral regulation shifts from relative dependence upon adult caregivers to relatively greater self-regulation.

In early childhood, all children are developing the ability to coordinate and organize their behavior in an autonomous fashion and to use internalized social rules and understandings. On the basis of current research, it is still not known (a) how to discriminate normative from psychopathological variation in disruptive, noncompliant, impulsive, and aggressive behavior, in terms of the development of stable problems, and (b) how to segregate children in terms of types of disinhibitory psychopathology and affective disorder. In fact, the factors that indicate some degree of distinction between ODD and CD in later childhood, notably rule violations such as status offenses and illegal acts, are rare in early childhood (Loeber et al., 1991). Overactivity, impulsivity, aggressivity, and noncompliance tend to cluster in preschool samples.

In sum, disruptive behavior disorders represent a category of various problems that have in common behaviors that are public, socially undesirable, and particularly irritating and disturbing for others. They are known to be stable over time, to create risk for later mental health problems, and to be the most common cause of child mental health referrals. There is considerable symptom overlap among the three types of disruptive behavior disorders, but over the course of development there is some degree of differentiation that emerges. There is evidence for the stability of disruptive behavior even in young children.

Childhood disruptive behavior disorders are traditionally not regarded as affective disorders. Stated in the extreme, affective disorders are treated primarily as "emotional" problems while disruptive behavior disorders, particularly conduct and oppositional disorders, are more likely viewed as moral failure, and attention deficits as cognitive disabilities. That is, antisocial behavior is often regarded as behavior that requires adjudication and punishment rather than reflective of a type of emotional difficulty requiring mental health services. Nonetheless, all disruptive behavior disorders are mental health problems, inseparable from their affective components, although these components have tended to be underestimated.

The traditional segregation of behavior and affective disorders

In the attempt to identify distinct, non-overlapping classes of disordered behavior, disorders of affect or mood have traditionally been segregated from behavioral disorders. Two trends in the classification of psychopathology have led to this conceptual segregation. One trend stems from the practical clinical need for a diagnostic classification system in the absence of conclusive research, and the call within psychiatry for a working system that is reliable across diagnosticians. The second trend emerges from empirical efforts to differentiate types of symptom patterns in children.

Affective and behavior disorders in psychiatric classification

Although depression has been a category of mental disturbance since the earliest efforts of the Greeks to classify psychopathology, behavior disorders entered the nomenclature later. Psychiatric classification first identified behavior disorders during the 1889 International Congress of Mental Science (Tuke, 1890) when "moral and impulsive insanity" were added to the list of disorders. This historical separation of the two classes persisted in the

American Psychiatric Association's Diagnostic and Statistical Manuals (DSM) and was extended to the classification of children. The 1968 DSM–II was first to add the category behavior disorders of childhood and adolescence, and in DSM–III childhood depression was acknowledged.

The DSM system has both a practical and a scientific mandate. Practical demands have required that classification schemes be devised in the absence of conclusive investigation. Originally, such schemes were influenced by medical and psychodynamic models of personality and psychopathology. As the science of human behavior evolved and models proliferated, the DSM system has had to respond to a demand for less theoretical bias and for increased interjudge reliability. In turn, these demands have necessitated movement away from inferences about underlying causes, and toward a descriptive, atheoretical approach with an almost exclusive focus on more discriminative, observable symptoms.

This course of events has influenced the role of emotion as a factor in distinguishing types. Emotions are not observable; the scientific criteria for determining that an emotion or mood is present are not established and they are at best highly inferential. In regard to the emotional profile associated with a given formal diagnosis, the descriptive trend in psychiatric classification limits itself to those salient emotions or moods that are reliable markers for discriminating one presentation from another. The terms affective disorder and mood disorder are used almost exclusively for a family of depression-related disorders, whose most salient characteristics are episodes of chronic dysphoria or anhedonia. The expressed emotion is the foremost observable feature and assumptions about underlying emotional dynamics are not necessary to achieve a reliable diagnosis.

Disruptive children's most salient characteristics are not those of *personal* distress, although they may often evince irritable or sad mood, but those of behaviors that go against the social grain. If a disruptive child also manifests dysphoria or anhedonia, then two diagnoses are given. Some clinicians, however, view the disruptive behavior alone as an expression of internal distress, even if overt sadness and anxiety are not displayed. If in fact certain disruptive children are depressed but do not manifest more classic symptoms, DSM–III–R does not allow a diagnosis of depression.

Empirically-derived distinctions between affective and behavior disorder

A related trend which has contributed to the segregation of affective and disruptive disorders is based on empirically-derived classification systems. This approach, which statistically examines multivariate correlational patterns among reported symptoms of children, usually based on maternal and teacher ratings, consistently generates two broad groups of symptoms: those that have been labeled as overcontrolled or internalizing, and which include many emotion-related symptoms (fears, poor self-esteem, guilt, sad mood, tension, somatic complaints), and those that have been labeled as undercontrolled or externalizing and emphasize behavior rather than emotion (aggressivity, opposition, noncompliance, overactivity) (Achenbach & Edelbrock, 1978; Quay, 1986). The first dimension is thought to reflect internal distress, while the other dimension reflects causing distress to others. Therefore, negative affective states (e.g., enduring depressed mood) and verbal expression of negative thoughts and beliefs (e.g., negative self-statements and feelings of hopelessness) that communicate internal distress to adults are regarded as internalizing problems. Hyperactivity, aggressivity, and noncompliance, which are the symptomatic heart of the externalizing problems, emerge as a distinct and separate dimension and are called externalizing because others are distressed by these symptoms. Again, the distinction is based on symptoms witnessed by parents and teachers.

Overlap between emotional distress and disruptive behavior

Despite this tradition of conceptually segregating affective and behavior disorders, there is considerable evidence of overlap between symptoms of each and of comorbidity of related disorders. The robust, reliable nature of the statistical distinction between internalizing and externalizing factors based on behavior ratings must be understood in the context of studies that show that the two dimensions are often moderately and positively correlated (Achenbach & Edelbrock, 1983; Rose et al., 1989). That is, while each set of symptoms tends to cluster more strongly within itself, a significant number of problem children are reported to display elevated rates of behaviors across both clusters of symptoms. These ratings suggest that adults tend to infer emotional disturbances to some degree in children with disruptive behavior, or at least for some children. Research on the interrater reliability of parent and child reports of symptoms indicates that children are likely to rate themselves as experiencing more internal distress than their parents attribute to them, suggesting a potentially even stronger relationship between internal distress and disruptive behavior (Loeber et al., 1989). At the same time, children hospitalized on psychiatric inpatient units reveal considerable overlap between aggressive and depressive symptoms (Kazdin, Esveldt-Dawson, Unis, & Rancurello, 1983).

Affective symptoms associated with disruptive behavior disorder

Within the DSM–III–R system, it is recognized that the emotional life of the child with disruptive behavior disorder is not typical. The list of associated features for the diagnosis of conduct disorder mentions many emotion-based symptoms — the child may show no concern for others, lack appropriate feelings of guilt and remorse, readily blame others, have low self-esteem despite an image of "toughness", and have poor frustration tolerance, irritability and temper outbursts (American Psychiatric Association,

1987, pp. 53–54). Oppositional defiant disorder, is largely composed of emotional, particularly angry, features — loses temper, argues with adults, actively defies adult requests or rules, deliberately [annoys] other people, blames others, is touchy or easily annoyed, is angry and resentful, is spiteful and vindictive, and swears (p. 57). Again, it is important to note that all of these characteristics of oppositional disorder can be present in conduct disorder, and that oppositional disorder basically characterizes the disruptive child who does not engage in *overt* violations of social rules and acts against the rights of others. For attention deficit disorder, the list of associated features includes low self-esteem, mood lability, low frustration tolerance, and temper outbursts (p. 51). Difficulties in the affective domain, especially the control of anger, are clearly a problem in the disruptive behavior disorders. The affective disturbance is recognized but has not been adequately conceptualized or understood in terms of its relation to the disruptive behavior.

Comorbidity of internalizing and externalizing disorders

Another perspective on the relation between affective disturbances and disruptive behavior emerges in diagnostic studies of clinical populations. This literature addresses the issue of difficulties with personal distress in the form of depression and anxiety in externalizing children. Comorbidity of disruptive behavior disorder and depressive disorder is reported in clinical studies using diagnostic criteria (Carlson & Cantwell, 1980; Geller, Chestnut, Miller, Price, & Yates, 1985; Kovacs, Feinberg, Crouse-Novak, Paulauskas, & Finkelstein, 1984; Marriage, Fine, Moretti, & Haley, 1986; Puig-Antich, 1982; Stewart et al., 1980). The pattern of findings is that anxiety and/or depression are present in considerable numbers of children with a diagnosis of conduct disorders. Also, children with conduct disorders are at heightened risk for suicide (Pfeffer, 1986; Shaffer, 1974). In fact, Schaffer reported that problems associated with externalizing problems (e.g., disciplinary problems, fighting with peers) were common precipitating events in adolescent suicide. A sense of hopelessness, rather than a diagnosis of depression, is a critical and specific precursor to suicide (Hawton, 1986; Kazdin, French, Unis, Esveldt-Dawson, & Sherick, 1983).

Comorbidity of externalizing and internalizing patterns appears to be associated with diverse outcomes. For example, there is evidence that children with early tendencies toward both externalizing and internalizing patterns may be at highest risk for chronic, serious mental health impairment (Kellam, Simon, & Ensminger, 1983; Kovacs, Paulauskas, Gatsonis, & Richards, 1988; Ledingham & Schwartzman, 1984; Milich & Landau, 1984). These outcomes include social isolation, peer rejection, dependency on adults, inattentiveness, substance abuse, and antisocial behavior, and have been interpreted in terms of risk for depression, anxiety, schizophrenia, and antisocial personality. However, not all studies find that the comorbidity of internalizing and externalizing symptoms are associated with more serious risk or psychopathology.

Research with diagnosed children suggests that the presence of comorbid diagnostic conditions (e.g., anxiety and ADD; depression and CD) are associated with less severe disruptive behavior (McBurnett, Lahey, Frick, Risch, Loeber, Hart, Christ, & Hanson, 1991; Walker, Lahey, Russo, Frick, Christ, McBurnett, Loeber, Stouthamer-Loeber, & Green, 1991; also see ADD studies below). Therefore, the presence of internalizing and externalizing patterns appears to lead to diverse outcomes, and it will be important to investigate the specific internalizing patterns (e.g., social withdrawal vs. depression and anxiety) that lead to more or less severe behavioral disturbance.

Within the conduct disorder category, emotion-related factors have been thought to distinguish subtypes. The ability to establish affectionate, caring relationships has been used to distinguish the solitary or undersocialized type from the group or socialized type (see Quay, 1987 for review). These various data suggest that internalizing features and various additional emotional qualities (hostility, anxiety, irritability, sadness, affection), and how these are evidenced in social relations (social withdrawal, inability to attach to others, display of remorse and guilt), are factors that have complex relations with defiant, aggressive, antisocial behavior.

A recent study (Cole & Carpentieri, 1990) examined comorbidity of child depression and conduct disorder in children from different socio-economic strata. Over 1400 non-referred fourth graders were assessed to determine whether comorbidity of depression and aggression is greater than one would expect by chance. A substantial correlation between depression and conduct disorder was found after accounting for shared method variance. Rejected children were particularly likely to show both depression and conduct disorder. Children rejected by peers tended to show high rates of aggressive, undercontrolled behavior and low rates of prosocial activity.

In the case of ADD, there is mixed evidence of diagnostic comorbidity between major depressive disorder and ADD (Barkley, DuPaul, & McMurray, 1990; Biederman, Munir, & Knee, 1987). Barkley (1990) advises that dysthymic disorder can often coexist with ADD and conduct disorder. Dysthymic disorder is a condition of chronic mood disturbance, and is basically distinguished from major depressive disorder in terms of the latter being episodic and dysthymia reflecting enduring depressive symptoms. Studies of depressed and anxious children report a higher rate of ADD and CD symptoms in these children (Last, Strauss, & Francis, 1987; McClellan, Rubert, Reichler, & Sylvester, 1990).

Although DSM–III–R revised the diagnosis of attention deficit disorder to always include hyperactivity (ADHD), there is still considerable debate about the existence of two forms of ADD, with and without hyperactive behavior. The presence of internalizing symptoms seems to distinguish the two groups (Barkley et al., 1990; Berry, Shaywitz, & Shaywitz, 1985; Edelbrock, Costello, & Kessler, 1984; King & Young, 1982; Lahey, Schaughency, Hynd, Carlson, & Nieves, 1987). In general, these studies found that ADD children with hyperactivity were more impulsive and aggressive, and showed more severe conduct disorders. The group without hyperactivity appeared more lethargic and sluggish, and were more likely to receive an internalizing disorder diagnosis (particularly anxiety disorder).

Studies that examine characteristics of depressed and conduct disordered children also indicate sources of overlap between the two clinical conditions. For example, depressed children differ from nonproblem children in terms of being more socially isolated but when they do interact with their peers they tend to be more aggressive (Altmann & Gotlib, 1988). Depressed and conduct disordered preschoolers tend to interact less with their mothers than do nonproblem children, and depressed and conduct disordered children report more depressive symptoms than nonproblem children (Field, Sandberg, Goldstein, Garcia, Vega-Lahr, Porter, & Dowling, 1987). Both aggressive and depressed school age children show a hostile attribution bias although they differ in their reports of how they behave when they perceive hostility in others (Quiggle, Garber, Panak, & Dodge, in press). This is not to say that depressed and disruptive children cannot be discriminated but that there is overlap between the groups in terms of the qualities of their everyday behavior. In the DSM–III–R manual, irritability, sulkiness, withdrawal from the family, reluctance to cooperate, aggression, and wanting to run away are described as symptoms commonly associated with depressive episodes in older children and adolescents. These symptoms often occasion consideration of disruptive behavior disorder diagnoses but may not be sufficiently problematic to qualify for dual diagnosis.

These various studies suggest that there are: (a) disruptive children who show evidence of internal distress and who are likely to be given a comorbid diagnosis of anxiety or depressive disorder; (b) depressed and anxious children who frequently display ADD and CD symptoms; and (c) disruptive children, who do not reveal sufficient evidence to qualify for a dual diagnosis, but who show many concomitant signs that their emotional lives are atypical and perhaps distressed.

In our opinion, it is necessary to conduct extensive research on the role of emotion in the development of disruptive behavior disorders. The role of early childhood negative affectivity, of interpersonal distress and conflict, and of irritable, resistant patterns that make adults perceive the children as difficult-to-manage, must be investigated in terms of the development of emotional dysregulation and risk for psychopathology (see Cicchetti, Ganiban, & Barnett, 1991). The laudable advances in attempting to discriminate symptom clusters may have led to an oversimplification of the distinction between affective and behavioral disturbances.

Therapeutic perspectives on affective and behavior disorder

A final vantage point for the issue of the emotional underpinnings of antisocial behavior and its links with internal distress is the therapeutic perspective. In attempting to treat children with disruptive behavior disorders, many clinicians assume underlying emotional difficulties, particularly the possibility of depression. The tendency for disruptive behavior disordered children to reveal low self-esteem, sense of worthlessness and hopelessness has been a longstanding focus of treatment (e.g., Glaser, 1967; Horner, 1984; Kernberg & Chazan, 1991; Siegel, 1991). One view is that depression is an *outcome* of prolonged disruptive behavior. Patterson and his colleagues, who have conducted extensive observational research with behavior problem children, state that depressed mood may be a logical secondary result of the academic and interpersonal failures that conduct disordered children experience (Patterson, DeBaryshe, & Ramsey, 1989). They suggest that membership in a deviant peer group may help to alleviate such feelings of inadequacy and worthlessness; while the group helps the child feel some sense of belonging and of personal value, at the same time this group promotes and reinforces the child's antisocial behavior.

Another popular clinical view is that depression, or depression-inducing experience, is a *precedent* of aggressive or antisocial actions, often as a result of experiences of disappointment and actual or symbolic loss due to disturbed family dynamics. This is related to the view of aggressivity, defiance, and acting out as an expression of masked depression (Bakwin, 1972; Cytryn & McKnew, 1972; Kovacs & Beck, 1977; Malmquist, 1977; Winnicott, 1958/1975), in which parental and teacher concerns about disruptive behavior are the presenting problem, but the clinician detects or infers the presence of underlying depression and treats the misbehavior with the depression in mind. Although masked depression is a problematic construct from a scientific standpoint, it is commonly used in clinical work and given credence on inpatient units where children with conduct and oppositional disorders often develop clear depression when the acting out patterns are eliminated by the treatment program. More recently, Trad (1989) offered the term "masked dependencies" as a means of understanding the aggressive activity of behavior-disordered preschool age children in play therapy. His viewpoint is that their acting out behavior is a cry for limits and authority and control; that is, the children are seeking help with their behavioral difficulty and not rejecting the therapy.

Despite the scientific concerns about "masked" features, the concept lingers and warrants empirical attention. If we examine symptoms only, it is more difficult to comment on underlying emotional tendencies among disruptive children. Assessment of depressed, conduct disordered, and nonproblem children's social constructions, self-understanding, and interactional patterns in regard to emotionally challenging events may, however, help to clarify the issue.

An emotional profile of the disruptive child

On the basis of research and clinical experience, it seems reasonable to hypothesize that there are affective disturbances involved in disruptive behavior, including symptoms of difficulty with anger regulation and symptoms that are depressive in nature. These children, in general, are not happy, lack self-esteem, and express resistance to the world around them through emotional displays and/or through behavioral resistance and rule violations. They feel inadequate in many of their relationships, and develop beliefs that they are unloved or unworthy.

In attempting to conceptualize the emotional profile of disruptive children, we are influenced by the hypothesis that there are discrete emotion systems (Gray, 1982, 1987; Izard, 1977; Tomkins, 1963), and that emotion is regulatory and regulated (Campos & Barrett, 1984; Izard, 1977; Frijda, 1986; Sroufe, 1983). These theories offer a starting point for appreciating the complex relationship between emotion and problematic behavior patterns. Although all children with disruptive behavior disorder are not alike, we suggest the following emotional profile as a relatively common portrayal:

(1) Anger plays a dominant role in the child's emotional presentation, and serves to trigger and maintain the violation of rules and acting against others. Among disruptive children, there is a greater quickness to anger and frustration under certain conditions such as limit-setting and goal frustration, a tendency for anger to be more intense and more closely related to aggressive acts, a tendency for anger to be more sustained and less easy to resolve, a tendency for more chronic irritable mood, and a tendency to respond angrily in situations that elicit more submissive emotion in other children. We should point out that some of the phenomenological aspects of anger that we have just described may not distinguish a disruptive from a depressed child, although associated expressive and instrumental behaviors may differ among children. One recent study reported that children experience depression as both sadness and anger (Renouf & Harter, 1990). Moreover, the anger associated with depression was directed toward *others* more often than self.

It is also important to consider that there may be different angers (Kagan, 1991). The anger that is associated with asserting one's position and defending one's property and person may be qualitatively different from other types of angers. The relationship between normative anger and feelings of rage and hate is not understood. Rage, often associated with feelings of shame and humiliation, may be an important component of chronic hostile, aggressive behavior (e.g., Tomkins, 1963).

(2) Sadness and anxiety, more vulnerable or submissive emotions, are underrepresented in some disruptive children's emotional presentations. For those children, this is seen in a relative lack of **displayed** sadness and tension when the child experiences loss, of empathic distress when others are hurt, and of guilt over wrongdoing. It is important to realize that the absence of

observed sadness or anxiety in the moment does not inform whether the child experiences these vulnerable emotions, or whether the child has them in the emotional repertoire. It does suggest, however, some form of dysregulation in these affect systems. One possibility is that some behavior problem children may actually feel sadness and anxiety to a lesser degree because they are simply less reactive in these emotion systems, perhaps even biologically less responsive. Among adult antisocial individuals, there is a literature to suggest an underresponsiveness in emotional arousal under conditions in which typical individuals experience heightened tension and anxiety (e.g., Hare, 1975). Another possibility is that certain disruptive children cope with feelings of sadness and anxiety in a different manner than the nonproblem or depressed child. For example, the onset of these feelings may trigger a coping response in which anger replaces sadness and anxiety, or vulnerable feelings are blunted such that a conscious or displayed emotion does not evolve and only indifference is communicated.

Yet another possibility is that certain disruptive children may be highly sensitive within the sadness and fear systems. This sensitivity might promote a tendency to hide or blunt these intense feelings and over time the child may appear indifferent or unaffected in situations that typically elicit some expression of sadness or anxiety. Clinicians often feel that disruptive children's responses to projective stimuli reflect confusion and conflict over feelings of loss and danger. One perspective is that the degree of sadness that the child could possibly feel, given life events and lack of alternative coping, would be akin to despair and that the maintenance of an angry posture may serve as a protection from hopelessness and depression.

Possibly, these emotion systems are also involved in or related to the development of the social emotion of empathy, in which one feels concern and tension when another is in distress. In a recent study we found that sadness was related to reparative attempts in toddlers (Cole, Barrett, & Zahn-Waxler, 1992). Possibly, deviations in the capacity for sadness are associated with the lack of empathy that accompanies antisocial behavior. We know that maltreated preschoolers, who are victims of poorly modulated aggression and anger in the home and who tend to develop disruptive behavior patterns, appear more indifferent to others' distress than nonmaltreated preschoolers (Howes & Eldridge, 1985; Klimes-Dougan & Kistner, 1990; Main & George, 1985), and they may even display anger (and aggression) toward a distressed other (Main & George, 1985). Hence, maltreatment may interfere with the normative empathic response in young children (see Zahn-Waxler & Radke-Yarrow, 1990).

If prolonged expression of sadness and anxiety and anger are all common in the child's presentation, the child is then likely to be classified as having an affective and/or anxiety disorder, due to the sustained display of negative affect, and a disruptive behavior disorder, if the negative affect is accompanied by noncompliance or aggression. But sadness and fear, emotions which are associated with vulnerability rather than power and control, may be masked by certain children who are oppositional and disruptive. If these "vulnerable" emotions are not displayed, it should not be assumed that they are not experienced or operative. We know that as early as three years, typical children show some capacity for minimizing the expression of negative emotions (Cole, 1986). We also know that children, who are the victims of poorly modulated parental anger and aggression, minimize the expression of negative emotions more than other children (Crittenden & DiLalla, 1988; Lynch & Cicchetti, 1991).

(3) Joy, which is typically diminished in depressive disorders, is often atypical in its intensity or situational appropriateness in the disruptive disorders. Joy may be overarousing for some children leading to overexcited activity associated with impulsive actions and inadvertent harm to others' belongings or persons. Some impulsive children may not be intentionally aggressive children although they may present as quick to anger, unable to regulate the intensity of anger, and apt to engage in destructive acts. These same children may also be quick and exuberant in their joy. They may not regulate any affect well but they may not be characterized by chronic negative mood, particularly during early childhood.

Joy, for some children, may be displayed in socially inappropriate circumstances, for example, laughing at another's distress when sadness or concern might be a more normative reaction. Additionally, joy might be displayed during aggressive or antisocial acts, such as taking pleasure in physical aggression, stealing or lying, or disobeying. Joy may also be displayed in concert with defiance and disrespect for authority. That is, joy may be substituted in situations where the more typical affective response would be guilt. Moreover, positive emotions associated with one's self-concept or pride can come to be based on disruptive behavior, a situation Erickson (1963) called "negative identity". That is, children who cannot value themselves because of their conformance with social rules can develop a sense of self or identity that stems from pride in their lack of conformity to the rules (cf. Patterson, 1982).

Emotional Antecedents of Disruptive Behavior Disorders

Thus far, we have argued that: (1) dysregulated affective patterns are associated with chronic disruptive behavior, and (2) these patterns can be understood in terms of anger dysregulation as well as disturbances in other emotion systems. Next we examine the evidence for emotional antecedents of disruptive behavior disorder in early childhood toward the goal of understanding the role of emotion in the development of affective dysregulation and the development of stable disruptive behavior patterns. There are several lines of developmental research that afford a means of examining the emotional correlates and antecedents of disruptive behavior disorders, including research on infant temperament, infant attachment, parenting practices, and exposure to distress.

The role of negative affectivity

Recent adult research has identified *negative affectivity* as a central dimension of individual differences in personality (Tellegen, 1982; Watson & Clark, 1984). A similar conclusion has emerged in infant developmental psychology in research on temperament (Goldsmith & Campos, 1990; Rothbart, 1988). Taken together, it appears that individuals vary in terms of the degree to which they experience distress, and that this trait may involve biological predispositions in regard to emotional reactivity and regulation. Temperament research has further suggested that distress or negative affectivity, at least in early childhood, may involve independent components, e.g., distress due to novelty (e.g., Rothbart, 1988), distress learned from prior fearful experiences (e.g., Bronson & Pankey, 1977), and distress due to restraint or goal frustration (e.g., Lewis, Alessandri, & Sullivan, 1990). Each of these tendencies appear to be stable (Bronson & Pankey, 1977; Kagan, Resnick, & Gibbons, 1989; Stifter & Fox, 1990). While these tendencies may be orthogonal, some children may tend to be reactive under combinations or all of these circumstances.

One hypothesis is that these basic individual differences may be associated with the degree of risk for mental health problems later in life. Moreover, if these distress patterns are distinct, reliable, and stable, they may have implications for different patterns of psychopathology. In the original work conducted by Thomas, Chess, and Birch (1968), infants with a "difficult" temperament were predicted to be more likely to develop behavior problems. Difficultness was then defined as a multidimensional concept including problems in rhythmicity, activity level, and other behaviors as well as emotionality.

Bates and his colleagues have shown that difficult temperament measured at 6 to 24 months predicted symptoms up to 3 to 6 years, and that two separate dimensions of temperament were systematically related to the nature of the symptoms in the preschool years (Bates & Bayles, 1984; Bates, Maslin & Frankel, 1985). Infant reactivity to novelty was related to preschool age internalizing symptoms, and infant resistance to control was related to preschool age externalizing symptoms. Infant difficultness was related to both patterns of symptomatology. The relationship weakened but was still present at age eight (Bates, Bayles, Bennett, Ridge, & Brown, 1991).

Another development in temperament research is the question of whether individual differences might actually reflect differences in patterns of self-regulation of distress, rather than reactivity. Particularly relevant to the development of emotional style and subsequent maladaptive patterns is the suggestion that certain patterns of temperamental negative emotion are associated with an inability to **shift** attention from the source of one's distress (Fox & Marshall, 1991). For example, the highly inhibited, fearful youngster remains vigilant and is less likely to self-distract or to be distracted by others when distressed (Derryberry & Rothbart, 1988; Rothbart, 1988). This regulatory aspect has not been studied in terms of distress due to limitations where an inability to shift attention away from the source of frustration and accept the limits may also be operating. Disruptive children may be particularly reactive to frustration and/or they may have difficulty distracting from anger.

Difficulty regulating fear is typically thought to serve inhibition, and therefore behavioral control, whereas difficulty regulating anger is thought to serve action. Recent longitudinal data suggest some interesting complexities in terms of the relation between infant inhibition and preschool age self-regulated behavior (Calkins, 1991). In a procedure to measure preschool age self-control, four-year-olds were given drawing materials but told they had to wait until the experimenter returned before they could play with them. Calkins found that four-year-olds who were classified as uninhibited as babies tended to have such a short latency to touching the objects that they often did so during the instructions. Four-year-olds who had been classified as inhibited as infants, however, showed restraint and listened compliantly to the instructions *until* the experimenter left and then they more quickly touched the materials, in contrast to control children (neither inhibited nor uninhibited as infants) who showed the most impulse control.

The temperament literature provides an interesting parallel to the child psychopathology literature in terms of the emergence of a dichotomy of problematic conditions. Presently, there is reason to believe that anger-based and fear-based distresses are distinct, and this view is consistent with biologically-oriented research (Gray, 1982, 1987; Henry, 1982) on distinct neurological and biochemical systems for these different emotions. At the same time, there is evidence that the predictive value of infant temperament may wane over time and that the relationship between different aspects of negative affectivity and later self-regulatory behavior may be complex. Temperament may be most important in facilitating our understanding of biological dispositions for displaying distress, both fear and anger, and, perhaps regulating negative affective states.

Temperamental negative affectivity, however, is only one source of influence that can contribute to eventual affect dysregulation and behavioral difficulties. We suspect that chronic negative affectivity is not sustained solely by internal predispositions but requires stimulation and maintenance by environmental demands if it is to develop into dysregulated patterns like those involved in psychopathology. In contributing to the development of child psychopathology, perhaps the most critical influence of temperamental difficulties are their impact on the parent-child relationship (Izard, Haynes, Chisholm, & Baak, 1991; Mangelsdorf, Gunnar, Kestenbaum, Lang, & Andreas, 1990; Miyake, Chen, & Campos, 1985). Infant negative emotionality is a litmus test for parental foibles, exacerbating the stress the family system undergoes with the accommodation of a new member and the feelings of insecurity and doubt that accompany the infinite decisions parents make about how to provide adequate care for their infant (see Dix, 1991). We now consider other emotional influences that contribute to difficulty regulating affect, negotiating control, and developing well-regulated social behavior. We begin with one of the earliest socioemotional events in childhood, the attachment relationship, and the role of insecure attachment in the development of disruptive behavior.

The role of insecure attachment

Attachment theory (Ainsworth, 1979; Bowlby, 1973; 1982; 1988) has yielded over a decade of substantive research. Insecurity in one's initial attachment relationship is thought to contribute to the risk for mental health problems. Bowlby suggested that different types of insecure mother-infant attachment could lead to different forms of psychopathology, with anxious resistant attachment being aligned with depression and anxiety disorders, and anxious avoidant attachment with personality disorders, including antisocial personality. In Bowlby's thinking, the attachment relationship serves as a rudder through the subsequent interactions and stresses that the individual experiences. The anxious resistant infant expresses its distress with its parent during separation and is less responsive to soothing. The anxious avoidant infant appears to distrust the responsiveness of the parent to child distress, fearing being rebuffed, and so avoids potential disappointment and frustration by being more emotionally "independent."

Attachment theory related research has indicated that infants who are securely attached to their mothers, as inferred from the Strange Situation procedure (Ainsworth, Blehar, Waters, & Wall, 1978), are more ego resilient, sociable and socially competent in early childhood (LaFreniere & Sroufe, 1985; Matas, Arend, & Sroufe, 1978; Park & Waters, 1989; Pastor, 1981; Sroufe, Fox, & Pancake, 1983; Waters, Wippman, & Sroufe, 1979). Insecurity of attachment has been linked to later problem behavior as measured by self-report, observations, and ratings (Cohn, 1990; Fagot & Kavanaugh, 1990; Sroufe, 1983). These findings support the theoretical position that insecure attachment creates risk for children, particularly in the areas of social competence and self-control (e.g., peer rejection, aggressivity, behavior problems, and poor social competence).

Do individual differences in early attachment patterns predict and discriminate types of problem behavior? Avoidantly attached infants, who seem to prefer to depend on themselves rather than seek emotional support from their caregivers, appear to be more emotionally demanding of others, antisocial, aggressive, and hostile (Fagot & Kavanagh, 1990; Sroufe, 1983). Infants with a resistant attachment, however, are also perceived as emotionally demanding, more easily frustrated and impulsive (Sroufe, 1983), although they are more tense than hostile. On the basis of limited research, insecurity of attachment relates to problem behavior in preschoolers but not specifically to an externalizing or internalizing pattern.

In a sample of preschool age children being evaluated in a clinic for externalizing problems, there was a threefold increase in the likelihood of an insecure concurrent attachment, particularly for boys (Speltz, Greenberg, & Deklyen, 1990). Also, infant attachment has predicted internalizing and externalizing behavior problems in preschool (Erickson, Sroufe, & Egeland, 1985) and first grade children (Lewis, Feiring, McGuffog, & Jaskir, 1984). Other studies have yielded less clearcut findings, suggesting that the prediction of specific problem patterns as a function of infant attachment has not been reliably achieved (Bates et al., 1985; Bates & Bayles, 1980, see also Sroufe, 1983).

Attachment seems important in our understanding of (a) the development of an internal sense of security and (b) the development of flexible control. Secure infant attachment seems to predict more harmonious, emotionally positive interactions between mother and toddlers during autonomy and control sequences (Bates et al., 1985; Londerville & Main, 1981; Main & Weston, 1981). Insecure infants appear to develop more resistance to control and more conflictual interactions emerge. In fact, in the Speltz et al. (1990) study, the most common insecure attachment classification for disruptive preschoolers was "insecure-controlling" in which the child behaved angrily or hostilely when the parent returned, ordering the parent to leave or to follow the child's instruction.

In the early years, the insecurity of attachment may be sustained and replayed in the parent-child relationship, and if the family situation is unfavorable or unchanging, the pattern of resistance and negativity may become entrenched. If the child then enters the world beyond the family with this set of experiences and expectations, these are likely to contribute to the child's continuing pattern of social problems, and to the development of beliefs about the social self that have a self-fulfilling influence. If the family situation worsens, and there are no extrafamilial influences that modify the pattern that the child is internalizing, then the path between insecure attachment and later psychopathology may be easier to trace.

Attachment may not be directly predictive of specific forms of psychopathology. Sroufe (1983) suggests that control issues and interpersonal negativity will be present in the later relationships of both types of insecurely attached children but that they will be manifested differently. If we can extrapolate from his suggestion to psychopathological behavior, a young adolescent with conduct disorder who is resistantly attached may misbehave in ways that draw the parent in (e.g., leaving evidence of rule violations like smoking or drinking), whereas the adolescent with conduct disorder who is avoidantly attached may misbehave and the parent may be unaware of the misbehavior. It remains to be seen whether failures in attachment differentiate the undersocialized and socialized conduct disorder types, as they theoretically should. If this is true, then attachment history may predict the likelihood of distress being communicated to others rather than the specific type of distress. Attachment appears to affect the child's manner of relationship; each type of insecure attachment may lead to different manifestations of problem behavior whether that behavior be predominantly depressive, aggressive or both. Future research should clarify the contribution of attachment to later psychopathology, hopefully with attention to both child and parent influences. Several tentative conclusions are possible. First, a tendency toward negative emotional reactions coupled with a parent who lacks the maturity or creativity to adapt to the unique needs of an emotionally demanding child, can evolve into a stable pattern of insecurity and resistance to control. Even without a predisposition toward negativity, failures in the emotional connectedness between parent and child can foster insecurity and risk for mental health problems.

Second, an impairment in the emotional bond between parent and child, when associated with interactions dominated by control issues, is a foundation for the creation and sustainment of lack of parental involvement, supervision, and acceptance. These gaps in emotional availability contribute to inconsistency and harshness in control interactions, and contribute to the child's behavioral choices about limit-testing and rule violations (cf. Patterson, 1982). At the same time this affects the sense of self that children who emerge from the first few years with a history of emotional dissatisfaction, insecurity, and power struggles develop (Cicchetti & Schneider-Rosen, 1986; Coopersmith, 1967; Schneider-Rosen & Cicchetti, 1991). It is understandable that some children would develop an arrogant sense of self, one that even they might construe as false, while some children might develop a sense of inefficacy immediately. Either child is primed for impulse control problems later in life, whether those be flaunted in the face of authority or more passively and discreetly executed. Either child is also primed for a profound lack of a sense of self as lovable or worthwhile, as well as for a lifetime of problems with self-esteem and identity.

The role of emotion in parenting practices

The childrearing patterns associated with disruptive behavior and compliant behavior are one of the few areas of research pertaining to developmental psychopathology that has a relatively long history of research and a substantive corpus of studies. In general, research on typical and atypical (conduct disordered, delinquent, ADD) children, has identified two main components of childrearing: parental control and parental warmth (see Hetherington & Martin, 1986; Loeber & Stouthamer-Loeber, 1986; Maccoby & Martin, 1983; Parke & Slaby, 1983; and Patterson, 1982 for reviews). A general view emerges that having a loving, involved, reasonable and consistent disciplinarian for a parent is associated with child competence. Child externalizing problems have been linked with a variety of negative child-rearing attitudes and activities such as parental rejection, inconsistent discipline, rigid control, harsh criticism, and lack of involvement or supervision. Parental control practices are an obvious starting point for examining parental contributions when one is interested in predicting behavior problems that are conceptualized as under- or overcontrolled. We know from research that the nature of control issues in the family is important but complex. Inept, inconsistent and lax control have been associated with disruptive, antisocial behavior (e.g., McCord, 1979; Olweus, 1980; Pulkinnen, 1983; Schmaling & Patterson, 1984; West & Farrington, 1973), and several studies (e.g., Baumrind, 1967, 1971; Block, 1971; Hetherington, Stouwie, & Ridberg, 1971; West & Farrington, 1973) indicate that overcontrolling, rigid parenting (e.g., intrusiveness, overinvolvement, coerciveness) is also associated with misconduct. Therefore, extremes in either direction (permissiveness vs. authoritarian control, lack of involvement vs. intrusiveness) are associated with child maladaptation. However, these parental behaviors are not necessarily precursors of problem behavior; they may well be correlates or effects of problem child behavior and contribute to the *maintenance* of disruptiveness.

We suspect that negative emotional qualities often precede or accompany the development of these types of parent-child interactions. Interestingly, Loeber and Stouthamer-Loeber's (1986) meta-analysis of research investigating family variables that correlate or predict conduct disorders and delinquency suggests that parental warmth factors are more predictive than parental control factors. They indicate that factors that involve a dearth of overall emotional investment of the parent in the child's life — lack of supervision (monitoring), lack of parent-child involvement, and parental rejection — have the most robust predictive power across studies. Discipline and control strategies are not as predictive. We interpret this as saying, not that discipline and control are unimportant in contributing to child social development, but that the basic emotional quality of the relationship is most important. The efficacy of discipline and control strategies may be predicated on the strength of the emotional relationship — trust, involvement, enjoyment.

Most children go through periods of heightened noncompliance and limit-testing, particularly during the third and fourth years. Individual differences in parenting practices during these years may contribute to the development of chronically problematic behavior. Prospective research (e.g., Baumrind, 1971; Zahn-Waxler, Iannotti, Cummings, & Denham, 1990) indicates that there are problematic control styles in very early childhood that precede and predict symptomatic problem behavior. One prospective study finds that internalizing and externalizing scores are higher at age 5 when mothers engage in more commands at age 2; the contribution of these maternal strategies holds even when compliance at age 2 is controlled (Kuczynski & Kochanska, 1990). Studies of the childrearing practices of parents of ADD children have not separated child and parent effects, but they show a tendency for parents of

ADD children to be more intrusive and interfering (Cohen, Sullivan, Minde, Novak, & Keens, 1983; Jacobvitz & Sroufe, 1987). The Jacobvitz and Sroufe study found that maternal intrusiveness during infancy was related to kindergarten hyperactivity. These studies do not rule out child characteristics that may elicit more parental activity, but they (a) suggest that problematic patterns can begin very early in the parent-child interaction, and (b) underscore that parental influences are powerful even in the face of individual child variation.

What is not known is the role of emotion in the course of these numerous exchanges, and how each party regulates the emotions that accompany them. Feelings of parental inefficacy (Bugental, 1985) and anger at the hard-to-manage child, and child frustration and feelings of failure in the parent-child relationship, repeated frequently over the first five years clearly pave a foundation for later child psychopathology, and well-rehearsed, easily triggered hostile confrontations.

The most detailed investigation of such automatized control interactions has been conducted by Patterson (1982). He describes the "coercive cycle", an insidious point-counterpoint of control efforts by parents and resistance by children that escalates in intensity and resistance, and is ineffective in reaching mutually satisfying solutions. The parent issues a command, the child refuses, the parent reiterates the command while becoming angrier, the child becomes more hostile and resistant, and the outcomes are either irresolvable or abusive.

The emotional tone of these control interactions is generally typified as angry; although Patterson has illustrated a powerful interactional mechanism by which disruptive, antisocial behavior is maintained, he also points out that this failure in the parent-child relationship promotes child depression (Patterson, et al., 1989). Although children react by displaying their own anger through defiance, rudeness, and misbehavior, over time they can come to feel devalued, ineffective and helpless. This condition sets the stage for either fending off or dwelling upon negative emotions and thoughts, patterns that are associated with depression. In clinical work, when parents are insisting that a child must change, they often do not realize that the problem is not merely a battle of wills, but that the child feels helpless and hopeless about how to change. The child perceives the parent as powerful (even if the parent does not), and it may be particularly frightening to realize that the parent is helpless to resolve the conflict between them (Fraiberg, 1959).

Analyzing the role of emotional tone in the development of particular parent-child socializing interactions will be complex. We suggest that it will not be a simple matter of the presence/absence of negative affect. Rather, it will be a matter of the contextual gestalt in which parental negative affect is communicated. It may be that effective parenting involves (a) a larger context of a positive emotional relationship, and (b) clear and reasonably well-regulated communication of felt anger. The contextual nature of the emotional tone of parenting is complicated and requires extensive research.

Consider, for example, data that suggest that the emotional tone in which commands and reprimands are delivered is important. A cajoling request or a gentle reprimand, each of which includes some degree of positive affect, can be ineffectual (Bugental, 1985; Pfiffner & O'Leary, 1989). This suggests that anger has a constructive role. We know, however, from the physical abuse literature that poorly modulated anger and aggression directed at children increase the likelihood of disruptive, aggressive, impulsive, oppositional behavior in those children (e.g., Egeland & Sroufe, 1981; Lahey, Conger, Atkeson, & Treiber, 1984; Trickett & Kuczynski, 1986). These child behaviors are paralleled by parenting practices that include parental feelings of anger and disgust in relation to discipline and generally negative feelings about self and others (e.g., Brunquell, Crichton, & Egeland, 1981; Pianta, Egeland, & Erickson, 1989; Trickett & Kuczynski, 1986).

Another important consideration is raised by the fact that not all difficult infants and hard-to-manage toddlers and preschoolers develop mental health problems. This suggests to us the importance of examining the positive attempts of parents in negotiating control with their children. We use the term, *proactive parenting*, to describe such efforts — attempts to anticipate potential problems, to structure situations to minimize conflict and to promote compliance without sacrificing child autonomy, to educate and promote internal control in the child (Pettit & Bates, 1989). Proactive parenting relates to the dimension of control but also includes the emotional availability between parent and child. To be creative in tailoring control or influence strategies, it is very helpful to feel relatively calm or positive and to be empathic with the child, understanding the child's emotional and cognitive state (Dix, 1991). We assume that such general emotional strength and balance is difficult if a parent is isolated and alone in their parenting, and that the support of the larger network of spouse, extended family members, friends, and neighbors is important (see also Coyne, Downey, & Boergers, this volume). Proactive parenting has been associated with social competence in young children (Pettit & Bates, 1989). Proactive parenting has been linked to decrements in behavior problems during the preschool years in longitudinal research. Mothers who anticipated the child's needs, exerted modulated control, and provided structure and organization during their toddlers' peer play, had children who showed decreases in externalizing symptoms across a three year period (Zahn-Waxler et al., 1990).

The role of exposure to distress

It is well-documented that exposure to distress is emotionally troubling to children and is associated with the development of mental health problems in some children. That is, it is not only direct child interaction that is important but also the overall emotional climate in which development takes place. The literatures on the effects of divorce (Emery, 1982; Hetherington, Cox, & Cox, 1982; Wallerstein, 1983), and of spousal abuse and marital conflict (Gottman

& Fainsilber Katz, 1989; Grych & Fincham, 1990; O'Leary & Emery, 1984) all indicate that these familial environments are emotionally challenging to children of all ages and types, and that they include a heightened risk of disruptive and depressive symptoms. Careful observational research suggests that exposure to angry conflict is emotionally arousing for children and can be followed by an increase in disruptive behavior (Cummings & Davies, this volume; Cummings, Iannotti, & Zahn-Waxler, 1985; Cummings, Zahn-Waxler, & Radke-Yarrow, 1981; El-Sheikh, Cummings, & Goetsch, 1989).

Children look to the family environment for a haven from the challenges of the world outside the home and as a social mirror of affirmation and value during the doubts and developments of childhood. Exposure to distress within the home disturbs the child at a very fundamental level, and increases negative affect and the likelihood of disruptive behavior. It is sometimes thought that disruptive behavior in this context is a regulatory strategy that pulls for the distressed parent to organize himself or herself and to resume control by responding to child misbehavior. A failure to do so represents a deviation in the socialization process and may interfere with or challenge the working model of a secure attachment. Young children exposed to very brief angry conflicts report feeling angry, as one might expect, but some also report feeling sad during those conflicts (Cummings, Ballard, El-Sheikh, & Lake, 1991). This suggests not a mere contagion effect of background anger but a psychological interpretation of the background as it relates to the child and, perhaps, a sense of loss and/or helplessness. It has been thought that the undersocialized conduct disorder child represents such a failure in attachment or early exposure to familial dysfunction. A recent study with mothers of incarcerated youth found that undersocialized conduct disordered youth had experienced significantly more stressful events during the first four years of their lives than socialized conduct disordered youth (Deutsch & Erickson, 1989). The authors report that interruptions in physical contact between parent and child during those early years and events that interfere with parental emotional availability may account for the findings.

A typically developing child with no particular predisposing vulnerabilities will find familial distress challenging. What leads to this challenge transforming into symptomatology? Various authors have discussed the importance of identifying protective factors (e.g., Cicchetti & Rizley, 1981; Garmezy & Rutter, 1983). We assume that the critical ingredient of any protective factor is its ability to provide some plausible, stable relief from chronic negative emotional conditions. The background anger research suggests that children feel relief when angry conflicts are resolved (Cummings et al., 1991). If a child cannot find sufficient relief, internally or externally, then the risk for psychopathology increases. We know from research on child sexual abuse that children exposed to overwhelming distress will dissociate or deny emotional events (Adams-Tucker, 1985; Putnam & Trickett, 1991) and that the development of such a coping style can have serious implications for later psychopathology (Cole & Putnam, 1992). If a child has been developing typical appropriate self-regulatory skills (delay of gratification, planful problem-solving, impulse control) prior to the onset of exposure to distress, we expect that these self-same skills can contribute to the development of internalizing symptoms (worry, reflection on self's unworthiness or inefficacy, belief that one's actions are futile).

Coping with an emotionally disordered parent. In general, emotional disorder in a parent influences childrearing practices in a negative way and creates a distressing familial climate, thereby creating risk for child maladjustment (Maccoby & Martin, 1983; Richman, Stevenson, & Graham, 1982; Rutter, 1966; Rutter & Quinton, 1984). We know that emotionally dysfunctional parents are more likely to be harsh and critical, to have difficulty in control exchanges, and that there is a greater likelihood of child misconduct in such families. In this section, we consider the presence of an emotionally dysfunctional adult in the home, a condition that is associated with a variety of unfavorable conditions, including separations from parents, financial distress, marital discord and disruption, and isolation from larger social networks.

Two studies examine the early childhood development of symptomatology and the role of the child's exposure to maternal depression and life stresses in the stability of problematic behavior. Zahn-Waxler et al. (1990) explored the role of maternal depression in the development of aggressivity, particularly hostile, dysregulated aggression, occurring between ages 2 and 5. They observed toddlers under challenging, sometimes stressful, conditions, and administered behavior checklists when the children were age five. The significant relationship between early dysregulated aggression and symptomatology at age 5 was particularly strong for offspring of depressed mothers. This relationship held for externalizing symptoms on behavioral checklists at age 5, and to a lesser degree internalizing symptoms. Rose et al. (1989) reported a similar pattern of stability for externalizing symptoms between age 2 and age 5, with strong correlations with maternal depression and life stresses, and with age two externalizing scores being correlated with later internalizing symptoms as well.

While some children may be predisposed to be negatively reactive to the changes associated with distress in the home, any child can become emotionally overwhelmed by a dysfunctional parent. Children who are generally sociable and who try to cope positively with problems are at risk, too, particularly for becoming overinvolved with parental distress. This pattern has been described as enmeshment, co-dependency or overfunctioning in the clinical literature, particularly the literature addressing adult children of emotionally disordered individuals, such as alcoholic, incestuous, depressed and personality disordered parents. Research on the development of empathy and guilt in risk and nonrisk children, where risk is defined by mother's depression, suggests that these are meaningful constructs, that the natural tendency to care for others and to feel responsible for their well-being can be suppressed or overdeveloped in some children (Zahn-Waxler, Cole, & Barrett, 1991; Zahn-Waxler, Kochanska, Krupnick, & McKnew, 1990).

In Zahn-Waxler and colleagues' naturalistic and experimental studies of the early development and socialization of empathic concern for others, they have shown that emotional arousal may be an important part of the development of empathy and guilt. Very young children show a range of emotional reactions in response to another's (simulated) distress: surprise, fear and wariness, concern and sadness, anger, interest, and amusement. By the end of the first year, most children show comfort to another person crying or in pain through simple physical gestures (touching, patting, hugging), and make an effort to comprehend what is going on. Children help, share, sympathize and comfort victims in distress, both when they cause others' distress and when they witness it (Zahn-Waxler, Radke-Yarrow, Chapman, & Wagner, 1992). Also, toddlers from homes with high parental conflict become angry and distressed during these episodes, and they intervene more than children from low conflict homes in efforts to get parents to stop, to comfort one of them, or to get them to make up (Cummings, Zahn-Waxler, & Radke-Yarrow, 1981). Thus, children as young as two begin to play the role of mediator or peacemaker.

This early capacity to care for others and to care about the consequences of one's actions is a landmark developmental step of major adaptive significance. When children help or comfort someone they have harmed, their acts have a reparative function and are part of the development of conscience and guilt. If similar acts are performed when children observe another's distress, the behaviors are interpreted as altruism or empathy. Early childhood then is also a time when emergent empathy and guilt patterns are vulnerable to becoming confused, as children's attributions of responsibility and causality are not necessarily accurate. Certain conditions in the family environment may encourage maladaptive patterns, in which either heightened or diminished empathy and guilt are fostered (Zahn-Waxler & Kochanska, 1990; Zahn-Waxler & Radke-Yarrow, 1990).

The literature on the offspring of dysfunctional mothers indicates that their offspring are at risk for both internalizing and externalizing problems, although we do not know why different children develop different kinds of problems. Rutter and Quinton (1984) suggested that exposure to hostile behavior was more important in accounting for child maladjustment than parental diagnosis. Research on the offspring of depressed parents has revealed a higher rate of both internalizing and externalizing symptoms in offspring, and similar patterns exist for children of abusive parents (Aber, Allen, Carlson, & Cicchetti, 1989).

Goodman and her colleagues (Goodman, Lynch, Brogan, & Fielding, in press) provide an interesting emotion regulation perspective to explain why children of depressed parents are at increased risk for both internalizing *and* externalizing problems. Children of depressed mothers may alternate between being withdrawn or compliant and aggressive in either systematic or random efforts to gain attention from an otherwise unavailable, inattentive or self-absorbed mother. Research on interactions of infants with their depressed mothers indicates that they become both withdrawn and distressed *and* more fussy, providing some support for the notion of shifting patterns of emotionality within individuals (e.g., Field, 1984).

On the other hand, another way to cope with the distress of a parent who fails to respond as expected, and who may anger the child by frustrating their goals for autonomy and harmony, is to be dismissive. As we know, this pattern is seen in some insecure infant attachments and is also believed to be one classification for adult internal working models for relationships (Main & Goldwyn, 1984). This trajectory has not been fully studied but we speculate that such a dismissive pattern early in life may interfere with the ability to be sensitive to others' emotions, and therefore to engage in acts that do not take into account the pain or inconvenience of others (e.g., George & Main, 1985; Troy & Sroufe, 1987). Patterns of excessive and diminished sense of responsibility, empathy and guilt are features of both depressive and aggressive disorders.

These data indicate that early difficulties in socioemotional development, particularly in a family environment where there may be difficulties that promote, or fail to respond effectively to, child disruptiveness, may set the stage for the development of stable patterns of symptomatology and the development of both disruptive and affective clinical conditions.

Summary and Conclusions

Disruptive behavior disorders have concomitant patterns that indicate the development of atypical regulation of anger, and the development of atypical patterns in the other affect systems (sadness, fear, and joy). Furthermore, disruptive behavior which distresses parents and teachers is associated with personal distress, including major depressive episodes, dysthymic disorder, anxiety disorder, and suicidality. Many different studies suggest that anger and sadness are both activated in the coping response. Both at the psychological and physiological level, the different patterns of response to emotional challenges may be separate but not mutually exclusive. There are separate and specific neurophysiological pathways that support a finite range of reactions to stressful events, and there is a dynamic but poorly understood relationship between the different emotions. It is likely that individuals vary within each of these systems and that it is possible for there to be symptomatic behavior in either or both systems. The polarized depictions of the antisocial person's angry, uncaring action against the world and the depressed individual's sad surrender to events now appear more as stereotypes than truths. In our present thinking, it is not a matter of one or the other system becoming dysregulated. Rather, we think that both anger and sadness are dysregulated in both disruptive and depressive disorders. The task ahead is to understand the transactional process by which individual differences in the child's biological dispositions and in the child's emotional experience come to lead to specific symptom presentations.

Personality research, both adult and child, indicates that negative affectivity is a core, stable dimension of personality, but we do not know how reactivity or difficulty regulating one negative affect system relates to or influences other affect systems. The implication is, however, that there may be varying patterns that contribute to the evolution of particular forms of psychopathology. A tendency to experience aversive negative states when linked with inhibition would suggest a potential path toward internalizing patterns, inhibition under certain social conditions, and difficulty with self-regulation of distress and behavior. The implications of a tendency toward distress due to limitations, its possible link with later noncompliant or aggressive behavior and potential for externalizing patterns merits study. For example, it is necessary to understand how individual variation in infant distress due to novelty and limitations influences (a) the amount of exposure to such distressing stimuli children receive, (b) individual differences in parental affect and practices, and (c) exploration beyond the family, particularly social exchange with peers and siblings. Temperament may be a construct that captures biologically predisposed tendencies to experience certain negative emotions and tendencies to have difficulty with self-regulation of these emotions.

Obviously, temperament alone is insufficient. Emotional distress and difficulty in one's environment and one's relationships in the early childhood years is an important influence in the development of childhood and adult psychopathology. We suggest that the negotiation of the parent-child relationship during the first five years, particularly in terms of affect-laden exchanges, is an important component of the predictive equation. The quality of attachment appears to have important implications for how a child will relate to others particularly in terms of sense of well-being and negotiation of control. The establishment of a secure base, in which parental control and discipline practices are embedded, diminishes the likelihood of later psychopathology. Emotional distress in the household (such as marital conflict, parental psychopathology), however, can tax the emotional and behavioral regulation of any child, exacerbating the already problematic child's behavior, and creating risk for the well-regulated child's further development.

In using emotional development as a model for charting trajectories toward disruptive and depressive disorders, we believe it is particularly valuable to consider the adaptive functions of the range of different emotions, their implications for how the stressed child is coping at any given point in time, and how these interact with environmental influences to contribute to the transactional process by which individual events are transformed into belief systems, coping styles, and chronic problems. It may be that in early childhood these seemingly separate paths are not so markedly differentiated and that children who are vulnerable or in distress may move more fluidly

between styles of coping than adults do. It appears, however, that an important part of the development of personality is the consolidation or constraint
of emotional style (Malatesta & Wilson, 1988).
Like the proverbial seekers of truth, we have apprehended the limbs of the
elephant but have not yet scientifically understood the larger dynamic, or-
ganic process of the development of psychopathology. Current research suggests many interesting risk conditions but the transactional process by which
such conditions emerge into specific, stable forms of coping and psychopathology remains to be revealed (Cicchetti & Aber, 1986). By examining
emotion-related phenomena in early childhood, we feel that the relationship
between depression and antisocial, disruptive behavior will be clarified.

REFERENCES

Aber, L., Allen, J., Carlson, V,. & Cicchetti, D. (1989). The effects of maltreatment on
development during early childhood: recent studies and their theoretical, clinical, and
policy implications. In D. Cicchetti & Carlson (eds.), *Child maltreatment* (pp. 579–
619). Cambridge: Cambridge University Press.
Achenbach, T. M., Conners, C. K., Quay, H. C., Verhulst, F. C., & Howell, C. T. (1989).
Replication of empirically derived syndroms as a basis for taxonomy of child/adoles-
cent psychopathology. *Journal of Abnormal Child Psychology, 17,* 299–323.
Achenbach, T. M., & Edelbrock, C. S. (1978). The classification of child psychopathology: A review and analysis of empirical efforts. *Psychological Bulletin, 85,* 1275–
1301.
Achenbach, T. M., & Edelbrock, C. S. (1983). *Manual for the child behavior checklist and
revised child behavior profile.* Burlington, VT: Department of Psychiatry, University of
Vermont.
Achenbach, T. M., Howell, C. T., Quay, H. C., & Conners, C. K. (1991). National
survey of problems and competencies among four- to sixteen-year-olds. *Monographs of
the Society for Research in Child Development* (Serial No. 225, Vol. 56).
Adams-Tucker, C. (1985). Defense mechanisms used by sexually abused children. *Child-
ren Today, 14,* 8–12.
Ainsworth, M. D. S. (1979). Mother-infant attachment. *American Psychologist, 34,* 932–
937.
Ainsworth, M. D. S., Blehar, M. C., Waters, E., & Wall, S. (1978). *Patterns of attachment:
A psychological study of the strange situation.* Hillsdale, New Jersey: Erlbaum.
Altmann, E. O., & Gotlib, I. H. (1988). The social behavior of depressed children: An
observational study. *Journal of Abnormal Child Psychology, 16,* 29–44.
American Psychiatric Association. (1987). *Diagnostic and Statistical Manual-III-Revised.*
Washington, D. C.: American Psychiatric Press.
Anderson, J. C., Williams, S., McGee, R., & Silva, P. A. (1987). DSM-III disorders in
preadolescent children: Prevalence in a large sample from the general population.
Archives of General Psychiatry, 44, 69–76.
Bakwin, H. (1972). Depression — A mood disorder in children and adolescence.
Maryland State Medical Journal, 55–61.

Barkley, R. A. (1990). *Attention deficit hyperactivity disorder: A handbook for diagnosis and treatment.* New York: Guilford.

Barkley, R. A., DuPaul, G. J., & McMurray, M. B. (1990). Comprehensive evaluation of attention deficit disorder with and without hyperactivity as defined by research criteria. *Journal of Consulting and Clinical Psychology, 58,* 775–789.

Bates, J. E., & Bayles, K. (1988). Attachment and the development of behavior problems. In J. Belsky & T. Nezworski (eds.), *Clinical implications of attachment* (pp. 235–239). Hillsdale, N.J.: Erlbaum.

Bates, J. E., Maslin, C. A., & Frankel, K. A. (1985). Attachment security, mother-child interaction, and temperament as predictors of behavior-problem ratings at age three years. In I. Bretherton & E. Waters (eds.), *Growing points of attachment theory and research. Monographs of the Society for Child Development,* (Serial Number 209), *50,* 167–193.

Bates, J. E., Bayles, K., Bennett, D. S., Ridge, B., & Brown, M. M. (1991). Origins of externalizing behavior problems at eight years of age. In D. Pepler & K. Rubin (eds.), *The development and treatment of childhood aggression* (pp. 93–120). Hillsdale, NJ: Erlbaum.

Baumrind, D. (1967). Child care practices anteceding three patterns of preschool behavior. *Genetic Psychology Monographs, 75,* 43–88.

Baumrind, D. (1971). Current patterns of parental authority. *Developmental Psychology Monographs, 4* (1, Pt. 2).

Berry, C. A., Shaywitz, S. E., & Shaywitz, B. A. (1985). Girls with attention deficit disorder: A silent minority? A report on behavioral and cognitive characteristics. *Pediatrics, 76,* 801–809.

Biederman, J., Munir, K., & Knee, D. (1987). Conduct and oppositional disorder in clinically referred children with attention deficit disorder: A controlled family study. *Journal of the American Academy of Child and Adolescent Psychiatry, 26,* 724–727.

Block, J. (1971). *Lives through time.* Berkeley, CA: Bancroft Books.

Bowlby, J. (1973). *Attachment and loss.* (Vol II) *Separation: anxiety and anger.* New York: Basic.

Bowlby, J. (1982). *Attachment and loss.* (Vol I) *Attachment* (2nd ed.) New York: Basic.

Bowlby, J. (1988). Developmental psychiatry comes of age. *The American Journal of Psychiatry, 145,* 1–10.

Bronson, G. W., & Pankey, W. B. (1977). On the distinction between fear and wariness. *Child Development, 48,* 1167–1183.

Brunquell, D., Crichton, L., & Egeland, B. (1981). Maternal personality and attitude in disturbances of child-rearing. *American Journal of Orthopsychiatry, 51,* 680–691.

Bugental, D. B. (1985). Unresponsive children and powerless adults: Cocreators of affectively uncertain caregiving environments. In M. Lewis & C. Saarni (eds.), *The socialization of emotion* (pp. 239–261). New York: Plenum.

Campbell, S., Breaux, A. M., Ewing, L., & Szumowski, E. (1984). A one-year follow-up study of parent-referred hyperactive preschool children. *Journal of the American Academmy of Child Psychiatry, 27,* 243–249.

Campos, J., & Barrett, K. C. (1984). Toward a new understanding of emotions and their development. In C. Izard, J. Kagan, & R. Zajonc (eds.), *Emotions, cognitions, and behavior* (pp. 229–263). New York: Cambridge University Press.

Carlson, G., & Cantwell, D. (1980). Unmasking masked depression in children and adolescents. *American Journal of Psychiatry, 137,* 445–449.

Calkins, S. (1991, March). *Temperament, attachment and self-regulation: A longitudinal perspective.* Paper presented at Conference on Research Issues in the Development of Emotion Regulation, Washington, D. C.

Cerreto, M., & Tuma, J. (1977). Distribution of DSM-II diagnoses in a child psychiatric setting. *Journal of Abnormal Child Psychology, 5,* 147–155.

Chamberlin, R. W. (1981). The relationship of preschool behavior learning patterns to later school functioning. In B. W. Camp (ed.), *Advances in behavioral pediatrics* (Vol 2, pp. 111–127). Greenwich, CT: JAI Press.

Cicchetti, D. & Aber, J. L. (1986). Early precursors to later depression: An organizational perspective. In L. Lipsitt & C. Rovee-Collier (eds.), *Advances in infancy, Volume 4* (pp. 87–137). Norwood, New Jersey: Ablex.

Cicchetti, D., Ganiban, J., & Barnett, D. (1991). Contributions from the study of high-risk populations to understanding the development of emotion regulation. In J. Garber & K. Dodge (eds.), *The development of emotion regulation and dysregulation* (pp. 15–48). New York: Cambridge University Press.

Cicchetti, D., & Rizley, R. (1981). Developmental perspectives on the etiology, intergenerational transmission and sequelae of child maltreatment. *New Directions in Child Development, 11*, 32–59.

Cicchetti, D., & Schneider-Rosen, K. (1986). An organizational approach to childhood depression. In M. Rutter, C. E. Izard, & P. Read (eds.), *Depression in young people: Clinical and developmental perspectives* (pp. 71–134). New York: Guilford Press.

Cohen, N. J., Sullivan, J., Minde, K., Novak, C., & Keens, S. (1983). Mother-child interaction in hyperactive and normal kindergarten-aged children and the effect of treatment. *Child Psychiatry and Human Development, 13*, 213–224.

Cohn, D. A. (1990). Child-mother attachment of six-year-olds and social competence at school. *Child Development, 61*, 152–162.

Cole, D. A., & Carpentieri, S. (1990). Social status and the comorbidity of child depression and conduct disorder. *Journal of Consulting and Clinical Psychology, 58*, 748–757.

Cole, P. M. (1986). Children's spontaneous expressive control of facial expression. *Child Development, 57*, 1309–1321.

Cole, P. M., Barrett, K. C., & Zahn-Waxler, C. (1992). Emotional displays in toddlers during mishaps. *Child Development, 63*, 314–324.

Cole, P. M., & Putnam, F. W. (1992). The effect of incest on self and social functioning: A developmental psychopathology perspective. *Journal of Consulting and Clinical Psychology, 60*, 174–184.

Coopersmith, S. (1967). *The antecedents of self-esteem.* San Francisco: W. H. Freeman.

Crittenden, P. M., & DiLalla, D. L. (1988). Compulsive compliance: The development of an inhibitory coping strategy in infancy. *Journal of Abnormal Child Psychology, 16*, 585–599.

Cummings, E. M., Ballard, M., El-Sheikh, M., & Lake, M. (1991). Resolution and children's responses to interadult anger. *Developmental Psychology, 27*, 462–470.

Cummings, E. M., Iannotti, R. J., & Zahn-Waxler, C. (1985). The influence of conflict between adults on the emotions and aggression of young children. *Developmental Psychology, 21*, 495–507.

Cummings, E. M., Zahn-Waxler, C., & Radke-Yarrow, M. (1981). Young children's responses to expressions of anger and affection by others in the family. *Child Development, 52*, 1274–1282.

Cytryn, L., & McKnew, D. H. (1972). Proposed classification of childhood depression. *American Journal of Psychiatry, 129*, 149–155.

Derryberry, D., & Rothbart, M. K. (1988). Arousal, affect and attention as components of temperament. *Journal of Personality and Social Psychology, 55*, 958–966.

Deutsch, L. J., & Erickson, M. T. (1989). Early life events as discriminators of socialized and undersocialized delinquents. *Journal of Abnormal Child Psychology, 17*, 541–551.

Dix, T. (1991). The affective organization of parenting: Adaptive and maladaptive processes. *Psychological Bulletin, 110*, 3–25.

Edelbrock, C., Costello, A., & Kessler, M. D. (1984). Empirical corroboration of attention deficit disorder. *Journal of the American Academy of Child Psychiatry, 23*, 285–290.

Egeland, B., & Sroufe, L. A. (1981). Attachment and early maltreatment. *Child Development, 52*, 44–52.

El-Sheikh, M., Cummings, E. M., & Goetsch, V. (1989). Coping with adults' angry behavior: Behavioral, physiological, and verbal responding in preschoolers. *Developmental Psychology, 25*, 490–498.

Emery, R. E. (1982). Interparent conflict and the children of discord and divorce. *Psychological Bulletin, 92*, 310–330.

Erickson, E. H. (1963). *Childhood and society*. New York: Norton.

Erickson, M. F., Sroufe, L. A., & Egeland, B. (1985). The relationship between quality of attachment and behavior problems in a high-risk sample. In I. Bretherton & E. Waters (eds.), *Growing points of attachment theory and research. Monographs of the Society for Child Development, 50* (1–2, Serial No. 209), pp. 147–166.

Fagot, B. I., & Kavanagh, K. (1990). The prediction of antisocial behavior from avoidant attachment classification. *Child Development, 61*, 864–873.

Farrington, D. P., Loeber, R., & Van Kammen, W. B. (1990). Long-term criminal outcomes of hyperactivity-impulsivity-attention deficit and conduct problems in childhood. In L. N. Robins & M. Rutter (eds.), *Straight and deviant pathways from childhood to adulthood* (pp. 62–81). New York: Cambridge University Press.

Faulstich, M. E., Monroe, J. R., Carey, M. P., Ruggiero, L., & Gresham F. (1986). Prevalence of DSM-III conduct disorders and adjustment disorders for adolescent psychiatric inpatients. *Adolescence, 21*, 333–337.

Field, T. M. (1984). Early interactions between infants and their post-partum depressed mothers. *Infant Behavior and Development, 7*, 517–522.

Field, T. M., Sandberg, D., Goldstein, S., Garcia, R., Vega-Lahr, N., Porter, K., & Dowling, M. (1987). Play interactions and interviews of depressed and conduct disorder children and their mothers. *Child Psychiatry and Human Development, 17*, 213–234.

Fox, N., & Marshall, T. (1991, March). *The role of the left vs right frontal lobe in the development of emotion regulation*. Paper presented at the Conference on Research Issues in the Development of Emotion Regulation, Washington, D.C.

Fraiberg, S. H. (1959). *The magic years*. New York: Scribners.

Frick, P. J., Lahey, B. B., Loeber, R., Stouthamer-Loeber, M., Green, S., Hart, E. L., & Christ, M. A. G. (1991). Oppositional defiant disorder and conduct disorder in boys: Patterns of behavioral covariation. *Journal of Child Clinical Psychology, 20*, 202–208.

Frijda, N. H. (1986). *The emotions*. Cambridge: Cambridge University Press.

Garmezy, N., & Rutter, M. (1983). *Stress, coping, and development in children*. New York: McGraw Hill.

Geller, B., Chestnut, E. C., Miller, M. D., Price, D. T., & Yates, E. (1985). Preliminary data on DSM–III associated features of major depressive disorder in children and adolescents. *American Journal of Psychiatry, 142*, 643–644.

Glaser, K. (1967). Masked depression in children and adolescents. *American Journal of Psychotherapy, 21*, 565–574.

Goldsmith, H. H., & Campos, J. J. (1990). The structure of temperamental fear and pleasure in infants: A psychometric perspective. *Child Development, 61*, 1944–1964.

Goodman, S. H., Lynch, M. E., Brogan, D., & Fielding, B. (in press). The development of social and emotional competence in children of depressed mothers. *Child Development*.

Gorenstein, E. K., & Newman, J. P. (1980). Disinhibitory psychopathology: A new perspective and a model for research. *Psychological Review, 87*, 301–315.

Gottman, J. M., & Fainsilber Katz, L. (1989). Effects of marital discord on young children's peer interactions and health. *Developmental Psychology, 25*, 373–381.

Gray, J. A. (1987). *The psychology of fear and stress*. New York: Cambridge University Press.

Gray, J. A. (1982). *The neuropsychology of anxiety*. New York: Oxford University Press.

Grych, J. H., & Fincham, F. D. (1990). Marital conflict and children's adjustment: A cognitive-contextual framework. *Psychological Bulletin, 108*, 267–290.

Hare, R. D. (1975). Electrodermal and cardiovascular correlates of psychopathy. In R. D. Hare & D. Schalling (eds.), *Psychopathic behavior: Approaches to research* (pp. 107–144). New York: Wiley.

Hawton, K. (1986). *Suicide and attempted suicide among children and adolescents*. Beverly Hills, CA: Sage.

Henry, J. P. (1982). The relation of social to biological processes in disease. *Social Science Medicine, 16*, 369–380.

Hetherington, E. M., Cox, M., & Cox, R. (1982). Effects of divorce on parents and children. In M. Lamb (ed.), *Nontraditional families* (pp. 233–288). Hillsdale, N.J.: Erlbaum.

Hetherington, E. M., & Martin, B. (1986). Family interaction. In H. C. Quay & J. S. Werry (eds.), *Psychopathological disorders of childhood* (2nd ed., pp. 247–302) New York: Wiley.

Hetherington, E. M., Stouwie, R., & Ridberg, E. H. (1971). Patterns of family interaction and child rearing related to three dimensions of juvenile delinquency. *Journal of Abnormal Psychology, 77*, 160–176.

Hinshaw, S. P. (1987). On the distinction between attentional deficits/hyperactivity and conduct problems/aggression in child psychopathology. *Psychological Bulletin, 101*, 443–463.

Horner, A. J. (1984). *Object relations and the developing ego in therapy*. Northvale, NJ: Jason Aronson.

Howes, C., & Eldridge, R. (1985). Responses of abused, neglected, and nonmaltreated children to the behaviors of their peers. *Journal of Applied Developmental Psychology, 6*, 261–270.

Huesmann, L. R., Eron, L. D., Lefkowitz, M. M., & Walder, L. O. (1984). Stability of aggression over time and generation. *Developmental Psychology, 20*, 1120–1134.

Izard, C. E. (1977). *Human emotions*. New York: Plenum.

Izard, C. E., Haynes, O. M., Chisholm, G., & Baak, C. (1991). Emotional determinants of infant-mother attachment. *Child Development, 62*, 906–917.

Jacobitz, D., & Sroufe, L. A. (1987). The early caregiver-child relationship and attention-deficit disorder with hyperactivity in kindergarten: A prospective study. *Child Development, 58*, 1488–1495.

Kagan, J. (1991, March). *Philosophical and empirical issues in the study of emotion*. Paper presented at Conference on Research Issues in the Development of Emotion Regulation, Washington, D.C.

Kagan, J., Reznick, J. S., & Gibbons, J. (1989). Inhibited and uninhibited types of children. *Child Development, 60*, 838–845.

Kazdin, A. E., Esveldt-Dawson, K., Unis, A. S., & Rancurello, M. D. (1983). Child and parent evaluations of depression and aggression in psychiatric inpatient units. *Journal of Abnormal Child Psychology, 11*, 401–413.

Kazdin, A. E., French, N. H., Unis, A. S., Esveldt-Dawson, K., & Sherick, R. B. (1983). Hopelessness, depression, and suicidal intent among psychiatrically disturbed inpatient children. *Journal of Consulting and Clinical Psychology, 51*, 504–510.

Kellam, S. G., Simon, M. B., & Ensminger, M. E. (1983). Antecedents in first grade of teen-age substance use and psychological well-being: A ten year community-wide prospective study. In D. F. Ricks & B. S. Dohrenwend (eds.), *Origins of psychopathology* (pp. 17–42). Cambridge, England: Cambridge University Press.

Kernberg, P. F., & Chazan, S. E. (1991). *Children with conduct disorders: A psychotherapy manual*. New York: Basic.

King, C., & Young, R. (1982). Attentional deficits with and without hyperactivity: Teacher and peer perceptions. *Journal of Abnormal Child Psychology, 10*, 483–496.

Klimes-Dougan, B., & Kistner, J. (1990). Physically abused preschoolers' responses to peers' distress. *Developmental Psychology, 26*, 599–602.

Kohlberg, L., LaCrosse, J., & Ricks, D. (1972). The predictability of adult mental health from childhood behavior. In B. B. Wolman (ed.), *Manual of Child Psychopathology* (pp. 1217–1284). New York: McGraw-Hill.

Kovacs, M., & Beck, A. T. (1977). An empirical clinical approach toward a definition of childhood depression. In J. G. Schulterbrandt & A. Raskin (eds.), *Depression in childhood: Diagnosis, treatment, and conceptual models* (pp. 1–25). New York: Raven Press.

Kovacs, M., Feinberg, T. L., Crouse-Novak, M. A., Paulauskas, S. L., & Finkelstein, R. (1984). Depressive disorders in childhood: I. A longitudinal prospective study of characteristics and recovery. *Archives of General Psychiatry, 41*, 229–237.

Kovacs, M., Paulauskas, S., Gatsonis, C., & Richards, C. (1988). Depressive disorders in childhood: III. A longitudinal study of comorbidity with and risk for conduct disorders. *Journal of Affective Disorders, 15*, 205–217.

Kuczynski, L., & Kochanska, G. (1990). Development of children's noncompliance strategies from toddlerhood to age 5. *Developmental Psychology, 26*, 398–408.

LaFreniere, P. J., & Sroufe, L. A. (1985). Profiles of peer competence in the preschool: Interrelations between measures, influence of social ecology, and relation to attachment history. *Developmental Psychology, 21*, 56–69.

Lahey, B. B., Conger, R. D., Atkeson, B. M., & Treiber, F. A. (1984). Parenting behavior and emotional status of physically abusive mothers. *Journal of Consulting and Clinical Psychology, 52*, 1062–1071.

Lahey, B. B., Shaughency, E., Hynd, G., Carlson, C., & Nieves, N. (1987). Attention deficit disorder with and without hyperactivity: Comparison of behavioral characteristics of clinic-referred children. *Journal of the American Academy of Child and Adolescent Psychiatry, 26*, 718–723.

Ledingham, J. E., & Schwartzmann, A. E. (1984). A 3-year follow-up of aggressive and withdrawn behavior in childhood: Preliminary findings. *Journal of Abnormal Child Psychology, 12*, 157–168.

Lerner, J. A., Inui, T. S., Trupin, E. W., & Douglas, E. (1985). Preschool behavior can predict future psychiatric disorders. *Journal of the American Academy of Child Psychiatry, 24*, 42–48.

Lewis, M., Alessandri, S. M., & Sullivan, M. W. (1990). Violation of expectancy, loss of control, and anger expression in young infants. *Developmental Psychology, 26*, 745–751.

Lewis, M., Feiring, C., McGuffog, C., & Jaskir, J. (1984). Predicting psychopathology in six year olds from early social relations. *Child Development, 55*, 123–136.

Loeber, R. (1990). Development and risk factors of juvenile antisocial behavior and delinquency. *Clinical Psychology Review, 10*, 1–42.

Loeber, R., Lahey, B. B., & Thomas, C. (1991) Diagnostic conundrum of oppositional defiant disorder and conduct disorder. *Journal of Abnormal Psychology, 100*, 379–390.

Loeber, R., & Stouthamer-Loeber, M. (1986). Family factors as correlates and predictors of juvenile conduct problems and delinquency. In M. Tonry & N. Morris (eds.), *Crime and justice* (Vol 7, pp. 29–149). Chicago: University of Chicago Press.

Loeber, R., Tremblay, R. E., Gagnon, C., & Charlebois, P. (1989). Continuity and desistance in disruptive boys' early fighting at school. *Development and Psychopathology, 1*, 39–50.

Londerville, S., & Main, M. (1981). Security of attachment, compliance, and maternal training methods in the second year of life. *Developmental Psychology, 17*, 289–299.

Loney, J., & Milich, R. (1982). Hyperactivity, inattention, and aggression in clinical practice. In D. Routh & M. Wolraich (eds.), *Advances in behavioral pediatrics* (Vol. 3, pp. 113–147). Greenwich, CT: JAI Press.

Lynch, M., & Cicchetti, D. (1991). Patterns of relatedness in maltreated and nonmaltreated children: Connections among multiple representational models. *Development and Psychopathology, 3,* 206–227.

Maccoby, E. E., & Martin, J. A. (1983). Socialization in the context of family: Parent-child interaction. In E. M. Hetherington (ed.), P. Mussen (Series ed.), *Handbook of child psychology: Vol IV. Socialization, personality, and social development* (pp. 1–101). New York: Wiley.

MacFarlane, J. W., Allen, L., & Honzik, M. P. (1962). *A developmental study of the behavior problems of normal children between twenty-one months and fourteen years.* Berkeley: University of California Press.

Main, M., & George, C. (1985). Response of abused and disadvantaged toddlers to distress in playmates: A study in the day care setting. *Developmental Psychology, 21,* 407–412.

Main, M., & Goldwyn, R. (1984). Predicting rejection of her infant from mother's representation of her own experience: Implications for the abused-abusing intergenerational cycle. *Child Abuse and Neglect, 8,* 203–217.

Main, M., & Weston, D. (1981). The quality of the toddler's relationship to mother and father: Related to conflict behavior and the readiness to establish new relationships. *Child Development, 52,* 932–940.

Malatesta, C. Z., & Wilson, A. (1988). Emotion cognition interaction in personality development: A discrete emotions, functionalist analysis. *British Journal of Social Psychology, 27,* 91–112.

Malmquist, C. P. (1977). Childhood depression: A clinical and behavioral perspective. In J. G. Schulterbrandt & A. Raskin (eds.), *Depression in childhood: Diagnosis, treatment, and conceptual models* (pp. 33–59). New York: Raven Press.

Mangelsdorf, S., Gunnar, M., Kestenbaum, R., Lang, S., & Andreas, D. (1990). Infant proneness-to-distress temperament, maternal personality, and mother-infant attachment: Associations and goodness-of-fit. *Child Development, 61,* 820–831.

Marriage, K., Fine, S., Moretti, M., & Haley, G. (1986). Relationship between depression and conduct disorder in children and adolescents. *Journal of the American Academy of Child and Adolescent Psychiatry, 25,* 687–691.

Matas, L., Arend, R., & Sroufe, L. A. (1978). Continuity of adaptation in the second year: The relationship between quality of attachment and later competence. *Child Development, 49,* 547–556.

McBurnett, K., Lahey, B. B., Frick, P. J., Risch, C., Loeber, R., Hart, E. L., Christ, M. A. G., & Hanson, K. A. (1991). Anxiety, inhibition, and conduct disorder in children: II. Relation to salivary cortisol. *Journal of the American Academy of Child and Adolescent Psychiatry, 30,* 192–196.

McClellan, J. M., Rubert, M. P., Reichler, R. J., & Sylvester, C. E. (1990). Attention deficit disorder in children at risk for anxiety and depression. *Journal of the American Academy of Child and Adolescent Psychiatry, 29,* 534–539.

McCord, J. (1979). Some child rearing antecedents of criminal behavior in adult men. *Journal of Personality and Social Psychology, 9,* 1477–1486.

Milich, R., & Landau, S. (1984). A comparison of the social status and social behavior of aggressive and aggressive/withdrawn boys. *Journal of Abnormal Child Psychology, 12,* 277–288.

Miyake, K., Chen, S., & Campos, J. (1985). Infant temperament, mother's mode of interactions, and attachment in Japan: An interim report. In I. Bretherton & E.

Waters (eds.), Growing points of attachment theory and research. *Monographs of the Society for Research in Child Development, 50* (1–2, Serial No. 209) pp. 276–297.

Moffitt, T. E. (1990). Juvenile delinquency and attention deficit disorder: Boys' developmental trajectories from age 3 to age 15. *Child Development, 61*, 893–910.

Moskowitz, D. S., & Schwartzman, A. E. (1989). Painting group portraits: Studying life outcomes for aggressive and withdrawn children. *Journal of Personality, 57*, 723–746.

Offord, D. R., Adler, R. J., & Boyle, M. H. (1986). Prevalence and sociodemographic correlates of conduct disorder. *The American Journal of Social Psychiatry, 4*, 272–278.

O'Leary, K. D., & Emery, R. E. (1984). Marital discord and child behavior problems. In M. D. Levine & P. Satz (eds.), *Middle childhood: Development and dysfunction* (pp. 345–364). Baltimore: University Park Press.

Olweus, D. (1979). Stability of aggressive reaction patterns in males: A review. *Psychological Bulletin, 86*, 852–875.

Olweus, D. (1980). Familial and temperamental determinants of aggressive behavior in adolescents: A causal analysis. *Developmental Psychology, 14*, 644–660.

Park, K. A., & Waters, E. (1989). Security of attachment and preschool friendships. *Child Development, 60*, 1076–1081.

Parke, R., & Slaby, R. G. (1983). The development of aggression. In E. M. Hetherington (ed.), P. Mussen (Series ed.), *Handbook of child psychology: Vol. IV. Socialization, personality, and social development* (pp. 547–642). New York: Wiley.

Pastor, D. L. (1981). The quality of mother-infant attachment and its relationship to toddler's initial sociability with peers. *Developmental Psychology, 17*, 323–335.

Patterson, G. R. (1982). *Coercive family process*. Eugene, OR: Castalia.

Patterson, G. R., DeBaryshe, B. D., & Ramsey, E. (1989). A developmental perspective on antisocial behavior. *American Psychologist, 44*, 329–335.

Pettit, G. S., & Bates, J. E. (1989). Family interaction patterns and children's behavior problems from infancy to 4 years. *Developmental Psychology, 25*, 413–420.

Pianta, R., Egeland, B., & Erickson, M. F. (1989). The antecedents of maltreatment: Results of the Mother-Child Interaction Research Project. In D. Cicchetti & V. Carlson (eds.), *Child maltreatment: Theory and research on the causes and consequences of child abuse and neglect* (pp. 203–253). New York: Cambridge University Press.

Pfeffer, C. R. (1986). *The suicidal child*. New York: Guilford.

Pfiffner, L. J., & O'Leary, S. G. (1989). Effects of maternal discipline and nurturance on toddler's behavior and affect. *Journal of Abnormal Child Psychology, 17*, 527–540.

Prinz, R., Conner, P., & Wilson, C. (1981). Hyperactive and aggressive behaviors in childhood: Intertwined dimensions. *Journal of Abnormal Child Psychology, 9*, 191–202.

Puig-Antich, J. (1982). Major depression and conduct disorder in pre-puberty. *Journal of the American Academy of Child Psychiatry, 21*, 118–128.

Pulkinnen, L. (1983). Finland: The search for alternatives to aggression. In A. P. Goldstein & M. H. Segal (eds.), *Aggression in a global perspective* (pp. 104–144). New York: Pergamon.

Putnam, F. W., & Trickett, P. (1991, May). *Dissociation in sexually abused girls*. Paper presented at the Annual Meeting of the American Psychiatric Association, New Orleans.

Quay, H. C. (1979). Classification. In H. C. Quay & J. S. Werry (eds.), *Psychopathological disorders of childhood* (pp. 1–34). New York: Wiley.

Quay, H. C. (1986). Conduct disorders. In H. C. Quay & J. S. Werry (eds.), *Psychopathological disorders of childhood* (pp. 35–72). New York: Wiley.

Quay, H. C. (1987). Patterns of delinquent behavior. In H. C. Quay (ed.), *Handbook of juvenile delinquency* (pp. 118–138). New York: Wiley.

Quiggle, N. L., Garber, J., Panak, W. F., & Dodge, K. A. (in press). Social-information processing in aggressive and depressed children. *Child Development*.

Reeves, J. C., Werry, J. S., Elkind, G. S., & Zametkin, A. (1987). Attention deficit, conduct, oppositional, and anxiety disorders in children: II. Clinical characteristics. *Journal of the American Academy of Child and Adolescent Psychiatry, 26*, 144–155.

Renouf, A. G., & Harter, S. (1990). Low self-worth and anger as components of the depressive experience in young adolescents. *Development and Psychopathology, 2*, 293–310.

Rey, J. M., Bashir, M. R., Schwarz, M., Richards, I. N., Plapp, J. M., & Stewart, G. W. (1988). Oppositional disorder: Fact or fiction? *Journal of the American Academy of Child and Adolescent Psychiatry, 27*, 157–162.

Richman, N., Stevenson, J., & Graham, P. (1975). Prevalence of behavior problems in three year old children: An epidemiological study in a London borough. *Journal of Child Psychology and Psychiatry, 16*, 277–287.

Richman, N., Stevenson, J., & Graham, P. (1982). *Preschool to school: A behavioural study.* New York: Academic.

Robins, L. N. (1966). *Deviant children grow up: A sociological analytic study of sociopathic personality.* Baltimore: Williams and Wilkins.

Robins, L. N. (1986). The consequences of conduct disorder in girls. In D. Olweus, J. Block, & M. Radke-Yarrow (eds.), *Development of anti-social and prosocial behavior: Research, theories, and issues* (pp. 385–414). New York: Academic.

Rose, S. L., Rose, S. A., & Feldman, J. F. (1989). Stability of behavior problems in very young children. *Development and Psychopathology, 1*, 5–19.

Rothbart, M. K. (1988). Temperament and development. In G. A. Kohnstamm, J. E. Bates, & M. K. Rothbart (eds.), *Temperament in Childhood* (pp. 187–248), Chicester, England: Wiley.

Rutter, M. (1966). *Children of sick parents: An environmental and psychiatric study.* London: Oxford University Press.

Rutter, M., Cox, A., Tupling, C., Berger, M., & Yule, W. (1975). Attainment and adjustment in two geographical areas: I. Prevalence of psychiatric disorder. *British Journal of Psychiatry, 126*, 493–509.

Rutter, M., & Quinton, D. (1984). Parental psychiatric disorder: Effects on children. *Psychological Medicine, 14*, 853–880.

Schachar, R., & Wachsmuth, R. (1990). Oppositional disorder in children: A validation study comparing conduct disorder, oppositional disorder, and normal control children. *Journal of Child Psychology and Psychiatry, 31*, 1089–1102.

Schmaling, K. B., & Patterson, G. R. (1984). *Maternal classifications of deviant and prosocial child behavior and reactions to the child in the home.* Unpublished manuscript, Oregon Social Learning Center, Eugene, OR.

Schneider-Rosen, K., & Cicchetti, D. (1991). Early self-recognition and emotional development: Visual self-recognition and affective reactions to mirror self-images in maltreated and non-maltreated toddlers. *Developmental Psychology, 27*, 471–478.

Schroeder, C. S., Gordon, B. N., Kanoy, K., & Routh, D. K. (1983). Managing children's behavior problems in pediatric practice. In M. Wolraich & D. K. Routh (eds.), *Advances in developmental and behavioral pediatrics* (Vol 4, pp. 25–86). Greenwich, CT: JAI Press.

Shaffer, D. (1974). Suicide in childhood and early adolescence. *Journal of Child Psychology and Psychiatry, 15*, 275–291.

Shapiro, S., & Garfinkel, B. (1986). The occurrence of behavior disorders in children: The interdependence of Attention Deficit Disorder and Conduct Disorder. *Journal of the American Academy of Child and Adolescent Psychiatry, 25*, 809–819.

Siegel, E. V. (1991). *Middle-class waifs.* Hillsdale, N.J.: Analytic Press.

Speltz, M. L., Greenberg, M. T., & Deklyen, M. (1990). Attachment in preschoolers with disruptive behavior: A comparison of clinic-referred and nonproblem children. *Development and Psychopathology, 2,* 31–46.

Sroufe, L. A. (1983). Infant-caregiver attachment and patterns of maladaptation in preschool: The roots of maladaptation and competence. In M. Perlmutter (ed.), *Minnesota symposium on child psychology* (Vol 16, pp. 41–81). Minneapolis: University of Minnesota Press.

Sroufe, L. A., Fox, N. E., & Pancake, V. R. (1983). Attachment and dependency in developmental perspective. *Child Development, 54,* 1615–1627.

Stewart, M. A., DeBlois, C. S., Meardon, J., & Cummings, C. (1980). Aggressive conduct disorder children. *Journal of Nervous and Mental Disease, 168,* 604–610.

Stifter, C., & Fox, N. (1990). Infant reactivity: Physiological correlates of newborn and five-month temperament. *Developmental Psychology, 26,* 582–588.

Tellegen, A. (1982). *Brief manual for the Differential Personality Questionnaire.* Unpublished manuscript, University of Minnesota.

Thomas, A., Chess, S., & Birch, H. G. (1968). *Temperament and behavior disorders in children.* New York: New York University Press.

Tomkins, S. S. (1963). *Affect, imagery, consciousness.* (Vol II.) *The negative affects.* New York: Springer.

Trad, P. (1989). *The preschool child: Assessment, diagnosis, and treatment.* New York: Wiley.

Trickett, P. K., & Kuczynski, L. (1986). Children's misbehavior and parental discipline strategies in abusive and nonabusive families. *Developmental Psychology, 22,* 115–123.

Troy, M., & Sroufe, L. A. (1987). Victimization among preschoolers: The role of the attachment relationship history. *Journal of the American Academy of Child Psychiatry, 26,* 166–172.

Tuke, H. (1890). French retrospective. *Journal of Mental Science, 36,* 117.

Walker, L., Lahey, B. B., Russo, M. F., Frick, P. J., Christ, M. A. G., McBurnett, K., Loeber, R., Stouthamer-Loeber, M., & Green, S. M. (1991). Anxiety, inhibition, and conduct disorder in children: I. Relations to social impairment. *Journal of the American Academy of Child and Adolescent Psychiatry, 30,* 187–191.

Wallerstein, J. (1983). Children of divorce: Stress and developmental tasks. In N. Garmezy & M. Rutter (eds.), *Stress, coping and development in children* (pp. 265–302). New York: McGraw-Hill.

Waters, E., Wippman, J., & Sroufe, L. A. (1979). Attachment, positive affect, and competence in the peer group: Two studies in construct validation. *Child Development, 50,* 821–829.

Watson, D., & Clark, L. A. (1984). Negative affectivity: The disposition to experience aversive emotional states. *Psychological Bulletin, 96,* 465–490.

Werry, J. S., Reeves, J. C., & Elkind, G. S. (1987). Attention deficit, conduct, oppositional, and anxiety disorders in children: I. A review of research in differentiating characteristics. *Journal of the American Academy of Child Psychiatry, 26,* **133–143.**

West, D. J., & Farrington, D. P. (1973). *Who becomes delinquent.* London: Heinemann.

Winnicott, D. W. (1958/1975). *Through paediatrics to psycho-analysis.* New York: Basic Books.

Zahn-Waxler, C., Cole, P. M., & Barrett, K. C. (1991). Guilt and empathy: Sex differences and implications for the development of depression. In J. Garber & K. A. Dodge (Eds.), *The development of emotion regulation and dysregulation* (pp. 243–272). Cambridge: Cambridge University Press.

Zahn-Waxler, C., Iannotti, R. J., Cummings, E. M., & Denham, S. (1990). Antecedents of problem behaviors in children of depressed mothers. *Development and Psychopathology, 2,* 271–291.

Zahn-Waxler, C., & Kochanska, G. (1990). The origins of guilt. In R. A. Thompson (ed.), *Socioemotional development: Nebraska symposium on motivation, 1988* (pp. 183–258). Lincoln, Nebraska: University of Nebraska Press.

Zahn-Waxler, C., Kochanska, G., Krupnick, J., & McKnew, D. (1990). Patterns of guilt in children of depressed and well mothers. *Developmental Psychology, 26*, 51–59.

Zahn-Waxler, C., & Radke-Yarrow, M. (1990). The origins of empathic concern. *Motivation and Emotion, 14*, 107–130.

Zahn-Waxler, C., Radke-Yarrow, M., Chapman, M., & Wagner, E. (1992). Development of concern for others. *Developmental Psychology, 28*, 126–136.

VI Depression in Families: A Systems Perspective

JAMES C. COYNE, GERALDINE DOWNEY, &
JULIE BOERGERS

It is apparent that depression is concentrated in particular families (Coyne, Burchill, & Stiles, 1991; Keitner & Miller, 1990). The reasons for this are complex and little understood. Genetic factors may provide a partial answer, but evidence of a genetic component to depression should not discourage vigorous exploration of the role of the family environment and larger social context. Underscoring this point, a recent community-based twin study found that the heritability of severe and moderate depression is modest. It is less than for hypertension, schizophrenia, or bipolar affective disorder, and similar to that for peptic ulcers or coronary artery disease, medical conditions that are known to have a large environmental contribution (Kendler, Neale, Kessler, Heath, & Eaves, 1992).

These observations suggest a strong environmental contribution to depression. Although the nature of this contribution is largely unspecified, a number of studies provide intriguing clues about how family functioning may be linked with the onset, course and outcome of depression. For example, marital problems (Rounsaville, Weissman, Prusoff, & Herceg-Baron, 1979) and marital status (Keller, Beardslee, Lavori, Wunder, & Samuelson, 1988) predict response to antidepressant medication and spousal criticism strongly predicts relapse in medicated patients (Leff & Vaughn, 1985). More generally, the presence of a depressed child or adult identifies a family environment that is otherwise troubled. Depression in adults is strongly associated with child psychopathology and family problems, and depression in children is associated with parental psychopathology and similar family problems.

Efforts to trace connections between families and depression have usually assumed simple unidirectional influences or focused on dyadic relationships, ignoring the larger family context. For example, most studies of affect regulation between depressed mothers and their infants do not address how the quality of interchange may be shaped by emotional exchanges among other family members (for an exception, see Zahn-Waxler & Kochanska, 1990). Growing numbers of studies are documenting a connection between parental depression and the diagnostic status of children, but until recently researchers have ignored the possibility that other family members may influence or even determine this association. Findings that marital distress may contribute to both the parenting difficulties of depressed mothers and their children's adjustment problems (see Downey & Coyne, 1990, for a review) and that mothers of depressed children often lack a confiding relationship with a spouse (Goodyer, Wright, & Altham, 1988) should sensitize us to the importance of context. We must also be aware that an exclusive focus on the depressed mother-child dyad may inadvertently result in mothers being blamed for child difficulties that reflect broader contextual influences such as the adjustment and availability of the father. Clearly, we need theoretical models that offer the possibility of capturing the complexity of depression in families.

In this chapter, we review a number of relevant literatures and describe a model explicating some aspects of the relationship between depression and the family system. In particular, we focus on the literature on families that include a depressed parent or a depressed child and suggest that there may be a generalized emotional dysregulation in these families. The literature on children of depressed parents receives particular attention because it is considerably more developed than that on parents of depressed children. However, some links between these literatures are clear. A significant proportion of children with a depressed parent are depressed themselves (Downey & Coyne, 1990), there are temporal associations between depressive episodes in mothers and children (Hammen, 1991), and one-half to two-thirds of parents with a depressed child are depressed (Brumbeck, Dietz-Schmidt, & Weinberg, 1977; Puig-Antich, Lukens, Davies, Goetz, Quattrock, & Todak, 1985a). We are often talking about the same families whether we identify them because of depression in parents or in children. Furthermore, depression in parents in just one source of the disadvantages and difficulties experienced by children of depressed parents, and depression is only one of the many problems that these parents face in dealing with their children (Downey & Coyne, 1990). We can use findings about the life course and current circumstances of depressed parents to suggest what to look for in families of depressed children who do *not* have a depressed parent. Similarly, we can use our knowledge about the additional adjustment problems of depressed children to suggest how their behavior can contribute to emotional dysregulation in their families. In this way we hope illuminate a neglected topic in studies of depressed parents, namely, the reactive characteristics of their children, whether or not the children are depressed.

We are undertaking an exercise in abduction (Peirce, 1955). We bring together several literatures that have progressed independently and attempt to draw connections among them. Our task is a difficult one and we begin our review by describing some methodological problems that stand as obstacles to achieving our agenda.

Methodological Issues

It is surprising how much research is conducted with parents and children who are not typical of the populations to which generalizations are made. Research is usually conducted in tertiary university hospitals and clinics that attract patients with depressions that are recurrent, severe, or treatment-resistant. These patients may be unrepresentative in other ways as well. Their attendance at a specialized setting may reflect limitations in social resources, an especially disruptive impact of their disorder on their family, or comorbidity of their depression with dysthymia or a personality disorder. An even larger body of research is based on adults and children recruited from nonclinical populations because of elevated scores on screening questionnaires. Most of these "depressed" persons would not meet standardized diagnostic criteria for depression and differ in significant ways from persons who would (Coyne & Downey, 1991; Depue & Monroe, 1986).

The majority of depressed people — those who meet formal diagnostic criteria but who are not in treatment or who are being treated in the community — are largely absent from family studies of depression. There is a pressing need for research with these clinically depressed adults and children and their families. There is limited evidence that children of nonreferred clinically depressed persons are socially impaired and prone to psychiatric disturbance (Beardslee, Keller, Lavori, Klerman, Dorer, & Samuelson, 1988). Nonetheless, we should be cautious about uncritical generalizations from a literature about severely-impaired persons with depression and about distressed persons who would not meet the criteria for clinical depression.

As we learn more about depression, we are beginning to appreciate how difficult it is to disentangle the interplay of personal background, social context, and depression (Coyne & Downey, 1991). Depression is a recurrent disorder and those who suffer from it can spend up to 20% of their adult life in a state of severe depression (Angst, 1986). It can profoundly influence how developmental tasks are accomplished and the life contexts in which depressed persons find themselves (Cicchetti, Toth, & Bush, 1988; Coyne & Downey, 1991). Childhood experiences that increase vulnerability for adult depression may similarily increase risk for problematic parenting, marriage to an undependable mate, and employment difficulties (Harris, Brown, & Bifulco, 1987; Quinton, Rutter, & Liddle, 1984). Depression in children also is a recurrent disorder with serious implications for development (Cicchetti & Schneider-Rosen, 1986; Harrington, Fudge, Rutter, Pickles, & Hill, 1990; Kovacs, 1989). However, some of its apparent effects on development may be more appropriately viewed as stemming directly from the enduring family adversity that fosters childhood depression.

When dealing with life course phenomena and correlated risk factors, conventional methodological strategies, such as the use of matching, control groups, and statistical controls, may be of limited efficacy in separating spurious from genuine causal influences (Coyne & Downey, 1991; Walker, Downey, & Nightingale, 1989). We cannot always tell when we have tricked ourselves with statistical legerdemain. For instance, suppose we eliminate the association between parental depression and child adjustment by controlling for marital distress or life events. Have we truly demonstrated that the apparent effects of parental depression on children are spurious? Or, have we fallen prey to a logical error that would be more readily recognized in someone's demonstration that Denver is not really at a higher altitude than Ann Arbor, once atmospheric pressure is controlled? There is a growing literature on social factors in depression in which multivariate statistical techniques are blindly used to draw conclusions that may be unwarranted.

When evaluating findings associated with conventional matching and statistical control procedures, we should be aware that unrealistic assumptions may limit their generalizability. In particular, we should be careful not to distort the phenomena of interest in order to more closely approximate a controlled experiment with random assignment (e.g., controlling for spousal characteristics as if it simulates giving depressed women new husbands who are emotionally accessible and involved with their children). Instead, we might learn more about the processes linking families and depression by observing the nonrandom patterning of relevant variables (Lieberson, 1985).

Depressed Parents and their Children

Children's risk for disturbance

Children of depressed parents show heightened rates of general problems in adjustment, social and academic impairment, physical health problems, potential markers of risk for depression, and diagnosable clinical conditions including depression (Downey & Coyne, 1990). Difficulties are found early, with infants of depressed mothers evoking more negative reactions from strangers than infants of nondepressed mothers (Field, Healy, Goldstein, Perry, Bendell, Schramberg, Zimmerman, & Kuhn, 1988). Problems emerge in peer, teacher, and observer reports as well as in self and parent reports (Beardslee, Bemporad, Keller, & Klerman, 1983; Cicchetti et al., 1988; Downey & Coyne, 1990). The general adjustment problems of children with a depressed parent include social and academic difficulties and internalizing and externalizing behavior problems.

In showing many of these problems children of depressed parents resemble other children who experience the stress and disruption that accompany serious parental psychiatric or medical illness. However, depression, and especially major depression, appears to be more specific consequence of having a unipolar-depressed parent. Depression is the only diagnosable condition for which children of depressed parents consistently show significantly heightened risk across studies (see Downey & Coyne, 1990, for a review). The rate of any affective disorder is three times higher in children of unipolar disorder parents than in control children and the rate of major depressive disorder is six times higher than in control children.

In addition to general adjustment difficulties and clinical depression, children of depressed mothers show what have been interpreted as markers of risk for subsequent depression. Specifically, they are more self-critical than other children (Hammen, Adrian, & Hirato, 1988) and they have difficulties with regulating emotion and social interaction (Zahn-Waxler, Ianotti, Cummings, & Denham, 1990; Zahn-Waxler & Kochanska, 1990; Zahn-Waxler, McKnew, Cummings, Davenport, & Radke-Yarrow, 1984). Because peers and adults react negatively to such inappropriate emotional and social behavior, children of depressed parents who show these problems will probably experience heightened levels of rejection and adversity in social interactions. This may further confirm their negative self-concepts and lead them to avoid social situations, limiting their opportunities for learning appropriate social and emotional expression. Difficulties in socioemotional development may accrue over time, as they simply fail to keep pace with peers. Thus, we can see a potential interactional process linking high-risk children and their social context in the accentuation of their difficulties.

Parenting by a depressed person

An obvious explanation for the difficulties of children with a depressed parent has been that their problems result directly from living with a depressed parent. Certainly, the explanation that has received the most attention from researchers is that there is something pathogenic in the parenting behavior of a depressed mother. It is plausible and has the virtue of parsimony, but, as we shall see, it is becoming clear that the processes linking depression in parents and problems in their children are considerably more complex.

Parenting is a highly complex form of social interaction. The many qualities of effective parenting include the capacity for sustained effortful interaction, strong negotiation skills, an ability to be authoritative without being authoritarian, interpersonal sensitivity, a capacity to anticipate and avert potential crises, the ability to project warmth and consistency, and a high tolerance for criticism and aversive behavior. Depression will undermine these qualities. Furthermore, Bronfenbrenner (1978) has suggested that all children need at least one adult who is irrationally enthusiastic about them, and depressed persons have difficulty sustaining enthusiasm about anything.

Depressed mothers have been described in the literature as experiencing the difficulties in the parenting role that would be anticipated from their symptoms and associated problems. Weissman and Paykel (1974) observed that "the helplessness and hostility which are associated with acute depression interfere with the ability to be a warm and consistent mother" (p. 121). Fisher, Kokes, Harder, and Jones (1980) have also suggested that "depressed mothers display a high-degree of non-acknowledgement such that they do not interact meaningfully with the child" (p. 354).

The picture emerging from observational studies is that depression reduces the effort that parents put into interacting with their children (see Downey & Coyne, 1990, for a review). During parent-child interaction, depressed mothers show lower rates of behavior and less positive affect. They respond more slowly, less contingently, and less consistently to their child (see also Cohn & Campbell, this volume). They speak less often and their speech to infants lacks the exaggerated intonation of nondepressed caretakers (Bettes, 1988). They rely on less effortful conflict resolution strategies, often vacillating between abdicating authority by withdrawing or unilaterally enforcing obedience. The author William Styron (1990), himself a sufferer of depression, likens this condition to a "brown out". One might summarize the observational studies of depressed mothers and their children as indicating that depression is associated with a "brown out" in parenting.

Despite traditional psychoanalytic views of depression as representing anger turned inward, depression is not incompatible with being overtly hostile. Overt anger, criticism and irritability are characteristic of the interactions between depressed parents and their children, especially when the children are older (Cole & Zahn-Waxler, this volume; Cox, Puckering, Pound, & Mills, 1987; Cummings & Davies, this volume; Gordon, Burge, Hammen, Adrian, Jaenicke, & Hiroto, 1989; Panaccione & Wahler, 1986; Radke-Yarrow, Richters, & Wilson, 1988). Hammen (1991) has conducted some fascinating work on the origins of self-criticism in children of depressed parents. She found only weak support for the hypothesis that they were modelling their mothers' self-criticism. Instead, children's self-criticism was strongly tied to the hostile criticism directed at them by the mother. Further evidence of the central role of parental criticism in child disturbance is provided by Schwartz, Dorer, Beardslee, Lavori, and Keller (1990), who found that child-directed criticism mediated the relation between maternal depression and child disturbance.

There has been surprisingly little attention to the effects of depressed mothers' expression of sadness and personal distress on children beyond infancy. The observational coding systems used by most investigators were developed for other purposes and their adaptation for studying depression has usually been inadequate. In one of the few studies giving attention to sad affect, Biglan, Hops, Sherman, Friedman, Arthur, and Osteen (1985) reported that depressed mothers expressed more sadness during family interaction and that this reduced subsequent expressions of hostility by other family members. In an important sense, by showing depressed affect, these mothers exert an aversive control over other family members' behavior, providing brief, though immediate, respite from their sarcasm and irritation with her.

There has been almost no attention to parenting practices by depressed mothers that reduce their children's risk for adjustment problems. One important exception is the longitudinal study reported by Zahn-Waxler et al.

(1990). They identified several practices when the children were aged two that predicted fewer externalizing problems three years later. Notably, the depressed mothers whose children subsequently showed the fewest externalizing problems were more effective at permitting their child a separate identity with rights and needs of their own. Specifically, they were better at anticipating the children's point of view, exercising respectful, modulated control, and providing more structure and organization in the children's play environment.

In conclusion, two cautions are warranted in interpreting the findings from observational studies that indicate reduced parenting effort and increased negativity and hostility in the parenting of depressed persons. First, most of these difficulties do not appear to be specific to depressed mothers. They also occur in other mothers experiencing high stress, marital distress, and psychological distress. There is evidence that some aspects of parenting may be more affected by these factors than by clinical depression per se (Downey & Coyne, 1990). Even among depressed mothers, behavior that is sensitive and appropriate is inversely related to life stress, marital discord, and lack of support (Teti, Gelfand, & Pompa, 1990). Second, we really cannot evaluate the contribution of depression to parenting difficulties or adjustment problems in offspring without a closer look at the life course and current social context of depressed persons and their spouses. These factors may help to explain why the parent becomes depressed, moderate the effects of parental depression, or even provide alternative explanation of the offspring's problems.

The life course and social context of depressed parents

The childhood of depressed persons. The primary focus of research on the childhood antecedents of adult depression has been on establishing the connection between early loss of a parent and adult disturbance. It is now clear that the link between losing a parent and adult depression is neither simple nor direct. Rather, loss of a parent increases the risk for adult depression through its association with prolonged adversity and inadequate parenting in childhood (Breier, Kelsoe, Kirwin, Beller, Wolkowitz, & Pickar, 1988; Harris, Brown, & Bifulco, 1990). This evidence converges with retrospective accounts of depressed adults who often describe a troubled childhood characterized by harsh, affectionless, or controlling parenting (Gerlsma, Emmelkamp, & Arrindell, 1990; Holmes & Robins, 1988; Parker, 1983).

Efforts to explicate how childhood adversity is tied to adult depression have focused on a variety of indirect influences. Akiskal (1989) has argued that early adversity may indirectly increase risk for depression through inducing the development of a stormy interpersonal style marked by immaturity, hostile dependency, manipulativeness, impulsiveness, and a low threshold for alcohol and drug abuse in adulthood. These characteristics may precipitate life events that trigger depression earlier in life and result in more frequent episodes of depression without directly affecting lifetime risk for depression. Thus, Akiskal is arguing that this style is a moderator of risk for depression, rather than the primary vulnerability factor, which he presumes to be constitutional (see Akiskal, 1991, for a clarification of this point). Interestingly, the tendency to experience life stress of an interpersonal nature seems to run in families, separate from risk for depression (McGuffin & Bebbington, 1988). Further, in what may respresent in part a more extreme expression of this style, about 40% of depressed patients have personality disorders. These patients have more frequent life events, as well as an earlier onset of depression and a poorer recovery (Black, Bell, Hulbert, & Nasrallah, 1988; Phofl, Stangl, & Zimmerman, 1984).

Childhood adversity may also contribute to adult depression by fostering a set of depressogenic life circumstances (Harris, Brown, & Bifulco, 1990). Children in troubled families are at increased risk for exposure to negative life events and for chronic stress as a result of dropping out of school early, subsequent employment difficulties and poverty, and being married an unsupportive spouse. Consistent with this scenario, Harris et al. (1987) identified a pathway linking inadequate care following loss of a mother with early premarital pregnancy, which in turn increased the risk of marriage to an undependable partner. They speculated that marriage to such a partner, in addition to being low in intimacy, increased the risk of serious life events such as legal troubles, discoveries of infidelities, and threats of eviction, as well as poverty. Support for this speculation comes from a study of women raised in institutions (Quinton & Rutter, 1988; Quinton, Rutter, & Liddle, 1984). Quinton and colleagues found that those women who were free of psychiatric and social difficulties had a supportive relationship with their spouse. Women with supportive spouses constituted only a minority, however, and spouse support was linked with whether the spouse was currently involved in substance abuse or criminal activities. In summary, there is evidence from a variety of sources that the link between early childhood adversity and adult depression is indirect and operates largely through setting in motion a chain of events that increase the probability of a life style replete with the type of events and experiences that promote depression.

Spouses of depressed persons. Spouses of depressed persons are an important influence on the vulnerability of their partners, the family climate, and the wellbeing of children. Among women who have experienced childhood adversity, having a supportive spouse substantially reduces the risk of becoming depressed (Birtchnell, 1980; Harris et al., 1987; Parker & Hadzi-Pavlovic, 1984; Quinton et al., 1984). However, there is evidence that, as a group, the spouses of depressed persons have heightened psychological and physical complaints during their partner's depressive episode, in addition to personal and family histories of psychopathology (see Coyne et al., 1991, for a more extensive review). About 40% of spouses of patients currently in a depressive episode have clinically significant symptoms of distress, in contrast with 17% of the spouses of patients who are not currently depressed (Coyne et al., 1987).

Depressed women are more likely than other women to have a spouse with a history of depression or substance abuse. Over 50% of depressed women drawn from clinical populations have husbands with a history of psychiatric disturbance, mostly affective disorders (Merikangas & Spiker, 1982). About 25% of a community sample of depressed women have husbands with a history of depression and a fifth have husbands with a history of substance abuse (Peterson, Coyne, & Kessler, 1991). These rates are substantially higher than for husbands of nondepressed women. This concordance for psychopathology does not reflect contagion effects or common life experiences. Rather, first episodes of disorder in both wives and husbands usually precede their marriage. There is suggestive evidence that persons at risk for psychopathology may be attracted to each other because of similarities in early childhood adversity and adolescent deviance rather than similarities in psychopathology (Coyne, 1990; Merikangas, 1981). Our studies in a psychiatric population suggest that similarities in early adversity is a key determinant of similarities between depressed persons and their spouses in conflict management (Coyne, 1990). The ensuing emotional climate of the family may be what directly effects the vulnerable spouse's risk for disturbance.

The marriages of depressed persons. The majority of depressed persons have serious marital problems or score in the dissatisfied range on marital adjustment scales (Coyne, 1990; Rounsaville, Prusoff, & Weissman, 1980). Interviews and home and laboratory studies of the marital interaction of depressed persons reveal a pattern characterized by overt hostility and anger on the one hand and inhibition, avoidance and withdrawal on the other (Arkowitz, Holliday, & Hutter, 1982; Biglan et al., 1985; Hautzinger, Linden, & Hoffman, 1982; Hinchliffe, Hooper, & Roberts, 1978; Kahn, Coyne, & Margolin, 1985; Linden, Hautzinger, & Hoffman, 1983). Spouses are often very critical of the character and prior behavior of depressed persons, and such criticism is a strong predictor of relapse in persons with both unipolar and bipolar disorders (Hooley, Orley, & Teasdale, 1986; Leff & Vaughn, 1985; Miklowitz, Goldstein, Nuechterlein, & Snyder, 1988; Vaughn & Leff, 1976). In fact, Brown, Bifulco and Andrews (1990) recently identified critical negative exchanges with family members as the best predictor of the onset of depression from among a large number of background and environmental factors. When such negative exchanges were absent, low self-esteem and subclinical dysphoria were only weak predictors of the onset of a new episode.

Brown and Harris's (1978) classic work on the social circumstances associated with the onset of a depressive episode had identified lack of a confiding spouse as a key vulnerability factor. It now appears that lack of intimacy *per se* may not be the crucial relational risk factor. Having a spouse in whom one cannot confide is considerably more of a risk factor than not being married (i.e., being separated, divorced, or widowed) (Weissman, 1987). Marital relationships that do not provide intimacy are a subset of those judged "bad" in quality, and being in a bad marriage, rather than lack of intimacy, poses the greatest risk for depression (Roy, 1978). Approximately 40% of depressed women have experienced marital violence and more have probably experienced verbal threats and intimidation (Andrews & Brown, 1988). Presumably this would affect ratings of intimacy, but living under the threat of violence is undoubtedly a risk factor in itself (Coyne & Downey, 1991). In addition, maltreating mothers are diagnosed as depressed significantly more frequently than non-maltreating mothers from comparably low economic circumstances. Thus, there is suggestive evidence of a link between family violence and depression.

Life events and depression. Recent research also has elucidated the kinds of life events that precipitate depression. Only severe life events requiring long-term adjustment predict subsequent clinical depression (Brown & Harris 1978), and most items on typical life events inventory do not carry such a risk (Brugha, Bebbington, Tennant, & Hurry, 1985; Dohrenwend, Shrout, Link, Skodol, & Martin, 1986). Contrary to the focus of current psychological theories of depression, Brown and his colleagues found "no evidence that depression is caused by combinations of minor stress and negative cognitions" (Brown et al., 1990, p. 242). Many of the severe events associated with depression involve important losses or disappointments; however, interpersonal crises are more common as "provoking agents" than bereavement (Brown et al., 1987). Serious ongoing, chronic difficulties such as having a husband who drinks heavily are a somewhat less important class of provoking agents than severe life events (Brown & Harris, 1978). Chronic stress tends to be more strongly associated with depressive symptoms than with actual clinical depression (Breslau & Davis, 1986).

Brown, Craig, and Harris (1985) reviewed the onset of caseness of depression in ten population studies of women in the general population and found that an average of 83% of the women had a severe life event before onset. Studies of female psychiatric patients found a somewhat lower rate, but, nonetheless, most onsets were preceded by a severe life event. Despite this association between life events and the onset of depression, most people who experience a serious life event do not become depressed. The efficacy of the event in triggering a depressive episode depends strongly on the life circumstances of the person experiencing the event. It is possible to identify combinations of events and circumstances that account for most new cases of depression. One such combination is when a serious life events threatens the strongly held committments of someone with low self-esteem (e.g., a devout Catholic housewife with low self-esteem whose husband leaves her after twenty years of marriage). The event thus destroys any sense of self-worth or security derived from the commitment. A second combination is when the life event reflects the culmination of serious chronic difficulties (e.g., a marital separation follows chronic conflict over a spouse's substance abuse).

Summary. Overall, this brief review of the literature suggests that depressed persons and their spouses bring considerable difficulties to their relationships and to their efforts to parent, and they are likely to experience conflict and dissatisfaction with each other. Adversity in the background of the spouses of depressed persons may be associated with problems in parenting and with limitations in their ability to compensate for the parenting difficulties of the depressed person. If we focus on clinical depression rather than on self-reported depressive symptoms, we find that depression occurs in the context of serious stressors that also directly threaten family and child well-being. Yet, the occurrence and subsequent management of the stressor may reflect enduring characteristics of the spouse or characteristics of the depressed mother aside from her depression (e.g., a stormy interpersonal style).

Contextual Influences on the Parenting Difficulties of Depressed Persons and their Children's Problems

Our discussion of the family background and current social context of depressed persons suggests that, in addition to exposure to parental depression, children of depressed parents risk exposure to chronic stress and family crises, marital conflict and family violence, and a disturbed second parent. Thus, having a depressed parent is a marker of risk for living in a family context characterized by considerable disadvantage, and this adversity may explain some of the putative effects of adult depression on parenting and child adjustment. Billings and Moos (1983) provide powerful evidence of the effects of these co-occurring risk factors on children's general adjustment problems: in families with a depressed parent where stress is low and support is high, and where the illness was not severe, only 10% of the children were disturbed compared with 25% in all families with a depressed parent.

These correlated risk factors can contribute to behavioral difficulties in the child in three ways. First, they may increase the length, severity, and frequency of parental depressive episodes. Second, they may directly undermine the quality of parenting and family interaction. Parenting difficulties similar to those reported in depressed mothers are found in mothers coping with several different stressors including premature infants (Crnic, Greenberg, Ragozin, Robinson, & Basham, 1983), divorce (Hetherington, Stanley-Hagan, & Anderson, 1989), poverty (McLoyd, 1989), and job stress (Downey, Tiedje, & Wortman, 1991). For example, following divorce, custodial mothers become self-involved, erratic, uncommunicative, inconsistent, and punitive in dealing with their children (Hetherington et al., 1989). Third, these risk factors may contribute directly to the child's behavioral difficulties. For example, exposure to marital conflict appears to have a direct effect on children that is not completely mediated by parenting difficulties (Emery, 1982).

Marital conflict is the correlated risk factor that has received most attention (Cummings & Davies, this volume). The link between marital conflict and child maladjustment, especially conduct disturbance, is well established (Hetherington et al., 1989; Long, Forehand, Fauber, & Brody, 1987). Marital discord is a particularly credible alternative explanation for the general adjustment problems of children with a depressed parent. Using families from the Stony Brook High Risk Study, Emery, Weintraub, and Neale (1982) found that marital discord accounted for the relation between parent depression and child competence. However, it does not appear to account for depression in children of depressed parents. In a study of children with a depressed mother, Hops et al. (1987) found that marital distress was related to aversiveness and irritability but unrelated to depression. Similarly, Fendrich, Warner, and Weissman (1990) found that parental depression was strongly linked with child depression, whereas marital discord was linked with conduct disorders.

Dadds and his colleagues have also provided some insight into the processes linking conflicted marriages, parental depression, parenting and child difficulties (Dadds, 1987). In these families, exchanges between parents are rarely supportive and often aversive, especially around issues posed by the children's behavior (Dadds, Sanders, Behrens, & James, 1987). Dadds argues that it is likely that fathers withdraw from parenting and mothers' exposure to coercive, emotionally taxing exchanges with the child increases. This increased exposure induces and exacerbates depressive mood states, further undermining effective parenting. The increasing withdrawal of fathers as children become more difficult is consistent with the view that fathers' involvement in child care continues to be more discretionary than mothers and that mothers' self-concept and well-being are more tied to the parenting role. The scenario outlined by Dadds and his colleagues may explain the link between marital conflict, maternal distress, parenting difficulties, and child externalizing difficulties but it is unclear whether it explains the increased rates of depression in children with a depressed parent.

From a family systems perspective, the work of Dadds and his colleagues also is important because it opens up consideration of more triadic, reciprocal influences in families (cf. Minuchin, 1985). Yet it can be argued that this work does not go far enough, in that fails to consider how marital problems can structure the parent-child relationship beyond an influence on the quality of parenting. As systems theorists have pointed out, parents may involve children in their conflicts actively and pivotally (Kerr & Bowen, 1988; Kitzmann & Rohrbaugh, in press). They may focus excessively on children, "triangling" them in, breaking down any affective distance between the children and the parents' distress. Parents in conflict may enlist the children as allies and sources of comfort, or cut them off when they appear to be favored by the other parent or when they otherwise prove disappointing as sources of gratification. Being in such a predicament can be a powerful influence on children's development, particularly given their sensitivity to parental affect (Cummings, Iannotti, & Zahn-Waxler, 1985). Such systemic hypotheses are readily operationalizable and testable (Kitzmann & Rohrbaugh, in press), but to date they have received little attention in studies of the effects of parental conflict on children.

Although researchers have identified a connection between marital discord, parental depression and child behavior difficulties, there has been virtually no attention to the impact of life events that precipitate parental depression on children. Yet, as the divorce literature illustrates, major life events also disrupt parenting and children's well-being (Hetherington et al., 1989). Parents' attention is diverted from effective parenting as they deal emotionally and instrumentally with life crises like divorce. Children's sense of the coherence of their world is challenged by the disruption in relations with their parents, in their living arrangements, and in their economic security. They react with limit testing to establish the parameters of their world. Their obnoxious behavior toward parents may reflect both their sense of vulnerability and their anger about the disruption. These behaviors further tax custodial parents, usually mothers, who are already distressed by their loss, and whose sense of self-worth and expectations about the future are compromised.

In sum, the contextual factors like marital distress and serious life events that have been implicated in parental depression also influence children's lives directly and, through their impact on parenting, indirectly. Nonetheless, children also react to their circumstances and contribute to their parents' distress and parenting difficulties.

Children's contribution to depression in parents and parenting difficulties

Evidence from multiple sources and across multiple situations shows that children of depressed parents pose a greater challenge to effective parenting than the average child. The literature examining the impact of children's behavior on depressed parents is not a large one, but there are reasons to believe that child disturbance helps maintain parenting difficulties and parental depression. First, there is evidence that declines in maternal distress and improvements in the quality of parenting parallel the successful treatment of their children's behavior problems (Forehand, Wells, & Griest, 1980; Lytton, 1990; Patterson, 1982). For instance, drug-induced improvements in hyperactive children's compliance and attentiveness are paralleled by declines in aversive, controlling parenting (Barkley & Cunningham, 1979). Second, there is evidence of reciprocal relations between maternal depression and child behavior problems (Hammen, Burge, & Stansbury, 1990; Radke-Yarrow et al., 1988). Depressed mothers report more hostile interactions with their children than with their spouses (Weissman & Paykel, 1974). Observational studies substantiate that depressed mothers and their children engage in a reciprocal pattern of negativity and hostility. These patterns are evident even in infancy. Paralleling their depressed mothers' interactional pattern, children as young as three months direct their behavior toward their mothers less frequently, smile and express happiness less often and are more irritable and fussy. This unrewarding interactional style generalizes to strangers, in whom it evokes a negative response (Field et al., 1988).

Whatever the origins of the problematic interactional style shown by infants and children of depressed parents, it is clear that the feedback available to depressed parents from interactions with their children may help maintain depression by validating feelings of ineptitude, worthlessness and rejection. It is not just a matter of depressed mothers being self-critical because they view their interactions with their children as unsatisfactory. Children are a major source of criticism directed at depressed mothers and, thus, undermine their mothers' self-esteem. With single depressed mothers, children may be the primary source of criticism (Brown et al., 1990).

Difficult child behavior also may indirectly contribute to the maintenance of depression by providing another source of marital conflict and opportunity for spouses to criticize and to undermine one another. Finally, child difficulties that extend to schools and that involve illegal activities (e.g., substance abuse, stealing) will foster depression through the additional stressors they impose on the family system. Thus, adequate models of depression in the family and of the links between parental depression and child adjustment must incorporate the reactive characteristics of children and the systemic nature of the family.

Depressed Children and their Family Circumstances

Depression in children

Childhood depression is by far the most uncharted area with which we must contend in our efforts to construct a family systems model of depression. In the late 1970s, an article in *Psychological Bulletin* concluded that there was "insufficient and unsubstantial evidence" for the existence of depression in children (Lefkowitz & Burton, 1978), and standard psychoanalytic sources traditionally have outlined why the syndrome could not occur in childhood (Rie, 1966; Rochlin, 1959). In the past fifteen years, the field has moved from debates over the existence of childhood depression to an acceptance that depressive disorders in children are in important respects identical to those in adults. The basic phenomenology of major depressive disorder is quite similar from age six to old age and longitudinal studies show similar rates of recurrence and chronicity for childhood and adult depression (Cantwell, 1983; Keller et al., 1988; Kovacs, Feinberg, Crouse-Novak, Paulaskas, & Finkelstein, 1984).

Although it is now clear that even young children can be clinically depressed, it is fortunately an infrequent diagnosis. Based on a review of 14 epidemiological studies, Fleming and Offord (1990) reported a prevalence of 2–3% for major depressive disorder in unselected prepubertal children and concluded that the rate increases in adolescence. Rates of minor depression and dysthymia are thought to be somewhat higher (Kovacs et al., 1989). Even so, depressive disorders are considerably less prevalent in childhood than among adults, and most depressed adults were not depressed as children. Moreover, the majority of depressed children recover. They respond well to changes in their environments, and many show prompt recovery when hospitalized without further specific therapeutic intervention (Kashani, Carl-son, Beck, Hoeper, Corcoran, McAllister, Fallahi, Rosenberg, & Reid, 1987; Puig-Antich, Perel, Lupatkin, Chambers, Tabrizi, King, Goetz, Davies, & Stiller, 1987).

Nonetheless, clinical depression in childhood can have serious develop-mental consequences. Despite high recovery rates from initial episodes, the majority get depressed again before adulthood. In addition, early depression appears to carry a specific risk for adult depression (Harrington et al., 1990) and portends more frequent and more severe depressive episodes in adult-hood. Depressed children are also likely to develop another psychiatric condi-tion if they do not already have one and pure depression in children is rare (Fleming & Offord, 1990). Anxiety disorder is the most frequent comorbid diagnosis, followed by externalizing disorders like attention deficit disorder and conduct disorder, and substance abuse. In cases of comorbidity, depressive symptoms are often more severe. Thus, it is not surprising that clinical samples of depressed children will show particularly high rates of comorbidity.

About a third of depressed children are conduct disordered (Kashani et al., 1987), but the nature of the relationship between comorbid depression and conduct disorders is controversial. Complicating matters is the fact that the same symptoms may warrant the diagnosis of both disorders. While some sources suggest that conduct disorders are milder when associated with de-pression and remit when the depression is treated (Puig-Antich, 1982), other sources suggest that conduct disorders are no different when co-occurring with depression and that they persist beyond the depressive episode (Kovacs, Paulauskas, Gatsonis, & Richards, 1988). Undoubtedly this controversy re-flects differences in diagnostic practices as well as the mix of cases seen in particular settings.

Depression impedes educational progress and is linked with poor social competence and marked difficulties with social relationships. Existing re-search (e.g., Mullins, Peterson, Wonderlich, & Reaven, 1986; Peterson, Mullins, & Ridley-Johnson, 1985) suggests that depressed children may get caught up in the same interactional processes that have been described with adults (Coyne, 1976a, 1976b). Namely, they make both adults and peers uncomfortable and get rejected. Even children with high self-reported de-pressive symptoms have more aversive interactions with peers, spend more time alone, and are rated more negatively by peers (Altmann & Gotlib, 1988; Goodyer, Wright, & Altham, 1989; Kennedy, Spence, & Henaley, 1988). Again, however, clinically depressed children present more problems than the sadness and negative self-concept emphasized in these checklist-based re-search programs. These studies probably underestimate the difficulties that depressed children face themselves and pose for others, particularly in terms of aggression and impulsivity. Clinical experience suggests that depressed child-ren can make nonsense out of the best-conceived caretaking strategies. They deny the influence and satisfactions for which parents and teachers strive so hard, precipitate anger control problems in adults usually characterized by self-restraint, and sometimes leave others shocked and guilty about the strong reactions they elicit.

Family context of childhood depression

There are important similarities in families identified because of parental depression and families identified because of depression in a child. First, one half to two-thirds of parents of depressed children are themselves depressed (Puig-Antich et al., 1985a, 1985b). Parental depression is probably the most prevalent etiological factor in childhood depression. The association of other parental disorders with childhood depression may be spurious. It may reflect either co-morbidity between depression and another disorder in the diagnosed parent or disorders in the nondepressed parent, a consequence of assortative mating for psychopathology. Thus, parental alcoholism may appear to be associated with childhood depression. However, this is true only if one of the parents is also depressed (Merikangas, Weissman, Prusoff, Pauls, & Leckman, 1985). In summary, the apparent specificity of the association between depression in parents and their children together with the high rates of depression in the parents of depressed children and in the children of depressed parents suggest that these ostensively separate literatures are based on the same families.

Second, families of both depressed children and of depressed parents show similar parenting difficulties. Studies of clinically depressed children and of children with elevated depressive symptomatology characterize their families as emotionally distant, lacking in warmth, poor in emotion regulation and conflict resolution, and their parents as inconsistent, controlling and sometimes abusive (Amanat & Butler, 1984; Asarnow, Carlson, & Guthrie, 1987; Cole & Rehm, 1986; Kashani et al., 1987; Kaslow, Rehm, & Siegel, 1984; Poznanski & Zrull, 1970; Puig-Antich et al., 1985b). This description resembles the retrospective accounts of depressed adults about their childhood (Holmes & Robins, 1988; Parker, 1981, 1983; Perris, Arrindell, Perris, Eisemann, van der Ende, & von Knorring, 1986).

The literature on the family context of childhood depression is still woefully inadequate, but findings to date encourage us in our efforts to integrate it with our knowledge of depressed parents and the family context of depression. Yet, there is also a need for restraint in our speculations. The relative infrequency of childhood depression implies that children are relatively protected against it and cautions against glib statements implicating common family stressors as precipitants of childhood depression. The strong association of depression in children and parents suggests a particular direction to our inquiry. But, the cause of this association remains elusive. We still do not know the extent to which childhood depression reflects a particular constitutional vulnerability, something about the quality of relationship provided by a depressed parent, the social context that affords parental depression, or some complex confluence of these factors.

A Case Study of the Social Context of Depression

A brief clinical vignette illustrates the complexity of interpersonal processes in families with a depressed member. Anna is a 32-year-old woman suffering from major depression with endogenous features. She has been receiving antidepressant medication and individual counseling for the past three years. She was severely physically abused as a child by her father, and there is a suggestion of sexual abuse. She has always been wary of relationships with men, and after unsuccessful relationships with men in college, she experimented with lesbian relationships, which she also found unsatisfactory. Shortly after this period, a male friend who had been infatuated with her since high school returned from the military and sought her out. She became pregnant by him without deciding whether she wanted a relationship with any man. When they both dropped out of college and married, she was the closer of the pair to graduation. Ten years later, the couple has serious financial problems, and her decision to settle for an entry-level position at a grocery store is a continuing source of conflict. The husband works considerable overtime while attempting to complete a second year of college. Much of the time, the wife has supported and appreciated the husband's efforts to improve their financial situation, but during arguments, she complains that he has abandoned the family for his work. They now have a ten-year-old son who is clinically depressed. His depression was first diagnosed after referral for aggressiveness and disruptiveness in kindergarten. They also have a six-year-old daughter who has not been identified as having psychological problems.

Interactions occurring around the woman's efforts to get her son to do homework before her husband returns from work reveal some of the important interpersonal dynamics in this family. She states that she attempts to get the boy's homework done because she fears her husband's punitive style, which reminds her of her father's style. The son is extremely sensitive to actual or implied criticism and often reacts to her requests to complete his homework with a temper tantrum that does not subside fully until the next day. On these occasions, she gets angry and punitive and is guilt-ridden, irritable and exhausted by the time the husband returns. The ensuing argument with her husband may center on her lack of a cheerful greeting, his charges about her incompetence as a parent, his yelling at the son, or her charges that she shoulders an unfair share of the parenting responsibilities. The argument often shifts to their financial predicament, her lack of ambition and direction in her life, his absorption in his work, and finally, to the reasons they married.

Despite her own aversive exchanges with her son, the woman is protective of him, and frequently shifts to the son's side when her husband gets involved in disciplining him. On occasion, she has exaggerated her son's progress on his homework and this has undermined her credibility with her husband. In contrast to other family members, the daughter appears calm and nurturing, and both parents seek her out and indulge her. The son is outspoken about his resentment of this, and it is a theme in his angry complaints of being unloved. His sister is a frequent target of his aggression, although she appears to instigate hostile exchanges with him more than the parents acknowledge.

A Systems Perspective on Depression in Families

Depression typically arises in the context of conflicted relationships and severe life stress. Yet an adequate account of it must acknowledge that these conditions and how they are handled are influenced by the reactive characteristics of all family members and by their individual and shared histories. Like other family processes, those linking depression to the family are complex and probably involve multiple reciprocal feedback loops. Our appreciation of this complexity increases as we become more aware of the need to view depression as a life-course phenomenon that is associated with other risks and adversities. The heterogeneity of depression probably reflects the diversity of individual and family circumstances associated with it.

Nonetheless, three concepts have considerable heuristic value in understanding this diversity. Namely, family systems associated with depression can be characterized by a lack of coherence and agency and a general emotional dysregulation (Coyne, 1990). In invoking these concepts, we draw on their previous usages, but we will attempt to give them an integration and a systemic interpretation that has been underdeveloped in previous discussions.[1]

Coherence refers to the extent to which the family context supports a pervasive, enduring though dynamic confidence that life is predictable and safe and that things will work out as expected. We are, of course, borrowing from Antonovsky's (1979) notion of a sense of coherence, but even more than he, we wish to emphasize that coherence is not just a matter of an individual's cognitive appraisal. It is a transactional or contextual concept, taking as its focal unit persons-in-context. We have to look *both* at what the key persons think and what the family system affords. Particularly in the context of relationships that are already conflicted or attenuated, the kinds of events that provoke depression also threaten the meaningfulness and organization of family life. As Brown and Harris's (1978) work has highlighted, it takes a severe life event to do this. In the face of such an event, long-term goals may become unattainable or their realization put into doubt, and key

---

[1] Our use of the concepts of coherence and agency in understanding the family dysfunction associated with depression was inspired by a brief theoretical note by Ransom (1985). He invoked these concepts in a discussion of the role of families in health promotion, but we have found them to be more generally helpful in understanding emotional dysregulation in families.

commitments may be threatened, along with the sense of security and predictability that they support. Brown's work also emphasizes how the unfolding of severe events entails revelations and disappointments about significant others and shared lives (Brown, 1982).

The resulting loss of coherence may be seen in the disruption of routines. Many everyday activities are neither intrinsically rewarding nor justifiable outlays of effort except as they are appreciated by others or viewed as steps toward shared, attainable goals. With the loss of coherence, family members can get at cross purposes. They may differ in how they selectively withdraw from or remain invested in goals and activities, and this can add to their disappointment in each other. With a loss of coherence, trust in the good intentions and dependability of others is lost; personal control is emphasized over interdependency; and individual, short-term goals preempt collective, long-term ones. Because others are undependable and disagreements cannot be readily resolved, consensus and cooperation are not effectively sought. Long standing differences in philosophy or preferred ways of doing things may become more salient now that they are no longer suppressed by the negotiated compromises operating before the event. This can become particularly apparent in childrearing, when what is perceived as one parent's indulgence, harshness, or expediency in dealing with the children becomes an issue of conflict. Children can add to the deterioration of the situation with side-taking, limit-testing, or exploitation of the decline in order.

Agency refers to the degree to which a context affords a reliance on other people and routines to provide the scaffolding that allows one to pursue one's own personal agenda (Totman, 1979). It, too, is a transactional concept linking individuals to the affordance of their circumstances. The severe life events that provoke depression may be linked with loss of agency in several different ways. First, the agency that comes from established routines may be lost. For example, a particularly destructive aspect of losing a spouse involves the disruption of established, dependable routines like knowing that one will have dinner at a certain time each day. Second, the event may annihilate long-term cherished goals by removing a sense of purpose from mundane daily activitives. For example, a mother who dreams of having her child go to college may lose her motivation for getting up at 5 a.m. to go to her part-time job when her child dies. Third, the event may indirectly affect routines as when a financial crisis consumes the resources needed to sustain an particular life style. Fourth, the connection between the event and agency may be even more circuitous, as when the effort required to cope with the event leads to the neglect of other matters. The consequences of this neglect accumulate and impede getting things done efficiently. For example, when parents are coping with separation from their partner, their attention is diverted from the daily effort of parenting and the consistency that underlies smooth family life is lost.

Emotional dysregulation. There is a certain breeding quality to the misunderstandings, overt conflict, and upset in a family that lacks coherence and agency. Such a family system may become characterized by a general emotional dysregulation so that negative interactions are not repaired, disagreements are not resolved, negative affect becomes contagious, and there is little chance for negative affect to be transformed into positive (see also, Cicchetti, Ganiban, & Barnett, 1991; Cicchetti & Howes, 1991). The concept of emotional dysregulation and its synonyms are already familiar to developmental psychologists (Tronick, 1989), but in contrast to previous usage, we want to emphasize that emotional dysregulation in families is systemic or contextual rather than just dyadic. Furthermore, how irritability, hostility, and anger are handled may be as crucial as the handling of sadness and depression. Most studies of affective or emotional dysregulation in mother-infant interactions have emphasized still faces, flattened affect, simulated depression or clinical depression in mothers (see Cohn & Campbell, this volume). Aside from ethical limitations on the kinds of interactions that can be encouraged in the laboratory, overtly angry interactions between mother and infant are relatively infrequent and unlikely to be captured when the mothers are being observed and videotaped. For various reasons, then, discussions of emotional dysregulation in interactions between depressed persons and their infants have slighted the role of hostility.

In addition to being depressing, living in a family lacking in coherence and agency is likely to be frustrating and disappointing, and the families and individuals that compose them differ greatly in how they deal with such conditions. Akiskal (1989) proposed that persons who have early and frequent depressions may have a stormy style of dealing with negative affect. This style may precipitate interpersonal crises and shape how they are handled and there may be assortative mating for this trait. The style may not be apparent when family life is going well, but emerges and fuels emotional dysregulation once family life is disrupted. Focusing on related characteristics, Patterson (1982; see also Wahler & Dumas, 1989) also suggested that, under stress, some persons experience highly generalized disruptions in the quality of their social interactions with others. It is particularly difficult for them to contain their anger and irritability in the specific interactions that evoke these feelings.

This stormy style can, in a limited sense, be functional. Getting upset, having tantrums or emotional confrontations can serve as ways of regulating one's involvement in an emotionally dysregulated family and legitimizing withdrawal from chronically tense and uncertain circumstances. It also provides a temporary respite in the shared apologies or reconciliation that follow particularly hurtful encounters. While this relational style may represent enduring individual traits that emerge or become exaggerated under stress, some of its apparent consistency may reflect the enduring presence of particular people in someone's life, the history that is accumulated, and the kinds of relationships that are negotiated over time. These ways of dealing with tension, upset, and conflict can be "co-traits" that are elicited and exaggerated when family members are dealing with each other, but are largely absent when outsiders are involved.

We have noted that communication in families of depressed persons is often characterized by overt hostility and anger, on the one hand, and inhibition, avoidance, and withdrawal on the other. This style is probably a more general feature of emotionally dysregulated families. Most observational studies of families with a depressed member have involved structured problem-solving interactions with limited opportunities for participants' withdrawal. Even home observations of family interaction at dinner require that no one flee to the living room or escape the tense silence by turning on the television, and this is more of a break with routines than is acknowledged. To a greater extent than these studies suggest, daily life in emotionally dysregulated families may be a matter of family members' inhibition and avoidance of each other, punctuated by occasional unproductive disagreements and confrontations. Depressed persons and their spouses may be involved in a cycle where unsuccessful efforts to resolve differences by discussion or confrontation lead to longer periods of withdrawal and avoidance during which there is a further accumulation of negative affect, misunderstanding, mistrust, and misgivings about each other (Kahn, Coyne, & Margolin, 1985). The cumulative effects of stalemates overwhelm family members when they again attempt to settle specific differences, increasing further their pessimism about the possibility of improving their relationships.

We should also be sensitive to more subtle but pervasive effects of the social environment in our efforts to understand the behavior of depressed persons. Depressed persons can be confusing and frustrating in their inhibited style of communication, and this characteristic seems to endure beyond an episode of depression (Weissman & Paykel, 1974). Yet, this also reflects the inhibitory effect of their close relationships. Depressed persons often have histories of being the recipient of intimidation, verbal and physical abuse in close relationships (Andrews & Brown, 1988; Andrews, Brown, & Creasey, in press). Even if abusive behavior occurs infrequently, it is likely to have a profound influence. Because abusive behavior is likely to be suppressed during observational studies, these studies may provide a misleading portrait of how family interactions associated with depression are maintained in a particular form.

Hostile criticism is an important element of the negative interactions in families with a depressed person. It also has a number of direct and indirect effects in emotionally dysregulated families. It leaves recipients feeling badly about themselves and about their critics. It can derail efforts at problem-solving and reconciliation. Once introduced into an ongoing disagreement, hostile criticism and the resulting rebuttals and counter-accusations can replace the topic at hand and strengthen patterns of avoidance in the future. More generally, destructive criticism increases family members' reliance on ineffective ways of dealing with their conflicts and negative feelings (Baron, 1988).

Besides the direct induction of negative affect in overt conflict and hostile critical exchanges, there may be more pervasive, moment-to-moment processes in emotionally dysregulated families that dampen positive and promote negative affect, even to the point of negative affect becoming predominant. Attention to emotional regulation between adults and its effect on offspring lags behind progress in understanding these processes in mother-infant dyads (for exceptions, see Gottman & Fainsilber-Katz, 1989; Gottman & Levenson, 1988). Most work on adult depression still retains traditional notions of mood and affect as internal states secondary to cognition rather than as social processes in which others participate. There is little sense of the richness of the diverse processes by which emotional experience is shaped and regulated by persons in the environment, how they determine the unfolding of an episode of emotion and its outcome, or of how members of a family are "participants in an affective communication system" (Tronick, 1989).

Some of the same processes that have been identified in emotional regulation between mothers and young children (Thompson, 1990) can be seen as aspects of the more systemic emotional regulation in the family. Namely, there are processes of *contagion* and *social referencing* that allow negative affect to resonate through the family. Again, the processes are less well-documented in adults, but the value of considering them is supported by findings that even brief encounters with depressed persons can leave others distressed (Coyne, 1976a; Strack & Coyne, 1982), that interviewing physicians reflect patients' depression in their own behavior (Frey, Jorns, & Daw, 1980), and that students rooming with a depressed person show elevated depressive symptomatology (Burchill & Stiles, 1988). Although the phenomenon is not well studied, human adults, like infants and infrahuman mammals, attune to each other's emotional state with facial expression and vocal tone. Zajonc has provided provocative data indicating that married couples come to resemble each other physically because of habitual attunement or empathic mimicry of each other's facial expressions (Zajonc, Adelmann, Murphy, & Niedenthal, 1987).

Another process relevant to emotional regulation in families is *flooding*. Ekman (1984) has used this term to describe processes occurring in emotionally taxed individuals, but it can be given a more family-systemic interpretation. The notion is that against a background of generally negative affect, the experience of any particular negative affect may evoke other overwhelming negative affect. Thus, sadness may evoke anger and vice versa in an emotionally primed environment, and minor upsets and frustrations may evoke major upheavals.

Involvement in an emotionally dysregulated family is an important determinant of family members' ability to regulate their own emotions, but it is not the only determinant. Even infants are not solely dependent on caretakers to control their negative affect. Infants can cope with the negativity or unresponsiveness of caretakers by looking away, self-comforting, and self-stimulation, thereby shifting attention away from a disturbing interaction, or substituting positive for negative stimulation (Tronick, 1989). Analogously, older children and adults can engage in compensatory self-regulation, but the emotionally dysregulated family may limit the use of such options. The loss of coherence and agency may reduce the occurrence of previously rewarding activities. One cannot depend on the positive affect or encouragement of others or enlist them in previously shared activities. Breaking away and engaging in activities that do not involve the family may be negatively sanctioned as signs of rejection or abandonment in a context that has been sensitized to such themes and in which guilt-induction has become a way of relating.

Perhaps the most powerful barrier to depressed persons disengaging from the emotional dysregulation of the family is that they have committed their wellbeing to the quality of family life and their self-concept to the opinions of family members. They thus allow their own wellbeing to depend on the resolution of family difficulties. The upset and conflict in their families become problems to be solved before depressed persons can tend to themselves. Depressed persons may lament that they are hopeless or helpless, but they persist in miscarried problem-solving as if holding on to a desperate hope that they can make a crucial difference.

In our society at least, females may be more responsive to other people's distress and more willing to subordinate their wellbeing to its resolution (Belle, 1982; Wethington, McLeod, & Kessler, 1987). For depressed mothers to do otherwise would be to accept failure as a parent and would involve the immense guilt of having renounced a fundamental commitment to be a caring person. Sadly, depressed mothers may be too invested in caring for their children and resolving the family's problems to take care of themselves in a way that would allow them to be effective in these tasks. On the other hand, their husbands may lack such a strength of commitment, construe family involvement as discretionary rather than mandatory, and find excuses in the unpleasantness of home life for escape into work or the local tavern. The literature on divorce and marital discord alerts us to ways in which some children, like depressed mothers, may assume an unrealistic sense of responsibility for family problems and ineptly intervene to solve them (Emery, 1982). Zahn-Waxler and Kochanska (1990) reported that even very young children are negatively aroused emotionally by exposure to conflict and distress in others. Two-year-olds become sad and angry, scold the parent they see as the aggressor and comfort the perceived victim. By early school years, they more actively try to end quarrels and reconcile angry parents. Like depressed adults, depressed children may be involved in struggles that they cannot resolve, but upon which their sense of security and well-being depends.

Role of the depressed adult

Depression can be seen as a reaction to being in an emotionally dysregulated family or a way of coping with it. But depression also contributes to the complex reciprocal processes that maintain family dysregulation. One consequence of depression researchers' preoccupation with mildly distressed college students is the neglect of the personal and social costs of clinical depression. Being depressed can be a pervasive negative influence on someone's life and a source of considerable impairment. Family members living with a depressed person can find it difficult to maintain their own wellbeing. For our purposes, three features of depression are particularly important: the anergia, displays of obvious distress, and changes in emotional reactivity.

In focus group discussions, persons who suffered from recurrent depression emphasized how different the experience is from being sad or upset (Coyne & Calarco, 1990). A common complaint was the enormous difficulty they had getting anything done when in an episode of depression. They may be facing stress and their family life may be troubled, but once they become depressed their depression could overshadow other family difficulties. In addition to the obstacles posed by their family circumstances, they felt slowed down, inefficient, disorganized, and easily tired. As one patient described it, life was like floundering in molasses. Simple tasks like planning and executing a meal become overwhelming. Once initiated, tasks seem more manageable, but proceed less efficiently than in the past, and the depressed person may be readily deterred by small obstacles, quickly feel exhausted, and derive little or no satisfaction from getting done. Being receptive and responsive to others, even to the extent demanded by a simple phone call, may feel overwhelming; being attentive or affectionate with a spouse or child, even more so. A family system that already lacks coherence and agency and is emotionally dysregulated can be further strained when a key person, particularly the wife and mother, becomes impaired by depression. The depressed person's dysfunction adds to the disorganization of the family, and the family's upset over what is inexplicable and seemingly willful ineptitude can precipitate open conflict and critical, accusatory exchanges that increase the depressed person's dysfunction.

As spelled out in earlier papers (Coyne, 1976a, 1976b), displays of obvious distress by depressed persons have the effect of engaging others, making them feel responsible, and thereby shifting the interactional burden onto them. Depressed persons' distress proves aversive to others and can put them in a negative mood. Yet, at the same time, it is also guilt-inducing and inhibiting. People around depressed persons may try to control the depressed person's aversiveness by seemingly providing what the depressed person wants, even while communicating impatience, hostility, and rejection. This subtle communication further validates depressed persons' sense of insecurity, and elicits renewed expressions of distress, escalating the pattern. Thus, others may become involved with depressed persons in ways that unwittingly perpetuate or aggravate their problems. An interactional stalemate may be the result. Aside from the direct effects of getting caught up in such a pattern, everyone involved may find it more difficult to be pleasant and responsive to each other, maintain a household, deal with other problems that they face, or simply hold the discussions necessary to renegotiate their relationships (Coyne, Burchill, & Stiles, 1991).

The Oregon Research Institute (ORI) group (Biglan, Hops, & Sherman, 1988; Hops et al., 1987) has done an excellent job of refining these notions and demonstrating the hypothesized processes with sequential analyses of observations of interactions in the families of depressed persons. Drawing on Patterson and Reid's (1970) coercion theory, the ORI group conceptualizes depressive behavior as a form of aversive control. Using videotapes of the families of depressed persons in their homes, they found that depressive behavior may, in the short run, inhibit hostile behavior and elicit compliance from others, even though it also serves to suppress caring behavior and increases the likelihood of subsequent hostility.

Patterson (1982) has suggested that people differ greatly in how they handle being depressed. Some depressed persons can be particularly aversive with their incessant displays of distress and discussion of their problems, so that interactions with them become unidimensional. On the other hand, depressed persons in our focus group at the University of Michigan Depression Program reported working hard to control their indications of distress, because they are well aware of its negative consequences for relationships (Coyne & Calarco, 1990). We suspect that in many circumstances they succeed, but in some families, family members, particularly children, become highly sensitive to subtle signs of distress, attempt to mind-read the depressed person and overreact to small fluctuations in the depressed person's mood. In other families, relationships are so attenuated and the isolation and rejection of the depressed person is so severe that to gain any attention or assistance the depressed person must maintain a high level of obvious distress. The depressed person is left with few other ways of getting acknowledgement and sympathy or of reducing other people's demands, even if the aversiveness of such depressive displays ensures that family members remain distant.

About 10–15% of depressed patients are not particularly sad or blue (Whybrow, Akiskal, & McKinney, 1984). They are identified instead by loss of the ability to experience pleasure or satisfaction or a general emotional numbing or blunting. The inability to register pleasure or to express enthusiasm and affection can fuel the emotional dysregulation of their families, particularly if family members personalize this or make their own mood contingent on getting a positive response from the depressed person.

Although they may report being emotionally numbed, depressed persons' emotional negativity is not usually as blunted as their positive affect. Indeed, the slightest provocation may elicit tearfulness or angry outbursts. Further, because of their emotional lability they may become frustrated and hostile as readily as they become sad. They may recognize the inappropriate emotionality of their response, and assert that their reaction is unjustified, and yet get further upset. The temper outbursts of depressed persons and their difficulty regulating the intensity of their anger has received little attention in the literature, but family members frequently complain about this aspect of their behavior. Depressed persons' temper tantrums can alternately intimidate or disinhibit family members. Particularly when family members have suppressed their own hostility for fear of further upsetting them, depressed persons' outbursts can unleash counterattacks in which family members' pent up frustrations are cruelly expressed.

Role of the nondepressed adult

In our review of the literature, we attempted to identify how the spouses of depressed persons are involved in the occurrence of depression in their families, in how it is handled, and in their children's lives. Adversity in spouses' background may be tied to their reactive characteristics and their current life circumstances. These, in turn, may limit the quality of the marital relationship and degree of intimacy that is achieved and, in addition, generate serious life events for the family. Following serious events, spouses may play a key role in how emotional dysregulation comes to characterize the family. Our purpose is not to imply that depressed women are the hapless victims of their husbands, but rather to suggest how characteristics of these men might help to explain how depression comes about and why depression is often a marker for a family with many other problems.

The relationship between depressed persons and their spouses may be characterized by both similarity and complementarity. Spouses may be similar in having pre-existing difficulties in handling issues of impulsivity, closeness and distance, anger and dependency. Both depressed persons and their spouses are more destructive and less constructive than control couples in their ways of dealing with conflict, and members of couples that include a depressed person show strong similarities in conflict management style (Coyne, 1990).

Complementarity refers to the tendency of interpersonal actions "to invite, pull, elicit, draw, entice, or evoke 'restricted classes' of reactions from persons with whom we interact, especially from significant others" (Kiesler, 1983, p. 198). For example, depressed women are often characterized as chronically insecure and lacking in self-confidence. Because depressed persons' difficulties have usually been viewed as "role impairments" (Weissman & Paykel, 1974), their spouses' involvement in evoking expressions of difficulty are obscured. Fears of loss and rejection and continual demands for reassurance, comfort and support are often evoked by a spouse's criticism, denigration, and threats of abandonment. As Leff and Vaughn (1985) have noted, "few depressed patients described as chronically insecure or lacking in self-confidence were living with supportive or sympathetic spouses . . . when this was the case, the patients were well at followup" (p. 95). Thus, it is easy to see how depressed persons are maintained in their fear of loss and rejection by their spouses.

Depression is likely to arise in the context of a troubled marriage, but even in the absence of prior marital distress, the marital relationships of depressed persons can become strained. Spouses who have not been educated about depression may find their depressed partners confusing and may take their problems personally. They may oscillate from being solicitous and indulgent to demanding that depressed persons immediately snap out of their state. Spouses also may shift from putting their own lives on hold to help their depressed partner recover to threatening to leave the relationship and with-drawing emotionally from it. They may find it difficult to accept that decisive action on their part will not cure their spouse, and inadvertently make every-one more miserable by trying too hard to fix things (Coyne, Wortman, & Lehman, 1988). From a family systems perspective, it is important to ask not only why or how problems come about, but also why they persist (Bateson, 1972; Watzlawick, Jackson, & Beavin, 1967). For instance, while it is under-standable that symptoms of depression would impede effective parenting, there is the obvious, but neglected, question of why the nondepressed parent does not fill in for the impaired partner. When the nondepressed parent is well-adjusted and available to the children, their risk for psychopathology is substantially reduced (see Downey & Coyne, 1990, for a review).

For the most part, however, theorists and researchers have gone easy on the spouses of depressed persons and have not considered why nondepressed partners do not more readily compensate for the limitations on depressed persons' functioning. Our review of the literature suggests a number of possi-bilities. First, the spouses of depressed persons often bring their own limita-tions to the family and may simply lack the skills and experience needed to become a more active parent. Indeed, they are more likely than the average father to be negatively involved with their children (Andrews et al., in press; Quinton & Rutter, 1988). Second, as we have argued, the apparent impair-ment and lack of skills of depressed parents may be seen more appropriately as a systemic problem. The inability to enforce rules and to maintain consistency may reflect a more general lack of coherence and agency in such families rather than a simple lack of parenting skill. The high rate of hostile, critical exchanges between the depressed parent and children may be a general char-acteristic of these emotionally dysregulated families. Indeed, conflict over parenting may become a salient marital issue and overt marital conflict may preclude effective parenting. The solution of the nondepressed husband may be to abdicate the tasks of parenting completely to the depressed mother (Dadds, 1987). This reflects societal acceptance that fathers' involvement in the daily tasks of parenting is discretionary. The implicit acceptance of this position by theorists and researchers is demonstrated in their neglect of fathers in efforts to explain the difficulties between depressed mothers and their children. Clearly, clinical evidence of the father's reduced involvement in parenting in families with a depressed mother needs more scrutiny from researchers: Does reduced involvement precede and foster the difficulties between depressed mothers and their children? To what extent do the ensuing child difficulties and both parents' inability to cope with the difficulties serve to justify the nondepressed parent's further withdrawal?

Role of the depressed child

Although some research has shown that even mildly depressed children make peers and teachers uncomfortable and consequently get rejected, there has been little attention to the nature of depressed children's involvement in their families. Aside from their sadness, symptoms such as their anergia, loss of pleasure in previously rewarding activities, and difficulty in concentration may go ignored except as expressed in refusals to do chores, ineptness in completing them, and, importantly, school problems. Power struggles frequently erupt around these symptoms. It can be difficult for parents and teachers not to see such behavior as spiteful and directed at them personally. Of course, depressed children may be indeed angry and defiant toward the adults in their lives, but adults' tendency to personalize their behavior and become upset may confer a power on the children that they did not know they had and may not even want. Already feeling badly about themselves and impaired in their behavior, they may find the criticism and even rage directed at them daunting and further disabling. Such reactions from adults only serve to validate the children's belief that they live in a harsh, unfair, unpredictable environment.

Even when depressed children do not meet criteria for a conduct disorder, they are generally intensely angry (Brumbeck, Dietz-Schmidt, & Weinberg, 1977). Their angry behavior can be more salient than their depression, and may distract adults from their primary mood disturbance. Teachers, parents, and clinicians who fall into the trap of concentrating on these children's anger while ignoring their depression, may find that their usually effective approaches do not work. Often there is no apparent pattern to fluctuations in a depressed child's level of anger and no apparent precipitant to angry outbursts.

Clinically, conduct disorders of depressed children often have a different quality to them. There is an emotionality to children with comorbid depression and conduct disorder that is qualitatively different from that in children with only a conduct disorder. Problems with anger control, intolerance for frustration, and temper outbursts are likely to fluctuate with mood or to be triggered by depressive themes of rejection and injustice. A clinical example illustrates this. After days of uncharacteristically good behavior and no reports of problems at school, a 10-year-old depressed boy's father asked him at dinner if he wanted to go shopping that evening to get some new clothes. The boy readily agreed, and his father mentioned that he should try on some recently purchased pants before they go. If the pants fitted him, he would get a matching shirt. Otherwise the pants would be exchanged. At this point, the boy threw his dinner on the floor, yelled at his father "You're the mean fat ass, just look at you", and ran to his room crying. It was not until the next week that the father realized how sensitive the boy was about the weight gain associated with his use of antidepressant medication and that the boy had interpreted his father's suggestion as criticism.

For their part, depressed children may sometimes appear irrational and self-defeating in their instigation of needless conflicts with parents, but there is often a pattern to their behavior. They may be extremely reactive to overt conflict between their parents, and a particularly intense parental argument or an overheard threat of separation may be followed by days of acting out. They may succeed in detouring the parental conflict and even in getting scape-goated. Depression researchers have given little attention to such triadic patterning of behavior, but family systems therapists frequently comment on it (e.g., Minuchin, 1985). Therapists sometimes offer the parents the interpretation that the child is intervening to unite them as parents; however, from the child's point of view, it may be simply be a matter of alternately being terrorized and exploiting the disagreements between the parents.

Despite an inattention to their children's internalizing symptoms, parents may intermittently be aware of their children's distress and it may deter them from effectively disciplining the child. A depressed child's distress may elicit consoling behavior and indulgence when limit-setting may be more appropriate. The mother of a depressed child, particularly when depressed herself, may have to struggle against her own empathic responses and urges to salve the child's hurt feelings and protect the child from punishment. Efforts to be an effective parent under these circumstances can be paralyzed as much by empathy as by anger. Conflict between the parents may be precipitated by one parent intervening to protect a depressed child from the disciplinary efforts of the other, or covertly restoring privileges that the other has withdrawn. Parental roles may be reversed when such concessions fail to increase compliance or cheer up the depressed child, and the previously indulgent parent overreacts in a way that brings the intervention of the other.

Extrafamilial influences

Even relatively isolated families remain to some degree open systems and susceptible to influences originating from outside the family. Wahler (1980), for instance, has shown that aversive exchanges between isolated single-parent mothers and persons in the extrafamilial environment reverberate in the mothers' negative interactions with their children. We can identify four key ways which the extrafamilial environment may influence the emotionally dysregulated families of depressed persons.

First, the extrafamilial environment may be a source of stress that further taxes the family. As we have noted, some of the accumulated disadvantages of depressed persons and their spouses may be reflected in environmental adversity and in troubled relationships beyond the immediate family. For instance, extended family members may share extensive histories of conflict and serve as major sources of stress. McGuffin and Bebbington (1988) have noted the familial transmission of the tendency to experience interpersonal stressors, and Hammen (1991) has commented on the stress-generating capabilities of the extended families of depressed persons. The extrafamilial environment also may react in an untimely and noncontingent fashion. For example, the family of a previously undiagnosed depressed adolescent received treatment during the summer so that when he returned to school in the fall his behavior problems at school were markedly reduced. However, largely because of his reputation from the previous year, he was expelled following a fight with a boy with whom there was a long standing animosity. The principal and irate parents of classmates prevailed over the boy's teacher and parents.

Second, the extrafamilial environment may make demands that are well within the capabilities of a normally functioning family, but that are major stressors for one that lacks coherence and agency and that is emotionally dysregulated. Meeting deadlines and being punctual for social obligations, or effectively advocating for their children at school may be beyond the capabilities of the families of depressed persons. Even subdromal depressive symptoms are associated with more days in bed and impairment in daily life than are chronic medical conditions such as diabetes, arthritis, and hypertension (Wells, Stewart, Hays et al., 1990). Clinical depression is likely to have an even more profound effect on daily life than subdromal depressive symptoms.

Third, the larger environment may legitimize the withdrawal of the nondepressed parent from the family. In our culture, gender-differentiated role expectations sanction husbands' withdrawal from family troubles into work and extrafamilial activities and they sanction the depressed women remaining isolated at home. Thus, cut off from outside influences, depressed women may become overwhelmed in their efforts to solve the family's problems on their own.

Finally, the extrafamilial environment may be a positive influence, even compensating for the negative effect of the family on its members' well-being by providing them with the means of withdrawing and developing self-regulatory capacities that are independent of the family's difficulties. Positive peer relationships, neighbors, and well-functioning members of the extended family may provide the support and stability that the family cannot. Depressed women working outside the home show less social dysfunction at work than at home and, overall, they appear less impaired than women who remain at home (Weissman & Paykel, 1974). Achievement at school and involvement in extracurricular activities may reduce some of the risk shown by children of depressed parents. Yet, the positive influences exerted by the extrafamilial environment may depend on the ability of family members to engage it, and those who are most in need may be least able to derive any benefit.

Summary and Conclusions

We began by observing that depression is concentrated in particular families and that both parental and child depression are markers for families with other problems and with other troubled family members. Our explication of these observations took us into an exploration of how the childhood and adolescent experience of both depressed persons and their spouses may be reflected in their families' current circumstances. We also considered the processes by which major life stressors may reverberate in families already characterized by conflictful and attenuated relationships. Finally, we explored the exchanges between these families and the larger environment. While contextualizing some problems that are usually reduced to the role impairments and other shortcomings of depressed persons, we were careful to highlight the difficulties that depressed adults and children pose for other family members. Although the presence of a depressed person may indeed be a marker for other family problems, we should not ignore the profound impact of depression on a family.

At the outset, we acknowledged some limits to the empirical data available for this exercise. These include the selectivity of samples that have been studied and the discrepancies between these samples and the typical depressed adults and children to whom researchers wish to generalize; the lack of attention to the spouses of depressed persons; and the limited literature on the family context of childhood depression. Yet, as we proceeded, other limitations on the available literature became apparent and we believe that several of these topics also should receive priority in future research. Namely:

1. In identifying possible reasons for the strong association between parental depression and problems in their offspring, we were able to generate ample alternative explanations for externalizing problems of these children; however, we made little progress in explaining the apparent specificity of their risk for clinical depression. More complex processes may be involved, and they may well involve a confluence of environmental and constitutional factors.

2. Although there has been progress in tracing some patterning of dyadic interactions in the families of depressed persons, exploration of triadic or more systemic patterns is needed. Family systems thinking has had little impact on research on depression.

3. There has been scant attention to how depressed parents interact with and affect their children beyond infancy in ways other than the administration of discipline and little·attention to any positive impact that depressed parents have on their children. Although we know that children of depressed parents vary considerably in adjustment, we have little sense of how some depressed parents manage to buffer their children from their circumstances whereas other depressed parents do not.

4. There has been little attention as to why nondepressed spouses do not more adequately compensate for the depressed persons' limitations as parents.

We also proposed a set of concepts to organize a perspective on the processes by which stress in the context of already troubled relationships might generate the proximal family conditions associated with depression. Specifically, we outlined how loss of coherence and agency might result in an emotionally dysregulated family and how, in turn, depression may contribute to the perpetuation of such family conditions. Our model is more clinical and descriptive than formal. We believe that there is a pressing need for concepts that will stimulate a broader sampling of the particulars of the lives of depressed persons. The most useful thing that new models can do is to guide our process of discovery, rather than constrain us to prematurely specific hypotheses. Too much of current theory and research fails to adequately convey a sense of what it is like to be depressed or to live with a depressed person. We need theory-informed, but phenomena-driven research (Coyne & Downey, 1991; Coyne et al., 1990). We must be conscious that there are limits to concepts and that our crisp theoretical distinctions may not map well into separable factors in the lives of depressed persons and their families. When one takes a life course perspective that is senstitive to how recurrent depression can shape the handling of adult developmental tasks, it should not be surprising that distinctions among personal background, stress, support, and coping become blurred.

REFERENCES

Akiskal, H.S. (1991). An integrating perspective on recurrent mood disorders: The mediating role of personality. In J. Becker & A. Kleinman (eds.), *Psychosocial aspects of depression* (pp. 215–236). Hillsdale, N.J.: Erlbaum.

Akiskal, H.S. (1989). New insights into the nature and heterogeneity of mood disorders. *Journal of Clinical Psychiatry, 50*, 6–12.

Altmann, E.O., & Gotlib, I.H. (1988). The social behavior of depressed children: An observational study. *Journal of Abnormal Child Psychology, 16*, 29–44.

Amanat, E., & Butler, C. (1984). Oppressive behaviors in the families of depressed children. *Family Therapy, 11*, 67–77.

Andrews, B., & Brown, G.W. (1988). Marital violence in the community: A biographical approach. *British Journal of Psychiatry, 153*, 305–312.

Andrews B., Brown G.W., & Creasey L. (in press). Intergenerational links between psychiatric disorder in mothers and daughters: The role of parenting experiences. *Journal of Child Psychology and Psychiatry.*

Angst, J. (1986). The course of affective disorders. *Psychopathology, 19*, 47–52.

Antonovsky, A. (1979). *Health, stress, and coping.* San Francisco: Jossey-Bass.

Arkowitz, H., Holliday, S., & Hutter, M. (1982). *Depressed women and their husbands: A study of marital interaction and adjustment.* Paper presented at the Annual Meeting of the Association for the Advancement of Behavior Therapy, November.

Asarnow, J.R., Carlson, G.A., & Guthrie, D. (1987). Coping strategies, self-perceptions, hopelessness, and perceived family environments in depressed and suicidal children. *Journal of Counseling and Clinical Psychology, 55*, 361–66.

Barkley, R., & Cunningham, E. (1979). The use of psychopharmacology to study influences in parent-child interactions. *Journal of Abnormal Child Psychology, 9*, 303–310.

Baron, R.A. (1988). Negative effects of destructive criticism: Impact on conflict, self-efficacy, and task performance. *Journal of Applied Psychology, 73*, 199–207.

Bateson, G. (1972). *Steps toward an ecology of the mind.* New York: Ballentine.

Beardslee, W.R., Bemporad, J., Keller, M.B., & Klerman, G.K. (1983). Children of parents with an affective disorder: A review. *American Journal of Psychiatry, 140*, 825–832.

Beardslee, W.R., Keller, M.B., Lavori, P.W., Klerman, G.K., Dorer, D.J., & Samuelson, H. (1988). Psychiatric disorder in adolescent offspring of parents with affective disorder in a non-referred sample. *Journal of Affective Disorders, 15*, 313–22.

Belle, D. (1982). The stress of caring: women as providers of social support. In L. Goldberger & S. Breznitz (eds.), *Handbook of Stress*. New York: Free Press (pp. 496–505).

Bettes, B. (1988). Maternal depression and motherese: Temporal and intonational features. *Child Development, 59*, 1089–1096.

Biglan, A., Hops, H., & Sherman, L. (1988). Coercive family processes and maternal depression. In R. J. McMahon & R. DeV. Peter (eds.), *Marriages and families: Systems approaches* (pp. 72–103). New York: Bruner-Mazel.

Biglan, A., Hops, H., Sherman, L., Friedman, L., Arthur, J., & Osteen, V. (1985). Problem solving interactions of depressed mothers and their spouses. *Behavior Therapy, 16*, 431–451.

Billings, A.G., & Moos, R.H. (1983). Comparison of children of depressed and nondepressed parents: A social environmental perspective. *Journal of Abnormal Child Psychology, 11*, 483–6.

Birtchnell, J. (1980). Women whose mothers died in childhood: An outcome study. *Psychological Medicine, 10*, 699–713.

Black, D.W., Bell, S., Hulbert, J., & Nasrallah, A. (1988). The importance of Axis II disorders in patients with major depression: A controlled study. *Journal of Affective Disorders, 14*, 115–122.

Breslau, N., & Davis, G.C. (1986). Chronic stress and major depression. *Archives of General Pyciatry, 43*, 309–314.

Breier, A., Kelsoe, J.C., Kirwin, P.D., Beller, S.A., Wolkowitz, O.M., & Pickar, D. (1988). Early parental loss and development of adult psychopathology. *Archives of General Psychiatry, 45*, 87–93.

Bronfenbrenner, U. (1978). Who needs parent education? *Teachers College Record, 79*, 773–774.

Brown, G.W. (1982). Accounts, meaning and causality. In G.M. Gilbert & P. Abell (eds.), *Accounts and action* (pp. 35–38). Aldershot: Gower.

Brown, G.W., Bifulco, A., & Andrews, B. (1990). Self-esteem and depression: 3. Aetiological issues. *Social Psychiatry and Psychiatric Epidemiology, 25*, 235–243.

Brown, G.W., Craig, T.K.J., & Harris, T.O. (1985). Depression: Disease or distress? Some epidemiological considerations. *British Journal of Psychiatry, 147*, 612–22.

Brown, G.W., & Harris, T. (1978). *Social origins of depression: A study of psychiatric disorder in women*. New York: Free Press.

Brown, G.W., & Harris, T.O. (1987). Stressors and aetiology of depression: A comment on Hallstrom. *Acta Psychiatrica Scandinavica, 73*, 383–89.

Brugha, T., Bebbington, P., Tennant, C., & Hurry, J. (1985). The list of threatening experiences: A subset of 12 life event categories with considerable long-term contextual threat. *Psychological Medicine, 15*, 189–91.

Brumbeck, R.A., Dietz-Schmidt, S., & Weinberg, W.A. (1977). Depression in children referred to an educational diagnosis center. *Diseases of the Nervous System, 38*, 529–35.

Burchill, S.A.L., & Stiles, W.B. (1988). Interactions of depressed college students with their roommate: Not necessarily negative. *Journal of Personality & Social Psychology, 55*, 410–419.

Cantwell, D.P. (1983). Depression in childhood: Clinical picture and diagnostic criteria. In D.P. Cantwell & G.A. Carlson (eds.), *Affective disorders in childhood and adolescence: An update* (pp. 3–18). New York: Spectrum Publishers.

Cicchetti, D., Ganiban, J., & Barnett, D. (1991). Contributions from the study of high risk populations to understanding the development of emotion regulation. In J.

Garber & K. Dodge (eds.), *The development of emotion regulation and dysregulation* (pp. 15–48). New York: Cambridge University Press.

Cicchetti, D., & Howes, P. (1991). Developmental psychopathology in the context of the family: Illustrations from the study of child maltreatment. *Canadian Journal of Behavioural Science, 23*, 257–281.

Cicchetti, D., & Schneider-Rosen, K. (1986). An organizational approach to childhood depression. In M. Rutter, C. Izard, & P. Read (eds.), *Depression in young people: Clinical and developmental perspectives* (pp. 71–134). New York: Guilford.

Cicchetti, D., Toth, S., & Bush, M. (1988). Developmental psychopathology and incompetence in childhood: Suggestions for intervention. In B. Lahey & A. Kazdin (eds.), *Advances in clinical child psychology* (pp. 1–71). New York: Plenum.

Cole, D.A., & Rehm, L.P. (1986). Family interaction patterns and childhood depression. *Journal of Abnormal Child Psychology, 14*, 297–314.

Cox, A.D., Puckering, C., Pound, A., & Mills, M. (1987). The impact of maternal depression on young children. *Journal of Child Psychology and Psychiatry, 28*, 917–928.

Coyne, J.C. (1976a). Toward an interactional description of depression. *Psychiatry, 39*, 28–40.

Coyne, J.C. (1976b). Depression and the response of others. *Journal of Abnormal Psychology, 85*, 186–193.

Coyne, J.C. (November, 1990). *Depression and marital problems.* Paper presented at the Annual Meeting of Association for the Advancement of Behavior Therapy, San Francisco.

Coyne, J.C., Burchill, S.A.L., & Stiles, W.B. (1991). An interactional perspective on depression. In C.R. Snyder & D.O. Forsyth (eds.), *Handbook of Social and Clinical Psychology: The Health Perspective.* NY: Pergamon (pp. 327–349).

Coyne, J.C., & Calarco, M. (1990). *The experience of recurrent depression: Themes from focus group discussions.* Unpublished manuscript. University of Michigan Medical Center.

Coyne, J.C., & Downey, G. (1991). Social factors in psychopathology. *Annual review of psychology, 42*, 401–425.

Coyne, J.C., Kessler, R.C., Tal, M., Turnbull, J., Wortman, C., & Greden, J. (1987). Living with a depressed person: Burden and psychological distress. *Journal of Consulting and Clinical Psychology, 55*, 347–352.

Coyne, J.C., Wortman, C.B., & Lehman, D.R. (1988). The other side of support: Emotional overinvolvement and miscarried helping. In B.H. Gottleib (ed.), *Marshalling social support* (pp. 305–330). New York: Sage.

Crnic, K.A., Greenberg, M.T., Ragozin, N., Robinson, N.M., & Basham, R.B. (1983). Effects of stress and social support on mothers of premature and full-term infants. *Child Development, 54*, 209–217.

Cummings, E.M., Iannotti, R.J., & Zahn-Waxler, C. (1985). Influence of conflict between adults on the emotions and aggression of young children. *Developmental Psychology, 21*, 495–507.

Dadds, M.R. (1987). Families and the origins of child behavior problem. *Family Process, 26*, 341–55.

Dadds, M.R., Sanders, M.R., Behrens, B.C., & James, J.E. (1987). Marital discord and child behavior problems: A description of family interactions during treatment. *Journal of Clinical Child Psychology, 16*, 192–203.

Depue, R.A., & Monroe, S.M. (1986). Conceptualization and measurement of human disorder in stress research: The problem of chronic disturbance. *Psychological Bulletin, 99*, 36–51.

Dohrenwend, B.P., Shrout, P.E., Link, B.G., Skodol, A.E., & Martin, J.L. (1986). Overview and initial results from a risk factor study of depression and schizophrenia. In J.E.

Barrett (ed.), *Mental disorders in the community: Progress and challenge* (pp. 184–215). New York: Guilford Press.

Downey, G., & Coyne, J.C. (1990). Children of depressed parents: An integrative review. *Psychological Bulletin, 108,* 50–76.

Downey, G., Tiedje, L.B., & Wortman, C.B. (1991). *Work stress, effortful parenting and child distress: A longitudinal study of mothers in demanding occupations.* Paper presented at the Annual Meetings of the National Council on Family Relations, Denver, CO., November, 1991

Ekman, P. (1984). Expression and the nature of emotion. In K.P. Scherer & P. Ekman (eds.), *Approaches to emotion* (pp. 319–343). Hillsdale, NJ: Lawrence Erlbaum.

Emery, R. (1982). Interpersonal conflict and the children of discord and divorce. *Psychological Bulletin, 92,* 310–330.

Emery, R., Weintraub, S., & Neale, J. (1982). Effects of marital discord on the school behavior of children of schizophrenic, affectively disordered, and normal parents. *Journal of Abnormal Child Psychology, 16,* 215–225.

Fendrich, M., Warner, V., & Weissman, M.M. (1990). Family risk factors, parental depression, and psychopathology in offspring. *Developmental Psychology, 26,* 40–50.

Field, T., Healy, B., Goldstein, S., Perry, S., Bendell, D., Schramberg, S., Zimmerman, E., & Kuhn, G. (1988). Infants of depressed mothers show "depressed" behavior even with nondepressed adults. *Child Development, 60,* 1569–79.

Fisher, L., Kokes, R.F., Harder, D.W., & Jones, J.E. (1980). Child competence and psychiatric risk: VI. Summary and integration of findings. *Journal of Nervous and Mental Disease, 168,* 353–355.

Fleming, J.E., & Offord, D.R. (1990). Epidemiology of childhood depressive disorders. *Journal of the American Academy of Child and Adolescent Psychiatry, 29,* 571–580.

Forehand, R., Wells, K., & Griest, D. (1980). An examination of the social validity of a parent training program. *Behavior Therapy, 11,* 488–502.

Frey, S., Jorns, U., & Daw, W.A. (1980). A systematic description and analysis of nonverbal interaction between doctors and patients in a psychiatric interview. In S.A. Corson (ed.), *Ethology and nonverbal communication in mental health* (pp. 231–298). New York: Pergamon Press.

Gerlsma, C., Emmelkamp, P.M., & Arrindell, W.A. (1990). Anxiety, depression, and perception of early parenting: A meta-analysis. *Clinical Psychology Review, 10,* 251–277.

Goodyer, I.M., Wright, C., & Altham, P.M. (1988). Maternal adversity and recent stressful events in anxious and depressed children. *Journal of Child Psychology and Psychiatry, 29,* 651–658.

Goodyer, I.M., Wright, C., & Altham, P.M. (1989). Recent friendships in anxious and depressed school age children. *Psychological Medicine, 19,* 165–74.

Gordon, D., Burge, D., Hammen, C., Adrian, C., Jaenicke, C., & Hiroto, D. (1989). Observations of interactions of depressed women with their children. *American Journal of Psychiatry, 146,* 50–5.

Gottman, J.M., & Fainsilber-Katz, L. (1989). Effects of marital discord on young children's peer interaction and health. *Developmental Psychology, 25,* 373–381.

Gottman, J.M., & Levenson, R.S. (1988). The social psychophysiology of marriage. In P. Noller & M.A. Fitzpatrick (eds.), *Perspectives on marital interaction.* Clevedon, England, & Philadelphia: Multilingual Matters.

Hammen, C. (1991). *Depression runs in families.* New York: Sprenger-Verlag.

Hammen, C., Adrian, C., & Hiroto, D. (1988). A longitidinal test of the attributional vulnerability model in children at risk for depression. *British Journal of Clinical Psychology, 27,* 37–46.

Hammen, C., Burge, D., & Stansbury, K. (1990). Relationship of mother and child variables to child outcomes in a high-risk sample: A causal modeling analysis. *Developmental Psychology*, 26, 24–30.

Harrington, R., Fudge, H., Rutter, M., Pickles, A., & Hill, J. (1990). Adult outcomes of childhood and adolescent depression. *Archives of General Psychiatry*, 47, 465–473.

Harris, T., Brown, G.W., & Bifulco, A. (1987). Loss of parent in childhood and adult psychiatric disorder: The role of social class and premarital pregnancy. *Psychological Medicine*, 17, 163–83.

Harris, T., Brown, G.W., & Bifulco, A. (1990). Loss of parent in childhood and adult psychiatric disorder: A tentative overall model. *Development and Psychopathology*, 2, 311–328.

Hautzinger, M., Linden, M., & Hoffman, N. (1982). Distressed couples with and without a depressed partner: An analysis of their verbal interaction. *Journal of Behavior Therapy and Experimental Psychiatry*, 13, 307–314.

Hetherington, E.M., Stanley-Hagan, M., & Anderson, E.R. (1989). Marital transitions: A child's perspective. *American Psychologist*, 44, 302–12.

Hinchliffe, M., Hopper, D., & Roberts, F. J. (1978). *The melancholy marriage*. New York: John Wiley.

Holmes, S.J., & Robins, L.N. (1988). The role of parental disciplinary practices in the development of depression and alcoholism. *Psychiatry*, 51, 642–647.

Hooley, J.M., Orley, J., & Teasdale, J.D. (1986). Levels of expressed emotion and relapse in depressed patients. *British Journal of Psychiatry*, 148, 642–7.

Hops, H., Biglan, A., Sherman, L., Arthur, J., Friedman, L.S., & Osteen, V. (1987). Home observations of family interactions of depressed women. *Journal of Consulting and Clinical Psychology*, 55, 341–346.

Kahn, J., Coyne, J.C., & Margolin, G. (1985). Depression and marital conflict: The social construction of despair. *Journal of Social and Personal Relationships*, 2, 447–462.

Kashani, J.H., Carlson, G.A., Beck, N.C., Hoeper, E.W., Corcoran, C.M., McAllister, J.A., Fallahi, C., Rosenberg, T.K., & Reid, J.C. (1987). Depression, depressive symptoms, and depressed mood among a community sample of adolescents. *American Journal of Psychiatry*, 144, 931–4.

Kashani, J.H., Shekim, W.O., Burk, J.P., & Beck, N.C. (1987). Abuse as a predictor of psychopathology in children and adolescents. *Journal of Clinical Child Psychology*, 16, 43–50.

Kaslow, N.J., Rehm, L.P., & Siegel, A.W. (1984). Social cognitive and cognitive correlates of depression in children. *Journal of Abnormal Child Psychology*, 12, 605–20.

Keitner, G., & Miller, I. (1990). Major depression and family functioning. *American Journal of Psychiatry*, 147, 1128–1137.

Keller, M., Beardslee, W., Lavori, P., Wunder, J., & Samuelson, H. (1988). Course of major depression in nonreferred adolescents: A retrospective study. *Journal of Affective Disorders*, 15, 235–243.

Kendler, K.S, Neale, M.C., Kessler, R.C., Heath, A.C., & Eaves, J. (1992). A population based twin study of major depression in women. *Archives of General Psychiatry*, 49, 257–266.

Kennedy E., Spence, S.H., & Henaley, R. (1989). An examination of the relationship between childhood depression and social competence amongst primary school children. *Journal of Child Psychology, Psychiatry, and Allied Disciplines*, 4, 561–73.

Kerr, M., & Bowen, M. (1988). *Family evaluation*. New York: W.W. Norton.

Kiesler, D.J. (1983). The interpersonal circle: A taxonomy for complementarity in human transactions. *Psychological Review*, 90, 185–214.

Kitzmann, K.M., & Rohrbaugh, M. (in press). The focused-on child: Testing Bowen's family systems theory. *Journal of Family Psychology*.

Kovacs, M. (1989). Affective disorders in children and adolescents. *American Psychologist*, *44*, 209–215.

Kovacs, M., Feinberg, T.L., Crouse-Novak, M.A., Paulaskas, S.L., & Finkelstein, R. (1984). Depressive disorders in childhood: I. A longitudinal prospective study of characteristics and recovery. *Archives of General Psychiatry*, *41*, 229–237.

Kovacs, M., Paulauskas, S., Gatsonis, C., & Richards, C. (1988). Depressive disorders in childhood III. A longitudinal study of comorbidity with and risk for conduct disorders. *Journal of Affective Disorders*, *15*, 205–17.

Leff, J., & Vaughn, C.E. (1985). *Expressed emotion in families: Its significance for mental illness*. New York: Guilford.

Lefkowitz, M.M., & Burton, N. (1978). Childhood depression: A critique of the concept. *Psychological Bulletin*, *85*, 716–726.

Lieberson, S. (1985). *Making it count: The improvement of social theory and research*. Berkeley: University of California Press.

Linden, M., Hautzinger, M., & Hoffman, N. (1983). Discriminant analysis of depressive interactions. *Behavior Modification*, *7*, 403–422.

Long, N., Forehand, R., Fauber, R., & Brody, E. (1987). Self-perceived and independently observed competence of young adolescents as a function of parental marital conflict and recent divorce. *Journal of Abnormal Child Psychology*, *15*, 15–27.

Lytton, H. (1990). Child and parent effects in boys' conduct disorder: A reinterpretation. *Developmental Psychology*, *26*, 683–697.

McGuffin, P., & Bebbington, P. (1988). The Camberwell collaborative depression study. III. Depression and adversity in the relatives of depressed patients. *British Journal of Psychiatry*, *152*, 775–82.

McLoyd, V. (1990). The declining fortunes of Black children: Psychological distress, parenting, and socioemotional development in the context of economic hardship. *Child Development*, *61*, 311–346.

Merikangas, K.R. (1981). *The relationship of assortative mating to social adjustment and course of illness in primary affective disorder*. Unpublished doctoral dissertation. University of Pittsburgh.

Merikangas, K.R., & Spiker, D.G. (1982). Assortative mating among in-patients with primary affective disorder. *Psychological Medicine*, *12*, 753–764.

Merikangas, K., Weissman, M., Prusoff, B., Pauls, D., & Leckman, J. (1985). Depressives with secondary alchoholism: Psychiatric disorders in offspring. *Journal of Studies on Alcohol*, *46*, 199–204.

Minuchin, P. (1985). Families and individual development: provocations from the field of family therapy. *Child Development*, *56*, 289–302.

Miklowitz, D., Goldstein, M., Nuechterlein, K., & Snyder, K. (1988). Family factors and the course of bipolar affective disorder. *Archives of General Psychiatry*, *45*, 225–231.

Mullins, L.L., Peterson, L., Wonderlich, S., & Reaven, N.M. (1986). The influence of depressive symptomatology in children on the social responses and perceptions of adults. *Journal of Clinical Child Psychology*, *15*, 233–240.

Panaccione, V., & Wahler, R. (1986). Child behavior, maternal depression, and social coercion as factors in the quality of child care. *Journal of Abnormal Child Psychology*, *14*, 125–35.

Parker, G. (1981). Parental reports of depressives: An investigation of several explanations. *Journal of Affective Disorders*, *3*, 131–140.

Parker, G. (1983). Parental 'affectionless control' as an antecedent of adult depression. *Archives of General Psychiatry*, *134*, 138–147.

Parker, G., & Hadzi-Pavlovic, D. (1984). Modification of levels of depression in mother-bereaved women by prenatal and marital relationships. *Psychological Medicine*, *14*, 125–135.

Patterson, G.R. (1982). *Coercive family process*. Eugene, OR: Castilia Press.

Patterson, G.R. & Reid, J.B. (1970). Reciprocity and coercion: Two facets of social systems. In C. Neuringer & J. Michael (eds.), *Behavior modification in clinical psychology* (pp. 133–177). New York: Appleton-Century-Croft.

Peirce, C.S. (1955). *Philosophical writings of Peirce.* New York: Dover.

Perris, C., Arrindell, C., Perris, H., Eisemann, M., van der Ende, J., & von Knorring, L. (1986). Perceived depriving parental rearing and depression. *British Journal of Psychiatry, 148,* 170–175.

Peterson, L., Mullins, L.L., & Ridley-Johnson, R. (1985). Childhood depression peer reactions to depression and life stress. *Journal of Abnormal Child Psychology, 13,* 597–609.

Peterson, P., Coyne, J.C., & Kessler, R.C. (1991). *Assortative mating for psychopathology in a community sample.* Unpublished manuscript, University of Michigan.

Phofl, B., Stangl, D., & Zimmerman, M. (1984). The implications of DSM III–R personality disorders for patients with major depression. *Journal of Affective Disorders, 7,* 309–18.

Poznanski, E., & Zrull, J.P. (1970). Childhood depression. *Archives of General Psychiatry, 23,* 8–15.

Puig-Antich, J. (1982). Major depression and conduct disorder in prepuberty. *Journal of American Academy Child Psychiatry, 21,* 118–28.

Puig-Antich, J., Lukens, E., Davies, M., Goetz, D., Quattrock, J.B., & Todak, G. (1985a). Psychosocial functioning in prepubertal major depressive disorders. *Archives of General Psychiatry, 42,* 500–7.

Puig-Antich, J., Lukens, E., Davies, M., Goetz, D., Quattrock, J.B., & Todak, G. (1985b). Controlled studies of psychosocial functioning in prepubertal major depressive disorders, II. Interpersonal relationships after sustained recovery from the affective episode. *Archives of General Psychiatry, 42,* 511–17.

Puig-Antich, J., Perel, J.M., Lupatkin, W., Chambers, W.J., Tabrizi, M.A., King, J., Goetz, R., Davies, M., & Stiller, R.L. (1987). Imipramine in prepubertal major depressive disorders. *Archives of General Psychiatry, 44,* 81–9.

Quinton, D., Rutter, M., & Liddle, C., (1984). Institutional rearing, parenting difficulties and marital support. *Psychological Medicine, 14,* 107–124. 124

Quinton, D., & Rutter, M. (1988). *Parenting breakdown.* Aldershot, England: Avebury.

Radke-Yarrow, M., Richters, J., & Wilson, W.E. (1988). Child development in a network of relationships. In R. Hinde & J. Stevenson-Hinde (eds.), *Individual in a network of relationships* Cambridge, England: Cambridge University Press.

Radke-Yarrow, M., Belmont, B., Nottelman, E., & Bottomly, B. (1990). Young children's self-conceptions: Origins in the natural discourse of depressed and normal mothers and their children. In D. Cicchetti & M. Beeghley (eds.), *The self in transition.* Chicago, IL: University of Chicago Press.

Ransom, D.C. (1985). Random notes: Health promotion and the family. *Family Systems Medicine, 3,* 250–256.

Rie, H.E. (1966). Depression in childhood: A survey of some pertinent contributions. *Journal of the American Academy of Child Psychiatry, 5,* 653–85.

Rochlin, G. (1959). The loss complex. *Journal of the American Psychoanalytic Association, 7,* 229–316.

Rounsaville, B.J., Prusoff, B.A., & Weissman, M.M. (1980). The course of marital disputes in depressed women: A 48-month follow-up study. *Comprehensive Psychiatry, 21,* 111–118.

Rounsaville, B.J., Weissman, M.M., Prusoff, B.A., & Herceg-Baron, R.L. (1979). Marital disputes and treatment outcome in depressed women. *Comprehensive Psychiatry, 20,* 483–490.

Roy, A. (1978). Risk factors and depression in Canadian women. *Journal of Affective Disorders, 3,* 69–70.

Schwartz, C.E., Dorer, D.J., Beardslee, W.R., Lavori, P.W., & Keller, M.B. (1990). Maternal expressed emotion and parental affective disorder: Risk for childhood depressive disorder, substance abuse, or conduct disorder. *Journal of Psychiatric Research, 24*, 231–50.

Styron, W. (1990). *Darkness visible*. New York: Random House.

Strack, S., & Coyne, J.C. (1982). Social confirmation of dysphoria: Shared and private reactions to depression. *Journal of Personality and Social Psychology, 44*, 806–814.

Teti, D.M., Gelfand, D.M., & Pompa, J. (1990). Depressed mothers' behavioral competence with their infants: Demographic and psychosocial correlates. *Development and Psychopathology, 22*, 259–270.

Thompson, R.A. (1988) Emotion and self-regulation. *Nebraska Symposium on Motivation, Socioemotional Development, 36*, 183–258.

Totman, R. (1979). *The social causes of illness*. New York: Pantheon.

Tronick, E. (1989). Emotions and emotional communication in infants. *American Psychologist, 44*, 112–119.

Vaughn, C.E., & Leff, J.P. (1976). The influence of family and psychiatric factors on the course of psychiatric illness. *British Journal of Psychiatry, 129*, 125–137.

Wahler, R. (1980). The insular mother: Her problems in parent-child treatment. *Journal of Applied Behavior Analysis, 13*, 207–219.

Wahler, R., & Dumas, J. (1989). Attentional problems in mother-child interactions: An interbehavioral model. *Psychological Bulletin, 105*, 116–130.

Walker, E., Downey, G., & Nightingale, N. (1989). The nonorthogonal nature of risk for psychopathology. *Journal of Primary Prevention, 9*, 143–163.

Watzlawick, P., Jackson, D.D., & Beavin, J. (1967). *Pragmatics of human communication*. New York: Norton.

Weissman, M.M. (1987). Advances in psychiatric epidemiology: Rates and risks for depression. *American Journal of Public Health, 77*, 445–451.

Weissman, M.M., & Paykel, E.S. (1974). *The depressed woman*. Chicago: University of Chicago Press.

Wells, K.B., Stewart, A., Hays, R.D., Burnam, M.A., Rogers, W., Daniels, M., Berry, S., Greenfield, S., & Ware, J. (1989). The functioning and well-being of depressed patients: Results from the Medical Outcomes Study. *Journal of the American Medical Association, 262*, 914–919.

Wethington, E., McLeod, J.D., and Kessler, R.C. (1987). The importance of life events for explaining sex differences in psychological distress. In R.C. Barnett, G.K. Baruch and L.B. Biener (eds.), *Gender & Stress* (pp. 144–158). New York: Free Press.

Whybrow, P.C., Akiskal, H.S., & McKinney, W.T. (1984). *Mood disorder: Toward a new psychobiology*. New York: Plenum Press.

Zahn-Waxler, C., Iannotti, R.J., Cummings, E.M., & Denham, S. (1990). Antecedents of problem behaviors in children of depressed mothers. *Development and Psychopathology, 2*, 271–91.

Zahn-Waxler, C., & Kochanska, G. (1990). The origins of guilt. In R. Thompson (ed.), *Thirty-Sixth Annual Nebraska Symposium on Motivation: Socioemotional Development* (pp.183–258). Lincoln: University of Nebraska Press.

Zahn-Waxler, C., McKnew, D., Cummings, E.M., Davenport, Y.B., & Radke-Yarrow, M. (1984). Problem behaviors in peer-interaction of young children with a manic-depressive parent. *American Journal of Psychiatry, 141*, 236–240.

Zajonc, R.B., Adelmann, P.K., Murphy, S.T., & Niedenthal, P.M. (1987). Convergence in the physical appearance of spouses. *Motivation and Emotion, 11*, 335–346.

VII   The Family-Environmental Context of Depression: A Perspective on Children's Risk

CONSTANCE HAMMEN

In the early 1980s we began a project at UCLA to study children of depressed mothers. As initially conceived, the work had straightforward goals: to improve on the methodologies of current studies of offspring of parents with affective disorders, and to test theoretical ideas about psychosocial contributors to depression (to supplement the fairly strictly genetic assumptions guiding then-current studies in this area). The theoretical perspective derived directly from adult psychopathology, with the idea that cognitive vulnerability, stressful life events, and dysfunctional relationships — variables that seemed to correlate admirably with adult depression — should also apply to children. The extent of our developmental perspective at that point was that if certain constructs predicted adult depression, they probably had a childhood origin.

It seems almost unfair that I have been so amply rewarded for such a naive developmental position. But, to fracture Shakespeare, some are born developmental psychopathologists, some achieve it, and some have a developmental psychopathology perspective thrust upon them. I fall somewhere in the latter two categories. This chapter is the report of an odyssey toward the historical, contextual, transactional, and multifaceted perspective on the acquisition of disorder that I consider to be consistent with the aims of developmental psychopathology (Cicchetti, 1990; Cicchetti & Schneider-Rosen, 1986).

At the same time, I am also an adult psychopathologist, and what we have learned over the years about adult depression seems critical as a guide to some of the issues and processes that need to be studied in children. Here are some of the "truths" and assumptions about depression that inform my work, creating a phenomenological-empirical approach to theory development. The review of supporting data for each of these issues is presented more completely in Hammen (1991) and Gotlib and Hammen (in press). It might be noted that although these issues are based on research on adult affective disorders, they have important implications for the developmental psychopathology of depression.

1. It is unclear whether there is a continuity between mild, normal depression, and clinically diagnosable depression. Duration of symptoms and impairment of functioning are critical characteristics of depression that may separate normal and clinical forms. Severity of symptoms can certainly be *scaled* on a continuum, but even high-end scorers may have fairly transitory symptoms. Mild but chronic symptoms may be clinically relevant, but at the low end it is not clear whether the phenomenon is best understood as depression, or as some nonspecific negative affectivity.

Questions about continuity certainly have relevance for selection of research samples — e.g., whether college students or community residents or children in classrooms with high scores on depression scales really test questions about psychopathology. At the same time, clinical samples obtained from treatment settings are not necessarily representative of the phenomena of depression, since the great majority of depression goes untreated.

2. One of the major reasons for the above assertion that continuity must be proved rather than assumed, is that depression affects lives. This is a simplistic statement, or a profound truth, depending on one's orientation. If you have a medical model orientation positing a disease process within the person, then depression is something a person *has*. Alternatively, a psychosocial perspective emphasizes what a depressed person *does*. The reality is that depressed persons with persisting and impairing levels of symptoms think about themselves and their depression, they cope with their symptoms and difficulties (or fail to cope), and either reduce their symptoms or contribute to stressful conditions that may further prolong or exacerbate their depression. The social and work lives of depressed people are impaired, and impairment of functioning — including the impact of depression on others and their reactions — is inextricably tied to understanding the disorder, its course, and its outcome.

3. For the majority of people with major depression, the condition is a recurrent one, or possibly chronic. An individual with a single episode of depression is likely to be quite different from someone whose disorder recurs, at least in part because of the consequences of depression as noted above. There is also a tendency for earlier-onset depression (such as those with childhood or early-adolescent onset) to recur. Also, due to the disruption of normal development, childhood onset of depression is likely to represent a particularly pernicious course whose characteristics may not generalize to later-onset forms of disorder.

4. New onsets of depression in never-before depressed adults are relatively rare. Even under fairly dire stressful conditions most individuals do not become significantly depressed, and may instead experience relatively mild or brief symptoms. Moreover, the factors that predict onset of depression in the first place may be quite different from those that predict relapses. In an unselected sample of depressed persons, mixing first onsets with recurrent cases may provide misleading results. Much depression in unselected samples

may in fact be due to people having recurrences of depression. In any case, it is essential to particularize our models of depression and its development to account for onsets, relapse, recovery, or other phases of the course of disorder.

5. Following from these points, we have come to realize that the most potent predictor of depression is past depression. Our work needs to grapple more vigorously with this reality. Why does this occur? It certainly could stem from continuing vulnerability due to whatever etiological factors exist, but it could also be due in part to the *effect* of depression itself. As noted, depression changes lives and frequently elicits or contributes to stressors that themselves deepen or prolong the depression. One implication is that whatever the biological models of etiology and vulnerability to depression might contribute to our knowledge, psychosocial models are critical for helping to explain the course of disorder.

6. Depression is a singular term for heterogeneous subtypes. There are probably different disorders, different vulnerabilities, different risk factors, and different treatments that apply only to specific subtypes. While most researchers acknowledge this reality, few observe it in their investigations, and there are few truly useful schemes and leads for identifying meaningful subtypes. This ought to be a priority, and it implies much more modest theories than our field has been accustomed to.

7. Complicating the understanding of depression is the reality of overlap with other clinical conditions and dysfunctions. Comorbidity is the rule rather than the exception, and we have been relatively lax in demonstrating the specificity of our models for depression as such.

8. Important demographic trends in the incidence and prevalence of depression need to be accounted for, and have important implications. For instance, why is depression especially prevalent in females from adolescence on? Also, why do the rates of depression appear to be increasing in young people (with increasing convergence of male-female rates of disorder)? One implication is that young women of child-bearing ages are especially at risk for depression (or for a recurrence of earlier-onset depression). In view of our findings of the consequences of maternal depression on youngsters, this contributes to a significant public health issue.

9. There are various depression high-risk groups, such as the young, females, those with previous depression, who might provide much useful information about the mechanisms of the course of disorder and risk factors. The vast majority of people with diagnosable depression never seek help, so that clinical (treated) samples — highly vaunted in psychopathology research — may poorly represent the range of depressive disorders and their features. Moreover, the high risk groups remind us of the need for prevention research, to supplement our intense, and generally successful, focus on effective treatments.

These issues highlight the need to understand depression in the context of environmental, developmental, and historical processes, and to view it as a dynamic process that *alters* people and their environments. With these issues in mind as an assumptive background, the conceptual and methodological framework of our research project on children of depressed mothers will be presented.

Overview of the Methods of the UCLA Family Stress Project

When the study was originally undertaken, there were relatively few studies of children at risk as offspring of parents with affective disorders, and those studies had been relatively simplistically designed. Ironically, the heritage of the richly conceived and executed high risk schizophrenia studies had been seemingly ignored. Thus, our study was unique for this field in including both unipolar and bipolar parents, as well as a medical comparison group to test the effects of chronic illness, and a nonpsychiatric normal group. Also, we included a variety of psychosocial variables, as well as outcomes assessed from various sources including school performance and direct interview assessment of psychopathology. Also, the study was unique in including a 3-year follow-up with six-month evaluations of the mothers and children. Complete details of the aims, theoretical rationale, and methods of the study are reported in Hammen (1991).

Sample characteristics. Women with affective disorders were recruited from the UCLA Affective Disorders Clinic and UCLA hospitals, community agencies, and specialty private practices. The women had to have onset of their disorders before the child's birth (or in its early years), and to have at least one child between the ages of 8 and 16. By definition, bipolar disorders are recurrent, but we also required that the unipolar women have recurrent depression so that the index episode was not their only episode. In order to see the families when the mother was not in an acute episode, the initial evaluations were not conducted until at least three months after admission to treatment for the index episode.

Table 1 presents the demographic characteristics of the families entering the study. The 16 unipolar depressed women had a mean of 11 lifetime episodes of major depression, and about half of them would be characterized as double depression, with chronic or intermittent dysthymia punctuated by acute episodes of major depression. Ten of the women had been hospitalized at least once for depression, with an average of 1.7 hospitalizations for the group as a whole. The mean age of onset of diagnosable depression was 18.2 years, with the majority reporting onset in childhood or adolescence. The 14 bipolar women were about equally divided between the bipolar I (mania and depression) and bipolar II subtypes (hypomania and depression), and reported a mean of 7.2 episodes of mania or depression. Only one had not been hospitalized, and the group reported a mean of 2.3 hospitalizations overall. Age of onset was 21.4 years of age, with half reporting childhood or adolescent onset.

Table 1. Demographic Characteristics of Mothers/Families

	GROUP				
Variable	Unipolar	Bipolar	Medical	Normal	Overall
Number of families	16	14	14	24	68
Race					
Percent white	68	93	100	71	81
Percent nonwhite	32	7	0	29	19
Marital status					
Percent married or cohabiting	25	43	71	75	56
Percent divorced or separated	75	57	29	25	44
SES[a] category					
Percent I–III	56	93	100	92	85
Percent IV–V	44	7	0	8	15
Maternal education					
Percent more than 1 year of college	69	79	93	79	79
Percent high school or less	31	21	7	21	21
Mean maternal age	38.4	37.9	40.2	37.1	38.2
Mean chronic stress[b]	2.9	3.3	3.4	3.7	3.4

Note   a = Based on Hollingshead ratings.
b = Higher scores represent lower levels of stress

From C. Hammen (1991). *Depression runs in families: The social context of risk and resilience in children of depressed mothers.* NY: Springer-Verlag. Copyright 1991 by Springer-Verlag. Reprinted by permission.

The chronically medically ill women were selected to represent conditions with similar courses to affective disorders: recurrent or acute exacerbations sometimes requiring hospitalization, with some level of chronic or intermittent symptoms, and onset before the child's birth. This profile was best fit by women with insulin dependent diabetes or rheumatoid arthritis. The medically ill women were recruited from UCLA Hospitals and Clinics, specialty private practices, a diabetes registry, and newsletters. The 14 medically ill women had been hospitalized a mean of 5.8 times for their illnesses, and had a mean age of onset of 17.4 years. Some of the medically ill women had experienced past periods of depression that would be diagnosable as adjustment disorders with depressed mood, and in our judgment excluding them would have yielded an atypical sample of chronically medically ill women. However, they were not currently diagnosable or in treatment for psychiatric problems.

The normal women were recruited from the same or demographically similar schools as children of mothers with affective disorders. The 24 such women were similar, in terms of race, age, and education to the other groups. The socioeconomic status of the unipolar group was rated lower, due to several women being on public assistance because of their affective disorder. None of the normal women of course, had psychiatric or significant medical problems, although a few had a past episode of depression that would be diagnosed as adjustment reaction with depressed mood. The only other major difference between the groups was marital status, in that the unipolar and bipolar women were significantly less likely to be currently married compared to the other groups. Difficulties in sustaining marital relationships are common in persons with affective disorders (e.g., Barnett & Gotlib, 1988).

Children's characteristics. There were 22 children of unipolar women, 18 of bipolar women, 18 of medically ill women, and 38 of normal women. The children were equally distributed by gender within each group, and by adolescent/preadolescent ages. The overall mean age of the children did not differ by group. If the family had more than one child in the age range of 8 to 16, two were included in the study. The psychiatric status of offspring not included in the direct study, and other family members, was assessed from maternal report using the Family History Research Diagnostic Criteria (FH–RDC; Andreasen, Endicott, Spitzer, et al., 1977).

Diagnostic assessments and functioning. Diagnostic evaluations of the mothers and children were conducted using the Schedule for Affective Disorders and Schizophrenia (and the Kiddie-SADS), modified to yield DSM IIIR diagnoses as well as the original RDC diagnoses. Interviews of the children were supplemented by interviews with the mothers about the children, and the two sources of information were combined to yield final diagnoses as recommended in the literature (e.g., Chambers, et al., 1985; Weissman, Wickramaratne, et al., 1987). Initial diagnostic evaluations included lifetime diagnoses, and at six-month intervals the diagnostic interviews included the period since the last assessment.

Children's functioning was additionally assessed by school and teacher reports, and by mothers' completion of the Child Behavior Check List (Achenbach & Edelbrock, 1983). A verbal IQ estimate was obtained from the Peabody Picture Vocabulary Test-Revised (Dunn & Dunn, 1981). The children also completed the Children's Depression Inventory (CDI; Kovacs, 1981).

Assessment of cognitions, interactions, and life stress. Theoretically relevant variables in each of three domains were hypothesized to mediate the effects of maternal affective disorder on children. Children's depressive cognitions were assessed using methods currently available as downward extensions to children from adult depression research, such as the negative items of the

Children's Attribution Style Questionnaire (Seligman, et al., 1984), and an incidental recall task to measure putative self-schemas (Hammen & Zupan, 1984). A different memory for recent incidents task was also developed to evaluate areas of particular vulnerabilty such as interpersonal or achievement domains (e.g., Hammen & Goodman-Brown, 1990). Finally, the Piers-Harris Self Concept Scale (Piers & Harris, 1969) assessed global self-attitudes in children. It was anticipated that depressotypic cognitions would be acquired through direct learning experiences with the depressed parent, as well as through observational learning of the mothers' expression of negativistic attitudes about herself, the world, and the future. In addition to group differences that were predicted, therefore, we also expected that children who evidenced such negativistic thinking would be at risk for future depression as measured in the follow-ups.

Dysfunctional interpersonal relationships between depressed mothers and their children were also predicted from previous studies of the childhood recollections of depressed adults and from clinical assessments of depressed women or depressed children (e.g., reviewed in Burbach & Borduin, 1986; Puig-Antich, et al., 1985; Weissman & Paykel, 1974). The major assessment involved a direct observation task, in which the mother and child were asked to identify a common topic of disagreement (such as chores, curfew, allowance) and to discuss it for five minutes with a goal of reaching agreement. At the time of the original study there were very few such direct observation tasks involving clinically depressed women and their school-age youngsters. The conflict discussion task was then coded into approximately twenty content categories derived from the Peer Interaction Rating System (Whalen, et al., 1979) and supplemented to include depression-relevant content (such as self-criticism). Due to relatively low frequency of some of the categories, and conceptual similarity of others, most of the analyses were based on combined categories. Two of the dimensions that were theoretically expected to differentiate between the groups were *affective quality* (positive and negative comments to the children) and *involvement* (task productivity and ability to sustain a focus on the task with the child).

Finally, *stress* was predicted to be a mediator of depression in both mothers and children, based on the considerable body of research showing a presumed causal link between stressful life events and depression. An interview method for assessing chronic stressful conditions in the mothers was developed, covering domains of social/marital relations, finances, work, relations with family members, and health (see also, Hammen, Ellicott, Gitlin, & Jamison, 1989). Interview procedures for assessing episodic stressors were developed for the women, and also for children, based on George Brown's contextual threat assessment (Brown & Harris, 1978). In this procedure, information surrounding the event and its aftermath is elicited, and a detailed narrative summary is prepared for an independent rating team. The raters are blind to diagnostic group status and the subject's own reported reactions to the event, but attempt to evaluate the magnitude of the stress as an objective threat rating, from the point of view of how a typical person under identical conditions might experience the event. The raters also determine the extent to which the event occurs independent of the person, or might be partly or wholly due to characteristics or behaviors of the person. For children's events, both the mothers and children were interviewed separately, and all information was combined prior to the ratings.

Follow-up procedures. At six-month intervals the mothers and children were separately contacted and interviewed, covering symptoms and life events since the last evaluation. The interviews were typically conducted by telephone, owing to the enormous practical limitations of scheduling face to face interviews of families dispersed over a wide geographic area. Previous research has confirmed the reliablity and validity of telephone diagnostic evaluations, and our experiences indicated no reason to doubt the accuracy or completeness of the information obtained in this way.

In terms of retention of the samples, of the original 96 children, 90 were included for at least one year, and 79 for two years. Seventy children completed all three years. The attrition was relatively evenly distributed across groups except for a disproportionate loss in the bipolar group. Typical reasons for discontinuation were moving out of the area, or refusal. Several families entered the study relatively late and were not followed for the full three years.

Overview of Findings of the Original Hypotheses

The initial hypotheses of the study led to tests of the impact of specific factors on children's functioning. Some of the most interesting issues arose, however, as the interplay between different variables, and these will be discussed later. First, however, the main findings and hypotheses will be presented briefly.

Children's outcomes. The basic but least exciting question was whether children of women with affective disorders would be at greater risk for negative outcomes, not only compared to normal, nonpsychiatric families, but also compared to children of women with similarly disruptive conditions such as chronic medical illness? We also wondered if the negative outcomes would be apparent both in diagnostic evaluations based on direct clinical interviews and across other domains of functioning using diverse methods and informants. The answer is that children of unipolar women, in particular, have extremely high lifetime rates of all disorders, including major depression (Hammen, Gordon, et al., 1987). These rates of diagnosis include disorders that persist or recur over the follow-up period (Hammen, Burge, Burney, & Adrian, 1990). The rates of diagnosis of unipolar children and bipolar children are higher than for the medically ill kids, who have moderate rates of disorder. In general, the unipolar children are impaired across a variety of domains including social functioning, and school and academic performance. Somewhat surprisingly, the children of unipolar mothers were significantly more impaired in social and school functioning than were the bipolar offspring, whose rates of major disorder are also lower (Hammen & Anderson, 1990). The children of the manic-depressive mothers, despite moderate rates of symptoms, appeared to have mastered essential competencies that permitted them to function relatively well socially and academically.

This grim picture especially for the unipolar offspring, is made even more vivid by high rates of hospitalization or institutional care for psychiatric disorder, and even for suicides of youngsters that occurred in two of the unipolar families.

Cognitive vulnerability. As predicted, children of women with affective disorders evidenced more negative cognitions about themselves, and more negative attribution style (Jaenicke, et al., 1987). Negative self-concept, but not attribution style, appeared to be a vulnerability factor predicting increased depression over time (Hammen, 1988; Hammen, Adrian, & Hiroto, 1988).

Stressful life events. As noted, chronic family stress such as having a medically ill mother, is associated with elevated rates of disorder in the children. Within all of the groups, the families differed in levels of ongoing stressful conditions in social-interpersonal, financial, occupational, family, and health domains. In turn, levels of ongoing stress in the family were significantly associated with children's outcomes both concurrently, and over a follow-up period (Hammen, Adrian, et al., 1987). Children's own stressful life events, assessed in the follow-up interviews, were also found to be specific predictors of increased symptoms in the children (Adrian & Hammen, in press; Hammen, 1988; Hammen, Adrian, & Hiroto, 1988).

Characteristics of the mother-child relationship. It had been predicted that children of women with depression would have more negative relationships with their mothers, based on earlier descriptive reports by Weissman on women's impaired parental functionig. Direct observations of mothers and children having a discussion about an area of disagreement indicated that unipolar depressed women, in particular, were significantly more negative, disconfirming and critical in their interactions (Gordon, et al., 1989). Also, such mothers were significantly less involved in the task in the sense of making more off-task comments and less task-productive remarks. In turn, negative quality of interacting and low task involvement were associated with more negative outcomes in the children (Burge & Hammen, 1991).

Relationships Among Variables: A Contextual-Environmental Perspective

Many of the especially interesting results arose from the application of a contextual-environmental perspective, a general question of what are the determinants of the main effects, and how do the main variables relate to each other. What follows is an effort to note some of the points that emerged from such a perspective.

The context of women's depression. Many offspring or psychiatric studies appear to proceed with the implicit assumption that the diagnostic status of the patient is the cause of whatever outcomes are noted. While genetic/ biological substrates of affective disorders are relevant and vitally important to pursue, the medical model attributes outcomes to what the person *has* instead of what the person *does*. In the case of a clinically depressed woman, for instance, we have argued that her diagnosis is comprised of at least three overlapping ingredients that themselves may affect outcomes: severity/chronicity of psychiatric state, chronic stress, and current depressive symptoms. For instance, Hammen, Adrian, et al. (1987) showed that lifetime history of depressive diagnoses, current BDI, and chronic stress level were separable factors that had somewhat different contributors to children's outcomes. In particular, we noted that lifetime psychiatric history predicted very little, while chronic stress and especially, current depressed symptoms, were more significant factors with different correlates. Had we simply stopped at the point of comparing groups, our finding that worse outcomes were associated with unipolar depression might have led us to conclude that it is the depressive illness, possibly transmitted to the child, that is the source of risk. In trying to tease apart the separate factors, however, there are different implications. One is that current mood and chronic stress are not specific to affective disorders, so that the effects that unipolar women have on their children might be effects that other women without that diagnosis also have. Another implication is that we need to study more about what it is that chronic stress does to women in terms of their parenting, and what depressive symptoms are associated with what behaviors and outcomes (see also Downey & Coyne, 1990).

There is some suggestion in our analyses of the predictors of women's interaction behaviors, for instance, that women's affective negativity and criticism toward their children in the observation task was predicted by chronic stress, whereas uninvolvement was more associated with higher levels of depressive symptoms (Burge & Hammen, 1991). Thus, stressors might make women irritable and less tolerant, while depressed mood may contribute to withdrawal and even avoidance of conflictful interactions. In any case, since affective disorders, especially chronic and recurrent ones, are accompanied by stress and disruption, and by fluctuations in mood state and the types of depressive symptoms experienced, simple categorization of patients as having a depressive disorder or not contributes little to our understanding of what is actually going on.

There are additional facets of the context of women's depression that emerged as interesting propositions in our study. One concerns the role of her own family background, and there were four findings. First, most of the unipolar women (88%), and many of the other women as well, had psychopathology in their parents and siblings. The unipolar women in particular had parental major depression, as well as alcohol abuse. Second, the family loading for psychopathology was significantly correlated with her own severity of lifetime disorder. For example, the number of family members (parents, siblings) who were diagnosed correlated ($r = .41$ $p < .001$) with lifetime affective disorder ratings. Third, maternal family loading for psychopathology was related to the child's psychopathology. Table 2 presents correlations between

Table 2. Correlations Between Indices of Maternal Family
Psychopathology and Mother and Child Attributes

	Number of Mother's Ill First-Degree Relatives	Maternal "Loading" Index for Parent Diagnosis
Severity of Child Diagnoses		
Any Lifetime	.38	.34
Lifetime Affective	.46	.29
Average in Follow-Ups	.28	.16(n.s.)
Maternal Functioning		
Positive Quality of Interaction	−.20*	−.19*
Task Productivity in Interaction	−.46	−.21
Chronic Stress Index	−.43	−.24
Lifetime Severity of Depression	.41	.17

* $p > .05 < .10$. All other values significant at $p < .05$.

From C. Hammen (1991). Depression runs in Families: The social context of risk and resilience in children of depressed mothers. NY: Springer-Verlag. Copyright 1991 by Springer-Verlag. Reprinted by permission.

child diagnostic ratings and degree of mother's family pathology. Fourth, although these results are certainly generally compatible with a genetic explanation of intergenerational transmission of disorder (especially depressive disorder), there is also another possibility. Maternal family history was significantly related to maternal psychosocial characteristics that might themselves be mediators of the risk to children. Specifically, maternal family psychopathology was correlated with negative qualities of interaction with her own children, and with her own chronic stress. We might speculate a causal sequence here, postulating that women who were raised in dysfunctional families marked by parental psychopathology failed to acquire the interpersonal skills necessary for effective parenting, or at the very least, experience impairment in their own ability to deal with difficult children. As a result, their interactions with their children are marked by criticism and withdrawal or maladaptive avoidance of conflict. Thus, the historical context of maternal psychopathology and parenting includes intergenerational transmission of maladaptive skills.

Children's depressive cognitions in context. The above speculations rest on the assumption that effective interpersonal functioning (including parenting) requires the acquisition of adaptive representations of the self and object relations, and that these are acquired in the context of supportive, positive, and contingent parent-child relationships. To test this hypothesis in a microcosm, we explored the correlates of self-cognitions in the children in our sample, including self-concept, level of self-blaming attributions, and experimental measures of self-schemas. Of particular interest, we found a very high correlation ($r = .72$, $p < .001$) between children's Piers-Harris Self-Concept scores and their perceptions of the quality of their relationship with their mother. And, these associations were corroborated by a significant correlation ($r = -.28$, $p < .01$) between self-concept and *actual* negative interactions as observed in the mother-child tasks (see Jaenicke, et al., 1987). These relationships also obtained for the other cognitive measures of self-views. Also, in that study we wondered if children's negative cognitions about the self might be similar to their mothers' views of herself, with the idea that maybe negative self-views are modeled and acquired through observational learning. What we found instead, however, was that while mothers' and children's self-blaming remarks during the observation task were not correlated, there was a strong relationship between the child's self-blame and maternal criticism. That is, making self-blaming commmments was correlated $r=.51$ ($p < .0001$) with maternal criticism, and also children's self-reported self-blaming attribution style on the ASQ was correlated with maternal criticism on the observation task ($r = .42$, $p < .001$) (Jaenicke, et al., 1987). Thus, children's negative cognitions may be acquired in part through direct negative interactions with their mothers. This is hardly surprising, but what is surprising is that it has not been reported before in offspring studies. Negative cognitions about the self, moreover, may go on to have an impact on children's social behaviors, and their academic functioning. Indeed, we found strong associations between high self-concept scores and social competence and academic performance. We speculate that these are mutual, bidirectional effects. Children with positive views of themselves feel effective and worthwhile, and may achieve better in school and have more positive social relationships, which in turn help to build and support their views of themselves. According to a cognitive model of depression vulnerability, a negative self-schema tends to be self-perpetuating through selective perception and encoding of information that "fits" it. We might also add — and will discuss further below — that negative self-views may contribute to negative behaviors that are veridical, not distorted, reflections of the child's value and competence. Either view, however, implies a vicious cycle for a child with an early-acquired negative self-schema.

We have further speculated that negative views of the self are a specific vulnerability factor for depression. Cognitive research on adult depressives clearly supports the association between negative views of personal worth and depression, whereas cognitions about future danger and threat are especially associated with anxiety (e.g., Beck, Brown, Steer, Eidelson, Riskind, 1987; Clark, Beck, & Stewart, 1990). Therefore, situations or events that are interpreted as depletions of the sense of worth of the self might be especially likely to precipitate depression. A prospective analysis of the relation between negative self-cognitions and depression did indeed find that children who had negative self-concept scores became more depressed than children with more positive self-views, even controlling for initial depression (Hammen, 1988). A more refined prediction based on various models of adult depression (Beck, Arieti, Blatt), is that individuals may have particular areas of vulnerability on which their self-worth is especialled based. Only when negative events impinge on these areas will depression occur. This hypothesis has been supported in my work on adult depression (e.g., Hammen, Marks, Mayol, & de Mayo, 1985; Hammen, Ellicott, Gitlin, & Jamison, 1989). Extending the model of specific vulnerability to children in this sample, Goodman-Brown and I found that children were significantly more likely to become depressed if they experienced more stressful events that matched their vulnerability to either interpersonal or achievement domains. Actually, the effect was mostly accounted for by children who were interpersonally vulnerable assessed by our self-schema measure, who experienced negative interpersonal events (Hammen & Goodman-Brown, 1990).

Overall, therefore, we found that instead of a main effects model of depressive cognitions, it was more informative to explore the possible origins of negative cognitions, and the interaction between negative cognitions about the self and events happening in the child's world in an attempt to understand vulnerability to depression.

The context of stress. After nearly 1000 interviews with the women and children of these families, one of the phenomena that demanded attention was the enormous amount of stress to which these families were exposed, and the growing recognition that the women and children were contributing to the occurrence of stressors. Initially, our hypotheses were modest — and unidirectional: stress causes depression, and both mother stress and child stress ought to predict episodes of depression. We developed elaborate methods for assessing episodic stress using the contextual threat approach applied by George Brown in England, and our group was the first that we know of to extend them to children. We also developed in this and my other studies, a systematic measure of chronic, ongoing stressful conditions, noting as above, that such conditions are commonly an accompaniment of chronic psychiatric disorder. Both as consequences of symptoms, and as contributors to symptoms, chronic stressful conditions mark the social, relationship, and occupational disruption that occurs in depression.

As discussed above, chronic maternal stress was a specific, separable predictor of children's outcomes (Hammen, Adrian, et al., 1987; Hammen, Gordon, et al., 1987). Also, as Burge and Hammen (1991) found, chronic stress may have its effect in part by the negative impact it has on the quality of the mother-child interaction, and is especially associated with critical and disconfirmatory comments to the children in the Conflict Discussion task. We also noted that the chronic medical illness group, itself a test of the effects of chronic stressors, was associated with moderate levels of disorder and dysfunction in the children.

One of the factors that emerged to clearly characterize the groups was the amount of stress to which mothers and children were exposed. *Stress exposure,* in terms of our quantified measures of both chronic maternal stress and episodic stress for both mothers and children indicated that distinctive patterns occurred in the groups. Not surprisingly, the groups differed significantly on chronic stress, with the unipolar group having the worst levels, affecting marital/social, financial, occupational, and family relationships factors. Although personal health was worst for the medically ill women, the unipolar women had significant health problems, and the poor health of their family members also contributed to ongoing difficulties for them.

More surprising, however, was the observation of differences in exposure to episodic stressors (reported in Hammen, 1991). As Table 3 indicates, when the numbers of events, and the total objective threat ratings of various categories of events in the first year of follow-up are inspected, interesting patterns emerge. The unipolar women had significantly more total impact and more events than the normal women. Stress totals are comprised of both independent events that are "fateful" in the sense of being beyond the control or causation of the person, and those that are dependent or at least partly dependent on the person. The groups did not differ in exposure to independent events (although due to high rates of medical problems for themselves and family members, the medical group exceeded the others). However, in the *dependent* events, the unipolar group was the highest, significantly higher than normals and marginally significantly higher than the bipolar and medically ill women. But, the dependent events can be further subdivided into those that are primarily interpersonal and those that are not. Here we found a clear significant difference between the unipolar women and each of the other groups. It appears that the unipolar women are especially likely to experience negative interpersonal events that they at least partly cause. Moreover, although there were different kinds of content to these events, the most frequent characteristic of these events was conflict — conflict with husbands or boyfriends, friends, family members, teachers, and the like. Thus, we might speculate that one of the ingredients that contributes to recurring or chronic depression in these women is their difficulty in managing interpersonal relationships. This is certainly not a new thought in theorizing about depression (e.g., Barnett & Gotlib, 1988; Coyne, Kahn, & Gotlib, 1987), and it is not a new idea in the research on life stress and depression (e.g., Depue & Monroe, 1986). However, there is no empirical evidence in a longitudinal study like this that captures the dynamic, transactional flow between the person and environment. The stress generation process needs to be studied intensively to understand what is involved — whether it is a consequence of symptoms or characteristics of the person, poor interpersonal skills or dysfunctional cognitions about relationships, and whether it applies generally to people with recurring depression. Because our design included comparison groups for other chronic conditions such as bipolar disorder or medical illness, we are able to conclude that the patterns are unique to the unipolar women and not just to ill women. However, a lot more research needs to be done to clarify the range of application of stress generation and explain the mechanisms involved.

Table 3. Mean Objective Threat Rating Totals by Group

	TYPE OF EVENT CATEGORY			
Group	Total All Events	Independent	Dependent	Interpersonal
Unipolar n = 14	12.7 (12.5)	3.6 (3.2)	8.8 (9.6)	6.3 (7.0)
Bipolar n = 11	9.1 (6.0)	3.6 (2.7)	5.5 (4.8)	3.2 (3.2)
Medically Ill n = 13	11.6 (6.5)	6.6 (6.1)	5.1 (5.5)	3.0 (4.3)
Normal n = 22	7.6 (7.6)	4.4 (5.9)	3.3 (3.7)	2.0 (2.8)

Standard deviations are in parentheses.
Adapted from C. Hammen (1991). The generation of stress in the course of unipolar depression. *Journal of Abnormal Psychology.* Copyright 1991 by the American Psychological Association. Reprinted by permission.

An additional intriguing possibility that emerges from our study, is that the children of women with unipolar depression are themselves showing a stress generation tendency in the sense of exposure to more events and especially interpersonal events. For instance, my student Cheri Adrian (1990) examined children's stressors. Table 4 presents the means comparing the affective disorders groups with the other groups. Dr Adrian conducted analyses between groups using age as a covariate. The children of women with affective disorders differed significantly from the children of normal mothers in total stress across the 3-year follow-up, and the medically-ill children had moderate rates of stressors. As with their mothers, the groups differed on stress levels of events judged to be at least partly dependent on their behaviors or characteristics. The children of women with affective disorders differed from both the medically ill and normal groups on stress associated with dependent events. Thus, there was an excess of events to which they had at least partly contributed. When the content of the events was examined, there were significant group differences on three types of events: family conflict, peer conflict, and "other" (accidents and illnesses, for example). The first two categories were significantly higher for the children of women with affective disorders. Thus, much like their unipolar mothers, the children of unipolar mothers appeared to create stressors for themselves in their participation in conflicted interpersonal relationships — involving not only their families but also their peer relationships. The third category, "other" illness and accident

Table 4. Mean Three-Year Objective Threat Totals for Children's Stressors by Stress Type

	STRESS TYPE						
Group	Loss/ Bereavement	Family Conflict	Peer Conflict	Change/ Move	Other Negative	Overall Dependent	Overall Independent
Unipolar/ Bipolar	10.6 (6.4)	8.9 (6.6)	4.4 (3.7)	6.0 (4.6)	13.2 (9.9)	34.7 (18.4)	19.8 (10.4)
Medically Ill	8.3 (3.7)	7.3 (6.2)	1.4 (1.3)	3.8 (3.2)	19.6 (15.7)	21.3 (11.5)	23.7 (11.3)
Normal	7.1 (4.8)	2.8 (4.1)	1.5 (2.1)	5.3 (3.9)	7.6 (4.1)	8.8 (6.9)	18.1 (8.1)

Note. Figures in parentheses are standard deviations.
From C. Adrian, unpublished dissertation, UCLA, 1990.

stress, was highest in the medically ill mother group children, and they differed significantly from the normal group children.

One of the additional theoretically interesting issues about stress in children at risk is whether they have a particular vulnerability to stressors. That is, might they have a lower threshhold or tolerance for stress that is possibly biologically mediated as a genetically transmitted dysfunction in neuroregulatory mechanisms or as a consequence of neuroregulatory functioning being altered by early exposure to stress (e.g., Gold, Goodwin, & Chrousos, 1988; Gopelrud & Depue, 1985). This is an enormously difficult question to test in the real world since there is no control over the amount or sequencing of stressors children face at any given time. However, Adrian's dissertation (1990) was able to make use of the longitudinal design to define high-stress and low-stress periods for children and to observe subsequent symptomatology. She found that under high-stress conditions, the majority of children in all of the groups showed symptom increases. However, under low-stress conditions the picture was very different: 77% of the combined unipolar-bipolar group, but only 17% of normal and none of the medically ill children showed symptom increases. The results are generally compatible with other research indicating that most people do not react to stressors unless at high levels, or their reactions are fairly brief and mild (e.g., Gopelrud & Depue, 1985; Hammen, Mayol, et al., 1985). However, individuals who are vulnerable by virtue of prior symptomatology and/or family affective disorder may react with more prolonged symptoms to more mild stress provocation.

Another kind of vulnerability is cognitive vulnerability. We speculated, based on our prior research with adults and college students (e.g., Hammen, Marks, et al., 1985; Hammen, Ellicott, Gitlin, & Jamison, 1989), that the domain of self that is central to feelings of worth and competence must be affected by a stressor whose meaning is construed to be depleting or impairing of that sense of worth. Thus, children who are especially vulnerable in the interpersonal domain should become depressed only if they experience such events, but not if they experience non-relevant events. As noted, Hammen & Goodman-Brown (1990) observed that this pattern obtained in the children of this study whose cognitive self-schema vulnerabilities could be classified on the basis of a task of memories for recent events. However, the majority of the children who did become depressed when the events "fit" their vulnerability were interpersonally vulnerable, and were children of women with affective disorders. This raises the issue of whether children of such women are in fact interpersonally vulnerable, and why, or whether such events are more frequent and salient for children in general.

The complex context of stress in these families takes yet another form. We wondered what would be the role of maternal depression as a potential stressor in itself for the children. We asked two questions guided by the hypothesis that stress causes depression. The first question was whether the mother and child episodes of disorder would be temporally associated? The second question was what would be the relative contributions of maternal symptoms, along with their own episodic stressors, to children's depression?

The 3-year longitudinal follow-up gave us a unique opportunity to examine the relative *timing* of mother and child depressions. Although a genetic explanation could be invoked to explain children's risk for depressive disorders, such a perspective would certainly not predict that the timing of episodes would relate to each other. Instead, if such a pattern is observed, then a psychosocial explanation seems warranted. Hammen, Burge, & Adrian (1991) inspected the separate timelines of episodes of mothers and children, noting occasions when symptoms occurred within one month of each other. Symptoms were classified as onset, chronic/intermittent or none for the mother and child, and an overall chi-square analysis indicated that the distributions were significantly different from chance. Looking specifically at major depressive episodes over time, there were 11 children with such onsets, and only one of these occurred in the absence of maternal symptoms. Across the various episodes of disorder, sometimes the mother's preceded, but sometimes hers followed the child's onset. Thus, while there was a significant temporal association in symptomatology, both mother and child had an impact on the other.

The second issue concerned maternal disorder considered as a stressor, along with the children's other stressors during a six-month follow-up. Hierarchical multiple regression analyses were conducted, first entering the child's initial level of depression, then objective threat stress total and threat rating total for maternal symptomatology (rated by the independent team as any

Table 5. Hierarchical Regression Analysis to Predict Children's Depression at Six-Month Follow-Up

Variable	R^2 Change	Significance of R^2 change
Initial Depression	.21	$t = 4.0, p < .0001$
Event Stress Total	.03	$t = 1.76, p = .08$
Maternal Sympton Stress	.10	$t = 3.73, p < .001$
Events X Maternal Symptoms	.04	$t = 2.22, p < .05$
Overall F(4,79) = 11.75, $p < .0001$, Overall R = .61, R^2 = .37		

From Hammen, C., Burge, D., & Adrian, C. (1991). Timing of mother and child depression in a longitudinal study of children at risk. *Journal of Consulting and Clinical Psychology, 59*, 341–345. Copyright 1991 by the American Psychological Association. Reprinted by permission.

other stressors would be rated), and then the interaction of the two latter terms. Table 5 presents the results, indicating that not only was maternal symptom stress a significant predictor of child's subsequent depression, but also the interaction of child's stress and maternal symptom stress was an additional significant contributor. Figure 1 presents the interaction effect. What this depicts is that maternal symptoms seem to potentiate the ill-effects of children's own stressors. If the mother is not symptomatic, even high levels of stress do not appear to cause changes in depression in the children. We speculate that this effect in part represents the buffering effect that mothers would be expected to play to moderate the adverse impact of children's stressors. However, when the mother is not available because of her own symptoms to play such a supportive and buffering role, the child is relatively unprotected and becomes depressed.

Overall, therefore, our conceptualizations and assessments of stressful events and conditions were important elements in understanding the context of depression in the family. Stressors are a cause, and a consequence, of the individuals' characteristics. An ability to avoid stressful circumstances — or to deal with adversity in an effective and constructive fashion to mitigate its ill effects — is an important aspect of healthy development, and depression-resistence. Despite our emphasis on stress, however, we acknowledge that it is a complex and multifaceted topic, and believe that we, and others, have really only begun to explore such complexities.

Mother-child interactions in context. An enormous amount of conflict characterized mother-child relationships of women with depression, assessed both as stressful events when major fights occurred, and as ongoing strains. Such difficulties were apparently accurately captured in the brief mother-child Conflict Discussion task, that revealed more criticism and negative affective quality of communication between the unipolar women and their children

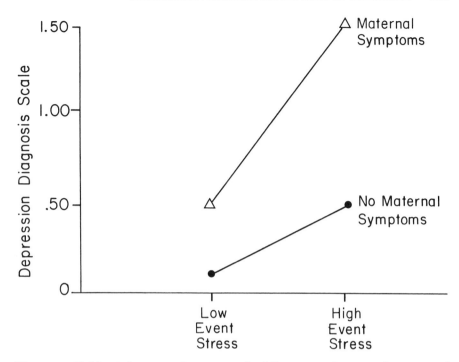

Figure 1. Children's depression diagnoses at the follow-up as a function of stressors and maternal symptoms. From Hammen, C., Burge, D., & Adrian, C. (1991). Timing of mother and child depression in a longitudinal study of children at risk. *Journal of Consulting and Clinical Psychology*, *59*, 341–345. Copyright 1991 by the American Psychological Association. Reprinted by permission.

compared to any other group. Such women were also highly likely to be uninvolved in the task, made efforts to avoid the discussion, or were otherwise unproductive. Interestingly, when we asked children what they understood about their mothers' conditions, and what characterized their mothers' conditions, most children of women with affective disorders readily perceived her depression but were especially likely to regard irritability as the most salient change they saw in her. Moreover, when she became irritable, the children tended to report that they became depressed themselves, and older children in particular, reported that they got angry.

It is important to examine the implications of this process: clearly, children and mothers react to one another, so that a static situation in which one affects an unchanging other simply does not occur. Instead, we think that it is profitable to consider the reciprocal effects of mothers and children on each other. Some earlier investigators suggested that depressed mothers might exaggerate the actual difficulties of their children (e.g., Griest, Wells, & Forehand, 1979; Griest, Forehand, Wells, & McMahon, 1980; Forehand, Wells, McMahon, Griest, & Rogers, 1982), but implied that the effect of the

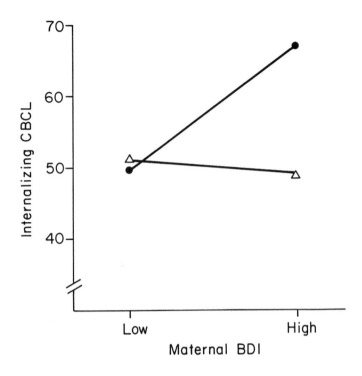

Combined Internalizing Variables

△ Less Symptomatic Children

● More Symptomatic Children

Figure 2. Maternal perceptions of child internalizing disorder as a function of maternal depression and symptomatology of the child. ("More symptomatic" children refers to those scoring above the median on a composite score of the Children's Depression Inventory and diagnosis of internalizing disorders. CBCL = Child Behavior Checklist. BDI = Beck Depression Inventory.) From Conrad, M., & Hammen, C. (1989). Role of maternal depression in perceptions of child maladjustment, *Journal of Consulting and Clinical Psychology, 57*, pp. 663–667. Copyright 1989 by the American Psychological Association. Reprinted by permission.

children's own conduct was somehow less of an issue than the distortion or intolerance due to maternal depression. In our study, Conrad and I compared the relatively depressed and nondepressed women in terms of how well their reports of children's symptoms agreed with external "objective" sources, such as interviewers and teachers. What we found, both for internalizing and externalizing disorders, is depicted in the example shown in Figure 2.

Depressed mothers made actual distinctions between children who did or did not have true difficulties; nondepressed women did not. It looks as if nondepressed mothers are showing the distortions, in terms of minimizing actual child problems (Conrad & Hammen, 1989). Moreover, in the same study we found that those mothers made a corresponding distinction in the quality of interactions with their children. Those women who perceived that their youngsters had difficulties interacted significantly more negatively with them in the Conflict Discussion task than did the women who did not perceive child problems. This suggests strongly to us that symptomatic children are probably also difficult children, eliciting more negative communications from their mothers, and that the two develop a reciprocal style of unsupportive and unproductive discussion of difficulties.

In addition to the overall group patterns suggesting that relatively depressed mothers have distinctive patterns of interacting with children who do and do not have problems, we also found such a distinction within the family. Heeding Plomin and Daniels' (1987) emphasis on "nonshared environments" that can account for differences between siblings in the same families, we examined a small group of families in which one child was diagnosed and one was not. The 10 discordant pairs differed not only on measures of competence and academic achievement, but they also differed in the Conflict Discussion task with their mother. The mothers were significantly more negative toward the more symptomatic, less competent sibling than toward the other (Anderson & Hammen, 1990).

Finally, to underscore our emphasis on reciprocal influences of the mother and children, Burge, Stansbury, and I specifically tested a statistical causal model of children's outcomes that included a reciprocal path in the model to reflect mother-child communications. And in turn both the interaction quality and characteristics of the child contributed to child outcomes (Hammen, Burge, & Stansbury, 1990).

Overall, therefore, we think that it is vitally important to think of children of depressed parents as having an important role in eliciting some of the negative interactions, and in turn, contributing to the parent's unhappiness and maladjustment as well. It is critical to take care not to imply that all of the psychosocial transmission of disorder is a one-directional path from a bad mother to the child. Instead, we see mothers and children both potentially locked into a mutually ineffective and provoking style of interacting. Both may be victims, and both may be perpetrators — and all should be targets of treatment efforts.

As with stress, mother-child interactions are enormously complex, and our methods were modest and highly limited. Still to be answered are questions about the mechanisms of influence: are depressed mothers less tolerant, do they have different needs and expectations of their children, are they (and the children) impaired in their actual communication and interpersonal negotiation skills? Although until very recently direct studies of the parent-child communication process in offspring/high risk populations have been rare, important and detailed work is ongoing to begin to answer such questions. For instance, the NIMH intramural project has yielded intriguing glimpses of maladaptive communications in mothers with affective disorders and their young children (e.g., Radke-Yarrow, Zahn-Waxler, and their colleagues). Goodman & Brumley (1990) reported on the behaviors of depressed and schizophrenic mothers with their infants or young children, and numerous investigations have begun to explore interactions between mildly or clinically depressed women and their infants (see Downey & Coyne, 1990 for a review, and the work of Cohn, Field, Lyons-Ruth, and their colleagues). Research by Cicchetti and other investigators studying interactions between maltreating women and their children are also relevant, and compatible with the present findings, especially since many such women have elevated depression levels (e.g., Cicchetti, 1990). It will be important to separate the specific types of depressive behaviors and their consequences, as well as to study descriptive qualities and interaction sequences.

A Developmental Psychopathology Model of Children's Risk for Depression in a Sample of Children at High- and Low-Risk

To me, developmental psychopathology implies an historical, contextual, transactional approach to studying changing processes over time that may eventuate in what we consider to be maladaptive outcomes. It is a strategy of multifaceted research, including reciprocal processes (e.g., Cicchetti & Schneider-Rosen, 1986).

One of the challenges of the UCLA Family Stress Project was to draw together into a coherent model the "nonorthogonal risk factors", as termed by Walker, Downey, and Nightingale (1989). In a high-risk sample such as ours, correlated risk factors are a terror to be reckoned with, and we attempted not only to analyze for the impact of separate factors, but also to explore what happens when they are combined in various ways. Two strategies were applied in our attempts to bring together the major variables of the project, that will help to organize our overall conclusions: a risk factors model, and a structural equation model.

For the risk factors model, we were guided by the strategy reported earlier by Rutter and colleagues (e.g., Rutter & Quinton, 1984), and made an attempt to identify a set of risk/protective factors. We came up with a list of eight potential resilience factors (or when absent or minimal could be considered risk factors) identified from the literature on high risk children: self-concept, paternal diagnosis, presence of father in the home, maternal current mood, level of maternal chronic stress, child's social competence, and academic performance. The relationship between number of risk/resilience factors and indices of children's diagnoses were significant. Figure 3 depicts the findings graphically. Clearly, the more such factors a child has, the less likely she or he is to have diagnosable depression, and effect is linear.

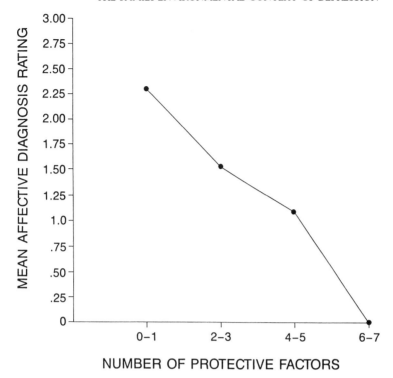

Figure 3. Lifetime affective disorder ratings by number of protective factors. (High risk random sample; excludes children of normal mothers). From C. Hammen (1991). *Depression runs in families: The social context of risk and resilience in children of depressed mothers.* NY: Springer-Verlag. Copyright 1991 by Springer-Verlag. Reprinted by permission.

A causal-modeling approach is a more elegant way to combine variables, indicating specific predicted relationships between variables and the extent to which the theoretical a priori model is actually fit by the covariance matrix of the variables. Because of a limited sample size (and the need to randomly include only one child per family), the model that we selected to test is a bare-bones model with as few variables as we could include and still have an interesting and meaningful model. The ingredients that we wished to test were the following:

1. three generations of effect (and we expect that if we followed the children into adulthood we would also see a fourth generation effect), and the impact on children's psychopathology is mediated by the effect of the mother's background on her parenting quality. We hypothesize that when the mother herself comes from a family with psychopathology, her own learning experiences in close interpersonal relationships are impaired, and she may have early onset of disorder that prevents acquisition of critical developmental

tasks involving problem-solving and other skills. As a result, she may have poor parenting skills in terms of a negative quality of interactions and ability to negotiate conflicts with her children.

2. a stress-generation effect as a way of capturing in part a mechanism by which families transmit depression. Specifically, we predict that women from dysfunctional (diagnosed) families of their own will tend to marry men with diagnoses (assortative mating, a highly stress-generative effect), as well as experience higher levels of chronic stress contributing to their negative relationships with the child. Additionally, the child will also show some stress generation effect in contributing to stressful life events that in turn contribute to depressive outcomes. We predict that impaired parenting has a direct consequence on children's social competence, which has a direct effect on symptomatology, and an indirect effect through the contribution of impaired social competence on children's tendency to generate stressors, particularly in the interpersonal domain.

3. specificity of the model for depression outcomes. The model is applied to children's depressive diagnoses over the 3-year follow-up period, and separately to nonaffective diagnoses, and to any diagnoses. If the model is unique to depression, then it would fit for such outcomes but not for other diagnosable conditions.

The model was tested using the EQS structural equation procedures developed by Bentler (1985). The model was first tested on children's depression diagnoses, and proved to be a significant fit as indicated by a nonsignificant chi-square showing that the actual and predicted covariances structures did not differ, X^2 (23) = 30.5, p = .14. Bentler (1990) has recently developed a Comparative Fit Index that is reliable for relatively small samples; its values range from 0 to 1.0, and indicate the extent to which the model is an improvement over the prediction of independent associations between variables. In the present model, the CFI was .95, indicating good fit to the data. Figure 4 presents the model and the standardized weights associated with each path. All of the predicted relationships were significant at least at p .025, one-tailed, with one exception. The direct path between the latent variables of maternal background and parenting quality failed to attain significance, although the path itself contributes to the fit of the overall model.

Application of the same model to nondepressive diagnoses, and to any diagnoses indicated that the model also fit those outcomes. In both cases the chi-square was nonsignificant, and the CFI values were .98 and .95, respectively.

Overall, therefore, it appears that the hypothesized model predicts children's psychopathology during a follow-up period, but it is not specific to depression. The fit of the model does not mean that other models would not also fit the data, or that different paths not included here are unimportant.

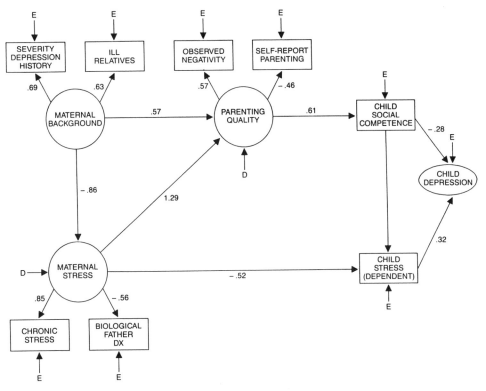

Figure 4. Structural equation model of the predictors of children's depression in a sample of children of women with affective disorders, chronic medical illness, or normal-women. Standardized solution with beta coefficients. E refers to error associated with measured variables, and D is the error associated with latent variable. From C. Hammen (1991). *Depression runs in families: The social context of risk and resilience in children of depressed mothers.* NY: Springer-verlag. Copyright 1991 by Springer-Verlag. Reprinted by permission.

Due to the small sample size and the subsequent limitations on the number of variables and paths that could be reliably tested, we did not include, for instance, a reciprocal path between parenting and child's social competence. In our work we have demonstrated through other analyses that mothers and children have a mutual impact on their interactions, but this reciprocity was not included in the present model. Also, due to the high level of comorbidity of symptomatology, this sample is not ideal for testing the specificity of the model for depression. Numerous other ingredients and variables that we did not include in our study might be important to include in future models. Thus, we emphasize that this is a working model, and not a final model, whose contribution ought to be evaluated in terms of its ability to provoke further elaborations and improvements. It is a unique model in its attempt to charac-terize the intergenerational transmission of depression in children through psychosocial paths indicating interpersonal disruption and generation of stressful conditions. The success of the current model in no way discredits the potential importance of genetic contributions to children's risk for disorder. However, our view is that such an emphasis has been overstated to the relative neglect of environmental transmission, and that ultimately, gene-environment correlation (Plomin, 1986) is probably the most valid way of thinking about the precursors of risk in children of parents with affective disorder. We included, but gave less attention than they deserve, to the fathers as well as the mothers, and to children's social competence. We have only scratched the surface of the complexities of children's interpersonal functioning and generation of, as well as coping with, stressful conditions. We recognize that this study has generated a great deal of information about what happens to children, but we think there are great gaps in understanding what the youngsters are *doing*.

Other limitations that we readily acknowledge include the relatively small sample size of separate groups, and the fairly wide range of children's ages studied (8 to 16) precluding more precise developmental formulations. Also, the unipolar sample included women who had serious clinical disorders including recurrent, if not chronic, symptomatology. In keeping with studies that suggest high rates of personality disorder in unipolar populations, probably many of the women would have Axis II disorders — not that such designation clarifies much except to say that they had long-standing, impairing disorders. Further studies with larger and more mildly depressed samples are needed to test the generalizability of the present findings. Also, of course, the current study is about only one model of children's depression — risk due to maternal characteristics. Whether the findings could be applied to populations of depressed children in general remains to be seen.

Overall, this study has proven to be rich in its yield of data, hypotheses, and suppositions. But now, much work lies ahead in more detailed and controlled studies that will help to clarify the processes and mechanisms about which we have bravely speculated.

Conclusion and Implications for Developmental Psychopathology

Cicchetti (1990; Cicchetti & Schneider-Rosen, 1986) has articulated central aspects of a developmental psychopathology perspective that have been influential in the present work: a transactional framework, historical and developmental continuities, and inclusion of multiple indicators of functioning. As noted at the outset, an understanding of the phenomenology and typical course of adult depression compel us to view the person in a context that includes the effect of the person on the environment as well as the environment's effects on the person. When applied to the development of depression in children, our study has emphasized the impact of the environment on the child in the form of mother-child interactions and the impact of stressors. It has also, however, emphasized the influence of the child on the environment — on the mother's moods and interaction quality, on peer and academic functioning, and on the occurrence of stressful events. The depressed mother and child carry on an elaborate, reciprocal process in which they not only have direct impacts on each other, but also influence the availability of each as a resource or liability in buffering the ill effects of stress.

The continuity and developmental process that are emphasized by Cicchetti are also captured in our approach, in the idea that early maladaptation or competence exerts an influence on subsequent functioning. The depressed mother's own background experiences appear to influence not only her depression but also her social and parental functioning. In turn, early interactions with the child appear to set the stage for his or her self-schema quality and for the acquisition of social skills and abilities to function in peer- and academic situations. Impairments of functioning in these critical domains are seen to further contribute to symptomatology, and presumably to further barriers to experiencing competence or compensatory achievements. The great majority of children who had early onset of symptomatology appeared to continue to have difficulties over the course of observation of up to 3 years, whereas those who seemed to have fared well early generally continued to develop skills and coping capabilities. We might speculate that children and adolescents that we observed to have difficult paths would continue to have difficulties, and even that some of them would go on to have maladaptive relationships that might lead to their own depressed parenting and its ill effects on their children.

The interplay between multiple levels of functioning cannot be overemphasized — the links between parenting, children's cognitions and representations of the world, relationships, and the self, and the actual skills and behaviors that reflect and support such underlying schemas — are all vitally important to pursue. An especially intriguing integrative approach that has considerable similarity to the present perspective, makes use of attachment theory as an explanatory mechanism linking early relationships, cognitions (working models), and behaviors to depression (Cicchetti, Cummings, Greenberg, & Marvin, 1990; Cummings & Cicchetti, 1990). These authors draw on theory and research findings to suggest intricate, transactional pathways in the developmental unfolding of maladaptive (depressive) outcomes in children. In our ongoing research, we are pursuing the study of attachments and their cognitive consequences in the forms of representations of the self and others, and how such schemas influence actual social behaviors and relationships, particularly as they may contribute to stressful events and use and availability of stress-buffering resources.

REFERENCES

Achenbach, T. M., & Edelbrock, C. S. (1983). *Manual for the Child Behavior Checklist Behavior Profile.* Burlington, VT: Thomas M. Achenbach, Department of Psychiatry, University of Vermont.

Adrian, C. (1990). *Differential vulnerability to stress in children of mothers with affective disorders and mothers without history of major psychopathology.* Unpublished doctoral dissertation, University of California, Los Angeles.

Adrian, C., & Hammen, C. (in press). Stress exposure and stress generation in children of depressed mothers. *Journal of Abnormal Psychology.*

Anderson, C. A., & Hammen, C. (1990) Sibling pairs of depressed women. Unpublished manuscript.

Anderson, C. A., & Hammen, C. (1992). Psychosocial functioning in children at risk for depression: Longitudinal follow-up. Manuscript under review.

Andreasen, N. C., Endicott, J., Spitzer, R. L., & Winokur, G. (1977). The family history method using diagnostic criteria. *Archives of General Psychiatry, 34,* 1229–1235.

Barnett, P. A., & Gotlib, I. H. (1988). Psychosocial functioning and depression: Distinguishing among antecedents, concomitants, and consequences. *Psychological Bulletin, 104,* 97–126.

Beck, A. T., Brown, G., Steer, R. A., Eidelson, J. I., & Riskind, J. H. (1987). Differentiating anxiety and derpession: A test of the cognitive content-specificity hypothesis. *Journal of Abnormal Psychology, 96,* 179–183.

Bentler, P. (1985). *Theory and implementation of EQS: A structural equation program.* Los Angeles: BMDP Statistical Software.

Bentler, P. M. (1990). Comparative fit indexes in structural models. *Psychological Bulletin, 107,* 238–246.

Brown, G. W., & Harris, T. (1978). *Social origins of depression.* London: Free Press.

Burbach, D. J., & Borduin, C. M. (1986). Parent-child relations and the etiology of depression: A review of methods and findings. *Clinical Psychology Review, 6,* 133–153.

Burge, D., & Hammen, C. (1991). Maternal communication: A predictor of children's outcomes at follow-up in a high risk sample. *Journal of Abnormal Psychology, 100,* 174–180.

Chambers, W., Puig-Antich, J., Hirsch, M., Paez, P., Ambrosini, P., Tabrizi, M., & Davies, M. (1985). The assessment of affective disorders in children and adolescents by semi-structured interview. *Archives of General Psychiatry, 42,* 696–702.

Cicchetti, D. (1990). The organization and coherence of socioemotional, cognitive, and representational development: Illustrations through a developmental psychopathology perspective on Down Syndrome and child maltreatment. In R. Thompson (ed.) *Nebraska symposium on Motivation, Vol. 36. Socioemotional development.* Lincoln, Nebraska: University of Nebraska Press.

Cicchetti, D., & Cummings, E. M. (1990). An organizational perspective on attachment beyond infancy. In R. Thompson (ed.) *Nebraska Symposium on Motivation, Vol. 36. Socioemotional development.* Lincoln, Nebraska: University of Nebraska Press.

Cicchetti, D., & Schneider-Rosen, K. (1986). An organizational approach to childhood depression. In M. Rutter, C. E. Izard, & P. B. Read, *Depression in young people* (pp. 71–134). NY: Guilford.

Clark, D. A., Beck, A. T., & Stewart, B. (1990). Cognitive specificity and positive-negative affectivity: Conplementary or contradictory views on anxiety and depression? *Journal of Abnormal Psychology, 99,* 148–155.

Conrad, M., & Hammen, C. (1989). Role of maternal depression in perceptions of child maladjustment. *Journal of Consulting and Clinical Psychology, 57,* 663–667.

Coyne, J. C., Kahn, J., & Gotlib, I. H. (1987). Depression. In T. Jacob (ed.), *Family interaction and psychopathology* (pp. 509–533). New York: Plenum.

Cummings, E. M., & Cicchetti, D. (1990). Toward a transactional model of relations between attachment and depression. In R. Thompson (ed.) *Nebraska Symposium on Motivation, Vol. 36. Socioemotional development.* Lincoln, Nebraska: University of Nebraska Press.

Depue, R. A., & Monroe, S. M. (1986). Conceptualization and measurement of human disorder and life stress research: The problem of chronic disturbance. *Psychological Bulletin, 99,* 36–51.

Downey, G., & Coyne, J. C. (1990). Children of depressed parents: An integrative review. *Psychological Bulletin, 108,* 50–76.

Dunn, L. M., & Dunn, L. M. (1981). Peabody Picture Vocabulary Test-Revised. American Guidance Service, Circle Pines, MN.

Forehand, R., Wells, K., McMahon, R., Griest, D., & Rogers, T. (1982). Maternal perception of maladjustment in the clinic-referred children: An extension of earlier research. *Journal of Behavioral Assessment, 4,* 145–151.

Gold, P. W., Goodwin, F. K., & Chrousos, G. P. (1988). Clinical and biochemical manifestations of depression: Relation to the neurobiology of stress. *New England Journal of Medicine, 319,* 413–420.

Goodman, S. H., & Brumley, H. E. (1990). Schizophrenic and depressed mothers: Relational deficits in parenting. *Developmental Psychology, 26*(1), 31–39.

Gopelrud, E., Depue, R. A. (1985). Behavioral response to naturally-occurring stress in cyclothymes, dysthymes, and controls. *Journal of Abnormal Psychology, 94,* 128–139.

Gordon, D., Burge, D., Hammen, C., Adrian, C., Jaenicke, C., & Hiroto, D. (1989). Observations of interactions of depressed women with their children. *American Journal of Psychiatry, 146,* 50–55.

Gotlib, I., & Hammen, C. (in press). *Psychological aspects of depression: Toward a cognitive-interpersonal integration.* NY: John Wiley.

Griest, D., Forehand, R., Wells, K., & McMahon, R. (1980). An examination of differences between nonclinic and behavior-problem clinic-referred children and their mothers. *Journal of Abnormal Psychology, 89,* 497–500.

Griest, D., Wells, K., & Forehand, R. (1979). An examination of predictors of maternal perceptions of maladjustment in clinic-referred children. *Journal of Abnormal Psychology, 88,* 277–281.

Hammen, C. (1991). Mood disorders (Unipolar depression). In M. Hersen & S. Turner (eds.), *Adult psychopathology and diagnosis,* Second Edition. New York: John Wiley.

Hammen, C. (1991). The generation of stress in the course of unipolar depression. *Journal of Abnormal Psychology, 100,* 555–561.

Hammen, C. (1988). Self-cognitions, stressful events, and the prediction of depression in children of depressed mothers. *Journal of Abnormal Child Psychology, 16,* 347–360.

Hammen, C. (1991). *Depression runs in families:The social context of risk and resilience in children of depressed mothers.* NY: Springer-Verlag.

Hammen, C., Adrian, C., Gordon, D., Burge, D., Jaenicke, C., & Hiroto, D. (1987). Children of depressed mothers: Maternal strain and symptom predictors of dysfunction. *Journal of Abnormal Psychology, 96,* 190–198.

Hammen, C., Adrian, C., & Hiroto, D. (1988). A longitudinal test of the attributional vulnerability model in children at risk for depression. *British Journal of Clinical Psychology, 27,* 37–46.

Hammen, C., & Anderson, C. (1990). *Longitudinal study of children of depressed mothers: Unipolar vs. bipolar comparisons.* Unpublished manuscript.

Hammen, C., Burge, D., & Adrian, C., (1991). Timing of mother and child depression in a longitudinal study of children at risk. *Journal of Consulting and Clinical Psychology, 59,* 341–345.

Hammen, C., Burge, D., Burney, E., & Adrian, C. (1991). Longitudinal study of diagnoses in children of women with unipolar and bipolar affective disorder. *Archives of General Psychiatry, 47,* 1112–1117.

Hammen, C., Burge, D., & Stansbury, K. (1990). Relationship of mother and child variables to child outcomes in a high risk sample: A causal modeling analysis. *Developmental Psychology, 26,* 24–30.

Hammen, C., Ellicott, A., Gitlin, M., & Jamison, K. R. (1989). Sociotropy/autonomy and vulnerability to specific life events in unipolar and bipolar patients. *Journal of Abnormal Psychology, 98,* 154–160.

Hammen, C., & Goodman-Brown, T. (1990). Self-schemas and vulnerability to specific life stress in children at risk for depression. *Cognitive Therapy and Research, 14,* 215–227.

Hammen, C., Gordon, D., Burge, D., Adrian, C., Jaenicke, C., & Hiroto, D. (1987). Communication patterns of mothers with affective disorders and their relationship to children's status and social functioning. In K. Hahlweg, & M. G. Goldstein (eds.), *Understanding major mental disorder: The contribution of family interaction research* (pp. 103–119).

Hammen, C., Marks, T., Mayol, A., & deMayo, R. (1985). Depressive self-schemas, life stress, and vulnerability to depression. *Journal of Abnormal Psychology, 94,* 308–319.

Hammen, C., Mayol, A., deMayo, R., & Marks, T. (1986). Initial symptom levels and the life event-depression relationship. *Journal of Abnormal Psychology, 95,* 114–122

Hammen, C., & Zupan, B. A. (1984). Self-schemas, depression, and the processing of personal information in children. *Journal of Experimental Child Psychology, 37,* 598–608.

Jaenicke, C., Hammen, C., Zupan, B., Hiroto, D., Gordon, D., Adrian, C., & Burge, D. (1987). Cognitive vulnerability in children at risk for depression. *Journal of Abnormal Child Psychology, 15,* 559–572.

Kovacs, M. (1981). Rating scales to assess depression in school children. *Acta Paedopsychiatrica, 46,* 305–315.

Piers, E., & Harris, D. (1969). *The Piers-Harris Children's Self-Concept Scale. Nashville: Counselor Recordings and Tests.*

Plomin, R. (1986). *Development, genetics, and psychology* (pp. 109–125). Hillsdale, NJ: Lawrence Erlbaum.

Plomin, R., & Daniels, D. (1987). Why are children in the same family so different from one another? *The Behavioral and Brain Sciences, 10,* 1–15.

Puig-Antich, J., Lukens, E., Davies, M., Goetz, D., Brennon-Quattrock, J., & Todak, G. (1985a). Psychosocial functioning in prepubertal major depressive disorders, I: Interpersonal relationships during the depressive episode. *Archives of General Psychiatry, 42,* 500–507.

Rutter, M., & Quinton, P. (1984). Parental psychiatric disorder: Effects on children. *Psychological Medicine, 14,* 853–880.

Seligman, M. E. P., Peterson, C., Kaslow, N. J., Tenenbaum, R. L., Alloy, L. B., & Abramson, L. Y. (1984). Attributional style and depressive symptoms among children. *Journal of Abnormal Psychology, 93,* 235–241.

Sroufe, L. A., & Fleeson, J. (1986). Attachment and the construction of relationships. In W. Hartup & Z. Rubin (eds.), *Relationships and development.* Hillsdale, NJ: Erlbaum.

Walker, E., Downey, G., & Nightingale, N. (1989). The nonorthogonal nature of risk factors: Implications for research on the causes of maladjustment. *Journal of Primary Prevention, 9*(3), 143–163.

Weissman, M. M., & Paykel, E. S. (1974). *The depressed woman: A study of social relationships.* Chicago, IL: Univeristy of Chicago Press.

Weissman, M. M., Wickramaratne, P., Warner, V., John, K., Prusoff, B. A., Merikangas, K. R., & Gammon, G. D. (1987). Assessing psychiatric disorders in children: Discrepancies between mothers' and children's reports. *Archives of General Psychiatry, 44,* 747–753.

Whalen, C., Henker, B., Collins, B., et al. (1979). Peer interaction in a structured communication task: Comparisons of normal and hyperactive boys and of methylphenidate (Ritalin) and placebo effects. *Child Development, 50,* 388–401.

VIII Parental Depression, Family Functioning, and Child Adjustment: Risk Factors, Processes, and Pathways

E. MARK CUMMINGS & PATRICK T. DAVIES

It is now well-established that children of depressed parents are at increased risk for the development of psychopathology (e.g., Beardslee, Bemporad, Keller, & Klerman, 1983; Downey & Coyne, 1990; Orvaschel, 1983). Until recently, however, empirical approaches in this area primarily focused on discovering genetic and biological factors involved in the relationship between parental depression and child difficulties. A common presupposition was that the primary bases for the transmission of psychopathology were to be found in biological structures contained within the individual. Although biological models have proven useful, at best they can only partially explain the association between depression in parents and maladjustment in children. Pertinent to this point, children of depressed parents are not only at specific risk for clinical depression, but are at risk for a full range of problems of adjustment (Downey & Coyne, 1990). Thus, an adequate model must account for the increased incidence of both externalizing and internalizing problems, including depression, in children of depressed parents. More complex models are clearly needed in order to obtain a complete picture of the transmission of psychopathology within families with parental depression.

Recent theoretical and empirical efforts have begun to address this problem by examining the role of contextual and environmental factors associated with depression in families. Instead of focusing on the intrapersonal factors that are characteristic of biological models, environmental approaches place emphasis on identifying interactional and interpersonal mechanisms associated with the development of psychopathology in families with parental depression. This chapter adopts such an environmental perspective in examining factors and processes that may be involved in the link between parental depression and child psychopathology, recognizing that biological factors, which are beyond the scope of the present chapter to review, are also elemental to a complete explanation. Our primary goal in the present chapter is to advance a process-oriented study of environmental effects of parental depression, focusing specifically on the role of two classes of environmental mechanisms, interparental conflict and parenting practices.

Relatedly, we outline key elements that should be considered for a process-oriented study of environmental elements associated with parental depression. Many of the investigations in the parental depression literature can be characterized as epidemiological in nature. Specifically, such studies have focussed on comparing rates of global, diagnostic disorders in children of depressed parents versus rates in children from other, including normal, groups (LaRoche, 1989). Implicit in such research is often the assumption that a significant association between parental depression and child maladjustment is adequate justification to conclude that depression in parents has directly "caused" child psychopathology. Diagnostic status, however, does not directly influence development, and is no more than a marker variable for the actual processes behind associations. From an environmental perspective, researchers must look beyond the diagnostic label of depression and examine the factors and processes associated with it. There have been increasing calls in the literature for more complex, process-oriented studies of the effects of family depression on children (e.g., Coyne, Downey, & Boergers, this volume; Hammen, this volume).

Pertinent to this issue, Cummings and his associates (Cummings & Cummings, 1988; Cummings & El-Sheikh, 1991) have recently outlined a process-oriented approach to the study of the effects of marital and family discord on children. In this chapter, we illustrate how such an approach, which is consistent with and incorporates key themes of the emerging discipline of developmental psychopathology (Cicchetti, 1984; 1990), might be extended to the study of the effects of depression in families. Adding to the pertinence of this approach for the present context, there is accumulating evidence for strong intercorrelations among marital discord, parental depression, and child maladjustment (see review in Downey & Coyne, 1990). Taking the study of relations among marital discord, parental depression, and child development a step further, that is, to begin to delineate process-relations between specific family environments and specific child outcomes, is thus a timely issue. As an approach, the process-oriented strategy developed to study the general effects of marital discord on children provides a rubric for the study of the effects of marital discord on children in the context of families with parental depression. Recent empirical findings from the process-oriented study of the effects of anger on children also would appear to have clear implications and relevance for the understanding of the impact of marital discord on children in families with parental depression. However, a consideration of only discord as a familial factor in the transmission of psychopathology within families with parental depression runs the risk of presenting an overly simple model of family process. As the approach develops, process-oriented strategies must continually expand the classes of family factors considered in ever more encompassing models, while at the same time fostering the development of more fine-grained, detailed examinations of relations within an individual class of variables. Consistent with this aim, in this chapter we examine the effects of another class of variables implicated in the effects of parental depression on children, that is, the child-rearing practices of parents.

The remainder of the chapter is organized into three parts. The first section considers a process-oriented analysis of children's responses to adults' angry behavior and relations with parental depression. Next, relations between child-rearing characteristics and parental depression are examined, including a consideration of interrelations between interparent anger, child-rearing practices, and parental depression. Finally, the general methodological and conceptual elements of a process-oriented approach are outlined and are specifically applied to the question of new directions for research in the study of the development of children in families with parental depression.

Parental Depression and Marital Conflict

Adult depression has been shown to covary to a substantial degree with marital hostility, distress, and anger (Ablon, Davenport, Gershon, & Adland, 1975; Coyne, Burchill, & Stiles, 1990; Davenport, Ebert, Adland, & Goodwin, 1977; Fendrich, Warner, & Weissman, 1990; Hay, Zahn-Waxler, Cummings, & Iannotti, in press; Rutter & Quinton, 1984). Furthermore, investigations that have simultaneously examined depression and marital conflict indicate that marital conflict may play a significant, and perhaps even focal, role in the intergenerational transmission of psychopathology in these families. For example, Emery, Weintraub, and Neale (1982) found that marital discord was the primary mediator in the transmission of difficulties from depressed parents to children. Subsequently, Shaw and Emery (1987) reported that the concurrent examination of depression and marital discord was a better predictor of child psychopathology than either factor alone. In a recent review of research on children of depressed parents, Downey and Coyne (1990) argue that the current evidence is strong enough to support a tentative conclusion that "marital discord is a viable alternative explanation for the general adjustment difficulties of children with a depressed parent" (p. 68). Finally, given the well documented relations between interparental anger and deleterious child outcomes in a variety of nondepressed samples (Emery, 1982; Grych & Fincham, 1990), it is not unreasonable to expect that such relations would also apply, at least in outline, to families with depressed parents, although differences in specific process relations in association with family contexts linked more-or-less uniquely with parental depression might be anticipated.

Until recently, few studies took into account or examined the multidimensional complexities of either interparent conflict or child behavior. Interparent conflict was typically treated as a unidimensional construct and child functioning was assessed in terms of global, questionnaire-based measures. Little was known of the effects of the numerous, constituent dimensions of family conflict (e.g., type of conflict, duration, intensity) or of the multi-level, multi-faceted nature of children's response systems (Cummings & Cummings, 1988; Cummings & El-Sheikh, 1991). However, more recent investigations have begun to shed light upon the complex nature of child functioning and parental discord, leading to corresponding progressions in the understanding of precise process relations between adults' conflicts and child outcomes. In the following sections, we consider: (a) the complex array of child responses and outcomes to interadult anger that must be considered for a process-oriented characterization of elements of responding; (b) the variable effects of specific dimensions of conflict on children; (c) evidence that children of depressed parents may be particularly likely to be exposed to certain severe and deleterious dimensions of marital conflict; and (d) how certain processes and mechanisms might contribute to the relationship between marital conflict and child pathology.

Children's Responses to Interadult Anger: A Detailed Analysis

Children's responses to interparental conflict can be examined across several levels of analysis, ranging from specific, microscopic assessments of specific behavioral responses to global, macroscopic analyses. An assumption of a process-oriented approach is that each level of analysis provides useful information, with a complete picture of effects only emerging from a complex consideration of all pertinent response data. The levels of response to be considered and reviewed here include: (a) specific assessments of single, isolated response domains (e.g., emotion or physiology or cognition); (b) coherent patterns or styles of responding extant across multiple response domains (e.g., hypersensitivity, appropriate sensitivity, hyposensitivity); (c) the stability and discontinuity of child responses across contexts and periods of development (e.g., stability of aggression in early childhood), and (d) diagnostic assessments such as adaptation and maladaptation, or more specifically, internalizing and externalizing difficulties. Because the marital discord literature has focused on the last, most global level of analysis, the following review emphasizes recent findings pertinent to the first three levels analysis.

Specific Response Domains

Interadult conflict has been shown to have powerful and predictable effects on children's emotions. Children most commonly respond to interadult conflict with anger (e.g., Cummings, Vogel, Cummings, & El-Sheikh, 1989; Cummings, Zahn-Waxler, & Radke-Yarrow, 1981; Grych, Seid, & Fincham,

1991), concern (e.g., Cummings, 1987; Grych et al., 1991; Shred, McDonnell, Church, & Rowan, 1991), and distress and fear (e.g., Cummings, Ballard, El-Sheikh, & Lake, 1991; Cummings et al., 1981). Other well-documented responses include sadness (e.g., Cummings, 1987; Cummings, Vogel, Cummings, & El-Sheikh, 1989; Cummings, Ballard, El-Sheikh, & Lake, 1991; Grych et al., 1991), shame (e.g., Grych et al., 1991), and helplessness (e.g., Grych et al., 1991). Although conflict between adults most reliably elicits negative emotions from children, both behavioral observations and children's self-reports indicate that "positive emotional expressions" may also increase during exposure to conflict. However, since positive emotions typically occur in concert with behaviors or expressions of negative emotional behaviors and feelings, it seems unlikely the correct interpretation is that children are made "happy" by others' anger (e.g., Cummings, 1987; El-Sheikh, Cummings, & Goetsch, 1989). More plausible is that the observed increases in positive, as well as negative, emotions indicates that adults' conflicts serve as an elicitor of general and nonspecific affective arousal in children.

In terms of children's social and interpersonal behavior, exposure to interadult anger has been shown to induce behaviors of aggression, social withdrawal, and prosocial intervention, with context being an important factor in children's specific behavioral expressions. Increases in aggressiveness have been reported in a number of studies, particularly when children are observed in play with peers following exposure to anger (e.g., Cummings, 1987; Cummings, Iannotti, & Zahn-Waxler, 1985; Klaczynski & Cummings, 1989), but more general increases in expressions of aggressiveness and anger also have been reported (Cummings, Hennessy, Rabideau, & Cicchetti, 1991). Younger children, in particular, often withdraw from social interaction and peer play when exposed to interadult anger (J. S. Cummings, Pellegrini, Notarius, & Cummings, 1989; Shred et al., 1991). Interparental anger also may elicit prosocial responses, such as mediation, distraction, and comforting, particularly when parents are involved in the fights (Cummings et al., 1981; Cummings, Zahn-Waxler, & Radke-Yarrow, 1984; J. S. Cummings et al., 1989).

Children's prosocial responses to interadult anger may take the form of "role reversal", that is, attempting to take care of the parent, in contrast to the more normative response of the parent taking care of the child. Child caretaking of the parent has been observed in response to naturally occurring episodes of marital discord in the home (Cummings et al., 1981; 1984) and laboratory simulations of conflicts involving the parents (J. S. Cummings et al., 1989; Cummings, Hennessy, Rabideau, & Cicchetti, 1991). Further, children's taking responsibility for parents' fights has been positively associated with the level of marital discord in the home. For a child, particularly a young child, to assume responsibility for the parents' welfare and feelings in this context surely places an undue burden on the child. In depressed families, further, the tendency of parents to depend on their children for comfort, support, and guidance may exacerbate these burdens (Davenport, Adland, Gold, & Goodwin, 1979; Davenport, Zahn-Waxler, Adland, & Mayfield, 1984). These children may frequently and perhaps grudgingly be placed in the parenting role, during interparental conflict and in other contexts as well. The stressful and difficult responsibility of caring for parents in high stress contexts, in combination with other factors in homes with depression, may increase children's internalizing symptomatology, including dysphoria, guilt, anxiety, and a sense of joylessness.

Children's cognitive processes both during and after observing episodes of anger have been less frequently and systematically examined. Nonetheless, the few studies that have been conducted underscore the potential significance of children's cognitive responses and the need for more study in this area (Grych & Fincham, 1990). Cummings and his collaborators, for example, have reported that an overwhelming majority of children interpret unresolved interadult conflicts as angry in content (e.g., Cummings, Vogel, Cummings, & El-Shiekh, 1989; Cummings, Ballard, El-Sheikh, & Lake, 1991; Cummings, Ballard, & El-Sheikh, 1991). A significant minority of children also perceive that conflicting adults are sad, especially when anger is expressed nonverbally (Cummings and Grogg, 1991). The emerging picture is that even very young children are extremely adept at detecting and labelling anger, but that some forms of anger expression (e.g., nonverbal anger) are seen by children as containing complex elements.

Recently, Grych et al. (1991) reported a study that examined 10–12 year old children's expectations, attributions, and beliefs about interparental conflicts. Children listened to audiotapes of interadult simulations of anger that varied systematically in terms of specific dimensions of conflict and then responded to a set of questions while imagining that the participants in the conflicts were their actual parents. Results indicated that children's beliefs and expectations about interparental conflict were shaped by specific dimensions of marital anger. For instance, conflicts in certain forms shaped children's expectations that the conflict would escalate (e.g., high intensity conflict), children's feelings of responsibility and guilt (e.g., high intensity conflict), and children's fears that they would be drawn into the conflict (e.g., high intensity conflict, child-related conflict). Conversely, other forms of conflict had a positive impact on the children by increasing their belief that they could effectively cope (e.g., child-related conflict).

Exposure to interadult conflicts also has been linked with changes in children's physiological response systems. For example, children may undergo hormonal changes in response to high levels of exposure to interparental conflict (Gottman & Fainsliber-Katz, 1989). More immediate physiological responses include consistent changes in systolic blood pressure and heart rate patterns during observations of background anger (Ballard, Cummings, & Larkin, in press; El-Sheikh et al., 1989).

Styles or Patterns of Responding

The study of specific response domains thus establishes that interadult anger is a stressor for children that effects a wide range of behavioral, emotional, and social systems. However, as with other stressors, most children cope successfully with exposure to even relatively high levels of interparental conflict along their way to normative developmental trajectories. Further, the examination of single response domains can make only a limited contribution to understanding of the general course and development of psychopathology associated with exposure to anger. Consistent with a basic tenet of the approach of developmental psychopathology (Cicchetti, 1984; Sroufe & Rutter, 1984), the study of individual patterns or styles of adaptation and maladaptation is more likely to be informative with regard to the prediction of developmental trajectories than group-based tendencies. Thus, another step along the way towards a process-oriented developmental psychopathology of angry environments is to look for individual coherences in responding across multiple response domains, based on the detailed study of these separate response dimensions.

With regard to this point, Cummings and his colleagues have identified coherent patterns or styles to interadult anger based on the assessment of multiple response domains (Cummings, 1987; El-Sheikh et al., 1989). Based on observations of children's social and emotional behavior, children's reports of feelings and thoughts, and a variety of assessments of children's physiological responding, children's responses to interadult anger were classified into one of three patterns or styles. *Concerned* responders exhibited behavioral signs of socioemotional distress and heart rate acceleration during exposure to interparental conflict. In later interviews, they also expressed empathic concern for the angry adults, that is, they said they felt sad for the adults and wished to help them. *Ambivalent* children, on the other hand, displayed generally greater rates of behavioral and emotional responding than other children, including *both* positive and negative affect, heart rate decleration with the onset of anger, and increased aggressiveness towards peers in play following exposure to anger. Finally, *unresponsive* children reported feeling angry and aroused by the adults' anger, but exhibited no overt behavioral or emotional reactions to anger. In other words, they apparently masked their underlying feelings of anger and arousal. In a subsequent study, Cummings and El-Sheikh (1991) found that the "more desirable" concerned pattern was linked with secure child-parent attachments as indicated by responses in a separation-reunion paradigm, whereas the other two "less desirable" patterns were associated with insecure parent-child attachments. Thus, the suggestion is that patterns of coping with anger might be linked with broader patterns of coping with stress (e.g., patterns of coping with separation), and thus may reflect more general and stable dispositions of individual normalcy or relatively problematic functioning in coping with everyday stressors during development. Several complex but differentiated patterns of responding to anger evidencing coherence across multiple domains of response thus emerged. While the evidence is surely thin at this point, and the interpretation of relations between behavioral and physiological domains, in particular, is not entirely straightforward (see El-Sheikh et al., 1989; Ballard, Cummings & Larkin, 1991; for discussion of these issues), one can conceptualize how these different behavioral styles may indicate antecedents of later developmental trajectories of normalcy and psychopathology. The empathy and distress associated with a concerned response pattern could be deemed as an "appropriately sensitive" style, and as a result, may promote normative development. An ambivalent style, on the other hand, could be a precursor of subsequent pathology. The behavioral dysregulation and tendency to act out may specifically facilitate the development of externalizing difficulties. Lastly, children identified as unresponsive to angry environments also may be at-risk for the development of psychopathology. Specifically, their apparent internalization and repression of arousal and anger might reflect risk for the development of internalizing disorders.

Behavioral Continuity Across Time and Context

The construct significance of a response disposition or style is increased if it can be shown that the response shows stability. Demonstrations of stability acquire significance for models of normal and psychopathological development if stability can be demonstrated for a substantial period of time in response to psychologically significant stressors that typically occur within the family. Pertinent to the construct validity and developmental significance of patterns of coping with anger, children's responses to interadult anger have been shown to be stable both for the short- and long-term in several studies, including studies of responding to actual marital discord in the home.

For example, Cummings et al. (1985) reported stable individual differences in response to interadult anger associated with two separate exposures to laboratory simulations of anger, with a one-month interval between exposures. Relatively high and significant correlations across exposures were found both for the distress induced in children by exposure to anger and for the aggressiveness shown by children in play towards peers. Stability in the tendency to respond emotionally to marital discord in the home has been reported in the short-term for both infants (Cummings et al., 1981) and school-age children (Cummings et al., 1984). Further, Cummings et al. (1984) reported long-term stability in children's tendency to respond emotionally to others' anger in the home for observations taken 5-years apart, with the first assessments taken when children were infants and with children observed again as school-age children. High levels of stability of aggression (rs as high as .76 for some dimensions of aggression) observed in the context of exposure to anger have been been reported for boys over a three year period (Cummings, Iannotti, & Zahn-Waxler, 1989).

Some of the results on this issue may be especially pertinent to issues of the developmental psychopathology of anger. Cummings (1987) reported evidence for long-term stability of responding to laboratory simulations of anger among children observed as toddlers and then again at preschool age. High levels of behavioral dysregulation, aggression, and emotional reactivity at 2 years of age were associated with the development of the ambivalent behavioral style when the children reached the late preschool years, a pattern characterized by similar, albeit more complexly organized, response dispositions (see the above description). By contrast, a low post-anger level of overt emotional reactivity in the toddler period was a precursor to an unresponsive behavior style at 5 years of age. Finally, toddler's displays of low levels of post-anger aggression and relatively moderate levels of emotional reactivity were associated with the concerned behavioral style when the children were exposed to conflict 3 years later. Given the aforementioned possible significance of these patterns to individual styles of coping with discord and more general coping styles, these findings suggest the intriguing notion that maladaptive styles of coping with stress may begin to find organization and stability quite early in childhood.

Pathways from Immediate Responding to Stable Dispositions

As the review of the process-oriented literature indicates, methodological recognition of the complexities of child behavior has advanced the understanding of children's responses to conflict. This work has not only begun to delineate the range of responses to anger but also has begun to delineate how specific responses to conflict may eventually develop into behavioral styles and pervasive dispositions. The evidence suggests that specific responses in one domain (e.g., emotional concern, physical aggression) are associated with responses in other domains (e.g., physiological responses such as heart rate and systolic blood pressure), that is, that domains of responding are interdependent. Over time such interdependent processes and influences may foster the development of behavioral styles or patterns of responding that are quite consistent across response domains.

These responses and behavioral styles in coping with exposure to background anger (i.e., anger in the family environment) may serve as general foundations or precursors of normative and psychopathological trajectories. Findings presented in the previous section indicate that there may be three **broad** developmental pathways that are roughly analogous to the courses of internalizing, externalizing, and normal trajectories. One pathway to internalizing difficulties may originate in children's responses to conflict that are indicative of low levels of overt emotional reactivity. These responses have been specifically associated with a subsequent behavioral style in which feelings of anger and negativity are repressed from overt displays of behavior. By contrast, behavioral dysregulation, aggression, or extremely high levels of emotional arousal in response to interadult anger lead to an ambivalent style of responding, which in turn, may be a precursor of later externalizing problems. Finally, moderate levels of emotional reactivity and behavioral self-control may be linked to an appropriate or normative style of coping with the stress of marital discord that is characterized by feelings of empathy, concern, and distress when exposed to interparental anger. Of course, it is recognized that multiple additional aspects of children's experience undoubtedly feed into the development of coping patterns and that children's own behavioral, and possibly genetically-based, styles are important elements of any developmental trajectory (e.g., see Dodge, 1990b; Lytton, 1990; Wahler, 1990).

Despite some recent progress in linking immediate responses of conflict to subsequent and more stable problems, exclusive focus on children's behavior precludes the identification of the precise dimensions of interparental anger that are contributing to these developmental pathways and child outcomes. In other words, only examining complexity in children's response processes leads to a limited picture; it also is necessary to examine variations in stimulus characteristics of anger. To address this issue, the following section reviews recent studies aimed at identifying relationships between specific stimulus dimensions of interparental anger and child response processes.

Dimensions of Interparental Conflict

Anger is a conceptually powerful and salient construct and, perhaps as a result, in both lay and professional literatures it is often explicitly or implicitly treated as if it were a single and unitary phenomenon. In fact, of course, anger is not a homogeneous stimulus, but can vary on a variety of dimensions and domains. Continued progress in understanding the effects of anger on children, both from the perspectives of developmental psychology and developmental psychopathology, surely requires a recognition of this fact. In this section we review recent findings on the effects of specific dimensions of anger on children and consider, when appropriate and feasible given current knowledge, issues of the effects of specific dimensions of anger in the context of parental depression.

Frequency

Greater frequencies of exposure to background anger have been associated with evidence indicating more emotional and behavioral difficulties in children. For example, Cummings et al. (1981; 1984) found that more frequent exposures to conflicts in the home were associated with heightened levels of distress, insecurity, and anger, suggesting that repeated exposure to interparental anger sensitizes children to conflict. Other studies also support a sensitization effect. Cummings et al. (1985) reported that a second exposure to interadult anger significantly increased children's levels of distress and aggression in response to anger. Over time and with very high levels of exposure, e.g., in families characterized by spousal abuse and / or physical abuse, one might expect outcomes that are even more enduring and intense. Eventually, this sensitizing process, in combination with other risk processes within the family, might produce enduring psychopathological dispositions, particularly with regard to aggression and other problems of undercontrol.

Cummings and Zahn-Waxler (in press) provide a detailed treatment of how increased levels of arousal associated with repeated exposure to marital discord might translate into increased risk for the development of externalizing disorders through related processes of sensitization, excitation transfer, and response disinhibition. A complete treatment of this issue, however, is beyond the scope of the present chapter.

Available evidence indicates that in comparison with children of normal parents, children of depressed parents are more likely to be repeatedly exposed to interparental conflict. The well documented comorbidity between marital conflict and parental depression (e.g., Coyne et al., 1990), is, in itself, support for the notion that conflicts are more frequent in depressed marriages. Further and more definitive evidence comes from detailed examination of the link between depression and anger (for more details, see Biglan, Hops, Sherman, Friedman, Arthur, & Osteen, 1985; Biglan, Rothlind, Hops, & Sherman, 1989; Hops, Biglan, Sherman, Arthur, Friedman, & Osteen, 1987). The data from these studies suggests that dysphoric behaviors of depressed wives serve as reinforcers by reducing the length of the husbands' anger episodes. In the long run, however, depressive behaviors are associated with an increase in the frequency of conflicts. Thus, the short-term reinforcing qualities of depression in reducing interparental hostility function, in the long run, to promote more frequent and explosive bursts of anger between parents. As noted above, frequent exposure to conflict is associated with high levels of emotional reactivity and behavioral dysregulation in children, and may contribute to the development of an externalizing coping style.

Mode of Expression

Physical expressions of anger. While depression is typically associated with the internalization of feelings, there is evidence that physical expressions of anger may, in fact, be more common in families with parental depression than in other families. Consistent with this hypothesis is evidence indicating that spousal abuse (Webster-Stratton & Hammond, 1988) and maternal maltreatment of children (Gilbreath & Cicchetti, 1991) are each significantly associated with maternal depression.

Observations of children's responses to interparental conflicts in the home indicate that physical conflicts elicit more distress from children than verbal forms of anger (Cummings et al., 1981). Another study found that children from homes with interparental violence reported feeling more distress than children without interparental violence in response to viewing videotaped conflicts between adults (Cummings et al., 1989). Further, comparisons of verbal anger with and without acts of physical aggression also indicate that children perceive conflicts containing physical aggression as being more negative (Cummings et al., 1989). Parental reports of physical conflict tactics also have been positively associated with children's emotional reactivity and concern during exposure to simulated expressions of anger involving parents (J. Cummings et al., 1989). The research thus indicates that children are most emotionally and behaviorally reactive to physical forms of conflict expression, which suggests that exposure to this form of anger expression may be most likely to be associated with risk for the development of patterns of behavioral dysregulation and an externalizing style of coping in children (Cummings, 1987). Consistent with this assertion, correlational investigations have shown that parental use of physical conflict tactics is most associated with externalizing disorders (Hershorn & Rosenbaum, 1985; Jouriles, Murphy, & O'Leary, 1989).

Nevertheless, it should not be assumed that physical anger between parents is not involved in the course of internalizing trajectories. Findings that children often respond to interadult physical anger with distress suggests that internalizing problems also could develop. Moreover, the intensity of physical anger is likely to elicit fear and anxiety; and such responses may be precursors of subsequent internalizing disorders. Consistent with this notion, recent research indicates that a pathway from interparental violence to child internalizing problems is a distinct possibility (Holden & Ritchie, 1991).

Nonverbal expressions of anger. The relatively few studies that have examined the impact of nonverbal modes of interparental anger on children have yielded an equivocal pattern of results. Jenkins and Smith (in press), for instance, reported that nonverbal forms of anger were not associated with the development of child behavior problems. At this juncture, however, it is surely erroneous to accept the conclusion of this study that children are not sensitive to nonverbal forms of conflict for at least two reasons. First, the results from this study were based solely on retrospective interviews with the parents and children; such measures may well not be sensitive to the relatively subtle characteristics and consequences of nonverbal anger.

Secondly, process-oriented studies designed to capture precise and subtle relations between nonverbal anger and children's responses suggest that children are, in fact, very sensitive to nonverbal conflicts. Children's emotional responses to nonverbal anger have generally been found to be quite negative (e.g., angry emotional responses), and virtually indistinguishable from responses to verbal anger in the negativity and anger induced in children (Ballard & Cummings, 1990; Cummings, Vogel, Cummings, & El-Sheikh, 1989; Cummings, Ballard & El-Sheikh, 1991), indicating that the immediate impact, at least, of nonverbal anger is comparable to that for verbal anger. One difference is that some forms of nonverbal anger expression are often perceived as sad as well as angry (e.g., anger shown by sighing) whereas verbal anger expressions and more demonstrative nonverbal anger expressions (e.g., anger indicated by angry facial expressions) are overwhelmingly perceived as angry (Cummings & Grogg, 1991). These findings illustrate that there are multiple dimensions even within specific modes of expression of anger such as nonverbal anger. Further, they begin to indicate how home environments characterized by nonverbal anger may differ in their impact on children from environments typified by verbal anger expression. Thus, these data are consistent with the notion that chronic exposure to high rates and levels of nonverbal forms of anger could contribute to the development of maladjustment.

Several factors underlying nonverbal anger can be seen as promoting internalizing styles of coping. For instance, the ambiguity and chronic tenseness in adults associated with nonverbal anger may act as a stressor for children in a number of ways, including increasing their arousal levels, feelings of anger, and uncertainties with regard to how to behave. Because feelings are not clear, out in the open, or resolved when adults express anger nonverbally, these environments may prevent the children from safely releasing their own anger and feelings of high arousal and tension, so that children resort to internalizing their feelings. However, these views are highly speculative at this point and more process-oriented research is clearly necessary before any conclusions can be made.

Nonverbal anger may be especially prevalent in families with parental depression, with relatively high rates of exposure to nonverbal anger in children from such homes. Clinical observations of Davenport and others (Davenport et al., 1979; 1984) suggest that families with a depressed parent are intensely preoccupied with controlling and avoiding expressions of anger and sadness. Avoidance of negative affect is particularly likely within the context of marital conflicts (Ablon et al., 1975). As an alternative to directly and appropriately expressing their anger, a depressed dyad may favor more subtle forms of hostility such as nonverbal anger (e.g., the silent treatment). Understanding of the effects of nonverbal anger thus may be particularly pertinent for a process-oriented analysis of relations between marital discord and children's adjustment in children from depressed families. Further, recent studies examining marital interaction of couples with a unipolar depressed spouse report that their conflicts qualitatively differ from conflicts of normal couples. Conflicts of depressed dyads contained interdependencies between anger and dysphoric expressions that are not as evident in conflicts of normal dyads (Biglan et al., 1985; Hops et al., 1987). Thus, children of depressed parents may be exposed to different forms of conflict that include substantial levels of both anger and dysphoria. While exposure to anger and hostility, in itself, may well be most directly linked to externalizing difficulties, the additional exposure of children of depressed parents to high levels of nonverbal anger and sadness, in conflict situations and more generally, may place children of depressed parents at particular risk for the subsequent development of internalizing difficulties, including depression, via contagion or a similar process. In short, the dysphoric nature of conflicts between depressed parental dyads may alter the impact of conflict on children and increase risk for internalizing as well as externalizing disorders associated with high levels of exposure to conflicts within families.

Intensity and Content

Conflicts also can vary in terms of intensity and content. During a verbal conflict, for example, parents could argue in an intensely negative manner; or alternatively, they could engage in a relatively calm and rational disagreement. It might be expected that, irrespective of differences in the forms of conflict, differences in intensity of expression would have differential impacts on children. With regard to content, in a recent review Grych and Fincham (1990) argued that the topic of the conflict may be a critical dimension of interparental anger; specifically, children may be become particularly distressed when exposed to child-related conflicts.

Although there appears to be good reason to believe that intensity and content are important dimensions of conflict, only the work by Grych et al. (1991) has addressed these issues. With regard to intensity, they found that, in comparison to low intensity fights, children reacted to high intensity conflicts with heightened levels of anger, sadness, concern, shame, and helplessness. In addition, children reported more fear, self-blame for the conflict, and reluctance to use direct intervention strategies to help end high intensity episodes of conflict. With regard to content, Grych et al. (1991) reported that when exposed to child-related conflicts children reported increased feelings of shame, self-blame, and fears that they would be drawn into the conflict. Thus, intense conflicts and child-related content would appear to be particularly associated with negative self-cognitions, and the feelings of helplessness, fear, and dysphoria associated with the symtomatology of depression.

Conflict Resolution

How conflicts end, particularly whether conflicts are resolved or not, may be as important, or more important, than how adults fight to child outcomes. The resolution of conflict repeatedly has been shown to significantly ameliorate the deleterious impact of conflict on children's emotions and behavior (Cummings et al., 1985; Cummings, Vogel, Cummings, & El-Sheikh, 1989; Cummings, Ballard, El-Sheikh, & Lake, 1991; J. S. Cummings et al., 1989; El-Sheikh et al., 1989). For example, Cummings et al. (1985) reported that children's aggression and distress reactions to interadult anger were reduced to baseline levels after the institution of a complete resolution. Cummings, Vogel, Cummings, & El-Sheikh (1989) found that children's feelings of anger and distress in response to adults' conflict were greatly mitigated by a subsequent resolution. In fact, children respond to a conflict followed by a complete resolution in a manner similar to their responses to entirely friendly interactions. A recent study (Cummings & Wilson, 1991) has shown that resolution significantly ameliorates children's distress regardless of the mode of expression of conflict, that is, whether conflicts were expressed nonverbally, verbally, or in a verbal-physical manner.

While resolution is often thought of as either being present or absent, it is not, in fact, a dichotomous factor, but is more accurately conceptualized along a continuum ranging from no resolution at one extreme to complete resolution at the other. Falling in between these two poles are various and numerous possible forms of partial resolution of conflict. Cummings, Ballard, El-Sheikh, & Lake (1991) reported that children were sensitive to relatively subtle variations in resolution, with the relative negativity of children's responses closely corresponding to the degree that fights were unresolved. For example, unresolved fights (continued fighting, the silent treatment) elicited more anger from children than partially resolved fights (submission, topic change), which, in turn, resulted in more anger than resolved conflicts (apology, compromise). Resolved conflicts and friendly interactions did not differ significantly in the anger induced in children. Conflict resolution is thus an important protective factor to consider when analyzing the effects of various rates of interparental conflict on children.

Depressive symptoms such as lethargy, withdrawal, and negative affect are likely to interfere with the effort and empathy required to resolve a conflict appropriately. Clinical studies suggest that depressed dyads are, in fact, substantially impaired in their abilities to communicate and resolve conflicts (Davenport et al., 1979). In a study that examined depressed mother-child dyads, Kochanska, Kuczynski, Radke-Yarrow, and Welsh (1987) reported that depressed mothers had substantial difficulties resolving conflicts with their children. Instead of attempting to reach a compromise, depressed mothers utilized less effortful strategies (e.g., power assertion, withdrawal) in order to end the conflict. Impairments in resolution abilities, however, may not be limited to the depressed spouse. Husbands of bipolar depressed wives, for example, have been characterized as passive and unresponsive in marital interactions (Ablon et al., 1975; Davenport et al., 1984). Other studies utilizing precise observational methods have found that depressed wives typically withdraw at the onset of a conflict while their husbands tend to become increasingly hostile (Biglan et al., 1985; Hops et al., 1987). This pattern of interaction precludes the utilization of an appropriate and empathetic approach necessary for resolution of conflict.

The chronic failure to resolve conflicts also may magnify the deleterious effects of exposure to interparental anger. Repeated failures at resolving conflicts may result in an accumulation of negative affect and unresolved issues, which might ultimately increase the frequency, intensity, and/or duration of subsequent angry episodes (Jenkins & Smith, in press). Thus, impairment in resolution abilities both fails to mitigate the immediate negative impact of interparental anger and also increases the cumulative adverse effects over time associated with exposure to marital discord.

Explanation

Whether parents explain marital conflicts to children, and the nature of these explanations, may also influence children's responses to conflict. With regard to this issue, Grych et al. (1991) reported that, in many cases, parental explanations absolving the child from blame for the parents' conflict appeared to buffer the child from feelings of fear and responsibility for conflict. Conversely, parental explanations imputing that the child was the cause of the conflict facilitated children's feelings of shame and distress. Thus, child-blaming explanations appear to increase children's negative self-cognitions and feelings, perhaps contributing to the development of a depressionogenic cognitive style, whereas explanations in which the child is absolved from blame may serve as a protective factor.

In another recent study on this issue, Cummings and Simpson (1991) found that adults' provision of explanations as to why they had fought and how they had made-up their differences had highly positive effects on children's emotional responding. Further, the benefits in this regard were as great as those obtained from showing adults actually engaging in a complete resolution of differences. This suggests that it may not be necessary for adults to actually resolve fights in front of children in order to ameliorate the effects of exposure to interadult anger on children, that is, a verbal account of the conflict and resolution process sometime later may accomplish the same ends.

Relatedly, Cummings and Wilson (1991) have found evidence to suggest that adults' resolving their differences "behind closed doors" also has highly beneficial effects. In this study children watched as adults fought (on videotape), left the room, and then came back sometime later interacting in a positive manner. Children's responses indicated that they inferred that adults had made up when outside of the room, that is, they responded to these fights in a non-negative manner quite similar to their responses to conflicts that they had actually observed being resolved. The message of recent work thus is that children do not need to be "hit over the head" with the fact that adults have resolved their conflicts in order to make this inference. However, it remains to be determined whether these conclusions apply to clinical (e.g., depressed) or high-risk (e.g., maltreated) families.

Unfortunately, depressed dyads may be impaired in their abilities to appropriately explain the causes and consequences of conflict to the child. Based on clinical observations Davenport et al. (1984) found that depressed parents go to great lengths to deny the occurrence of anger. Thus, the parents appear to foster further confusion in their children by not only refusing to provide an explanation but also denying that a conflict ever occurred. Other findings indicate that depressed parents are critical, provide less structure, and are relatively uninvolved during parent-child interactions (Goodman & Brumley, 1990; Gordon et al., 1989; Panaccione & Wahler, 1986). This is a further indication that depressed parents may refuse to reassure and support their child after marital conflicts.

In cases in which depressed parents do discuss the causes and consequences of conflicts to their children, the nature of the explanations may be critical, with some explanations having a more deleterious impact on children than failing to provide an explanation at all. Specifically, studies of parent-child interactions in a variety of contexts reveal that depressed parents often utilize critical and guilt-arousing parenting practices (Gordon et al., 1989; Zahn-Waxler, Iannotti, Cummings, & Denham, 1990). This negative style of parenting may use "explanation" as a means of placing the blame for the conflict on the child. Thus, the explanations provided by depressed parents could magnify negative outcomes associated with exposure to anger.

This review thus outlines dimensions of child response process and characteristics of anger stimuli pertinent to a process-oriented account for the observed relations among parental depression, marital discord, and child adjustment difficulties. Of course, elements of the family system associated with parental depression, in addition to marital discord, also are undoubtedly factors that increase the risk for the development of psychopathology in children from homes with parental depression. In the following section we consider evidence that another dimension of family functioning, namely, child-rearing practices, may be related to risk for the transmission of psychopathology in these families.

Parental Depression and Disruption in Child-rearing Practices

The comorbidity of parental depression and a variety of impairments in child-rearing practices is now well documented (Davenport et al., 1984; Gordon et al., 1989; Kochanska et al., 1987; Webster-Stratton & Hammond, 1988; Zahn-Waxler et al., 1990). Theoretical speculation coupled with some recent empirical work suggest that this association may develop out of several simultaneous processes.

An examination of the phenomonology of depression suggests that the presence of depressive symptoms alone can create a host of interpersonal difficulties for parent-child interactions. Depressive symptoms such as hostility, withdrawal, sadness, and passivity interfere with the capacity for parents to be responsive, sensitive, patient, consistent, and supportive towards children (Goodman & Brumley, 1990). Thus, the association between parental depression and parenting may, in part, result from a direct causal relation between the characteristics of depression and child-rearing practices (for more information, see Dix, 1991).

Depression also covaries with one or more variables that adversely affect child-rearing practices, irrespective of a diagnosis of depression, including low SES, lack of education about child development, and stressful life events (e.g., health problems, financial difficulties, marital conflict). For example, one study comparing families with depressed and well parents from poor socioeconomic conditions indicated that only one out of nine measures of childrearing significantly differentiated the two groups (Goodman & Brumley, 1990). At least in low SES families, other factors associated with environmental conditions may well be more robust predictors of child-rearing practices than the symptoms associated with depression.

Stressful life events may interact with depression, resulting in disruptions in parenting (Gordon et al., 1989; Hammen et al., 1987). Thus, depressive symptoms may increase the number and severity of environmental stressors through their deleterious influences on interactions with friends, co-workers, and others (Hammen, this volume). Environmental stressors, in turn, may exacerbate depressive episodes, setting up a vicious reciprocal cycle in which depression results in more stressful environmental events, and environmental stressors increase the severity of depression.

The identification of mediating processes in the link between depression and child-rearing impairments, however, does not suggest that child-rearing practices are unimportant, but rather indicates the complexity of relations between variables within family systems in which a number of simultaneous processes may be in operation. In the following section, literature is reviewed pertinent to the issue of whether and how impairments in child-rearing techniques may contribute to the transmission of psychopathology from depressed parent to child.

Emotional/Psychological Insensitivity

This dimension refers to parental behaviors that interfere with or are unresponsive to children's emotional needs. Various aspects of the behavior of depressed parents may have this effect. For example, bipolar depressed parents have been found to be more passive, unresponsive, withdrawn, and negative with their children when compared with normal parents, and also to suppress expressions of affect in interactions with their children (Davenport et al., 1984; Gaensbauer, Harmon, Cytryn, & McKnew, 1984). Similarly, unipolar depressed parents have been reported to be more negative, critical, unsupportive, intrusive, and less positive with their children when compared to both well parents and groups of medically ill control parents (Field, Healy, Goldstein, & Guthertz, 1990; Gordon et al., 1989; Panaccione & Wahler, 1986; Tronick, 1989; Webster-Stratton & Hammond, 1988).

Patterns of parental lack of responsivity, and resulting effects on children, associated with parental depression have been observed in parent-infant interactions. For instance, in studies of face-to-face interactions between mothers and infants, maternal displays of negativity, intrusiveness, and withdrawal have been found to elicit anger, reduced activity, dysphoria, and social withdrawal from infants (Cohn & Campbell, this volume; Cohn & Tronick 1983; Cohn and Tronick 1989; Field et al., 1990; Zekoski, O'Hara, & Wils,

1987). Prolonged exposure to such interactions has been associated with the development of depressive behavioral styles observed in contexts outside of mother-infant interactions (Cohn, Campbell, Matias, & Hopkins, 1990; Field et al., 1988). Further, parental insensitivity in caretaking situations has been associated with the development of passivity, lack of interest in the surrounding environment, and dysphoric mood (Ainsworth, 1979; Bell & Ainsworth, 1972; Watson, 1977). In addition, noncompliance and lack of self-control have been found to be more likely in children exposed to such parental behaviors (Ainsworth, Bell, & Stayton, 1974).

A particularly important finding in the literature is a consistent report of links between parental negativity and insensitivity and the development of insecure attachment relationships (e.g., Ainsworth, 1979; Ainsworth & Bell, 1974; Ainsworth, Blehar, Waters, & Wall, 1978; Blehar, Lieberman, & Ainsworth, 1977; Bowlby, 1988; Sroufe & Fleeson, 1986). Insecure attachment, in turn, has often been found to be a precursor of significant problems in social and emotional functioning in childhood (e.g., Arend, Gove, & Sroufe, 1979; Lewis, Feiring, McGuffog, & Jaskir, 1984; Main & Weston, 1981; Matas, Arend, & Sroufe, 1978). Further, parental depression also has been directly linked with the development of insecure and very insecure parent-child attachments (e.g., Radke-Yarrow, Cummings, Kuczynski, & Chapman, 1985; Spieker & Booth, 1988; Zahn-Waxler, Chapman, & Cummings, 1984).

In the literature concerned with the development of behavior problems, parental emotional insensitivity frequently has been associated with the development of externalizing disorders of aggression and acting out (Olweus, 1980, 1984; Parke & Slaby, 1983; Patterson, 1982, 1983), and internalizing disorders of withdrawal and passivity (Baumrind, 1966; Baumrind & Black, 1967). Some investigators have proposed pathways whereby parental depression leads to parental rejection and hostility toward the child, which in turn, results over time in increased risk for depression in children (e.g. Hammen, 1988).

Thus, the evidence suggests that emotionally insensitive parenting may contribute to the link between parental depression and psychopathology in children. An important next step in a process-oriented analysis of this issue is to identify the specific processes and mechanisms that might mediate the influence of this variable.

Dysregulation of Affect

A critical developmental task of infancy and early childhood is children's development of the ability to regulate affect and arousal. Tronick (1989) has suggested that parenting in the first couple of years importantly influences the child's emerging capacities to regulate affective arousal. Whereas warm, responsive, and sensitive parenting during parent-infant interactions elicit modest to moderate levels of arousal in infants, providing a mildly stressful context within which infants can learn to effectively regulate their arousal, intrusive, hostile, and insensitive parenting produces an environment that is excessively challenging and negatively arousing for children. The initial responses of children to insensitive parenting may include exhibitions of anger, distress, high activity, physiological arousal, and other indicators of affective dysregulation (Field, 1987). Over time this may result in more general effects, such as children learning to perceive their parents and even the larger social world as a threat to their own emotional and behavioral well-being, with one possible consequence that their arousal systems becoming sensitized to some or all social situations (Cummings & Cicchetti, 1990). While the specific processes whereby repeated arousal leads to sensitization are not clear, the child's ability to anticipate potentially threatening situations may intensify arousal states. Alternatively, to avoid the aversive state of dysregulation associated with insensitive parenting, children of depressed parents may resort to social withdrawal. Due to the successful dampening effect on the arousal system of withdrawal, children may come to rely exclusively and inflexibly on social withdrawal in almost any social context. Sensitization may again be a key process, but in this instance children may resort to a coping strategy of "internalization" rather than "externalization". Eventually this style of coping may result in a broader pattern of dysphoria and social unresponsiveness in children that places them at-risk for developing a larger and more severe constellation of symptoms linked with depression and other internalizing disorders.

Modeling

Field (1987) has proposed that simple mimicry of depressed mothers dysphoria, hostility, and withdrawal may also contribute to the development of infant interactive disturbances. Similarly, Cicchetti and associates have proposed that children may develop depressive symptomatology simply by emulating the dysphoria, withdrawal, and insensitivity of their depressed parents (Cicchetti & White, 1988; Cummings & Cicchetti, 1990). Alternatively, children may develop externalizing disorders through modeling processes by selectively mimicking the hostile and irritable behaviors of their parents. In this regard, children of bipolar depressed parents may be particularly at-risk due to the significant externalizing component that characterizes the phenomenology of bipolar depression.

Internal working models

The child's internal working models or representations of the self and the surrounding world have been hypothesized to begin to develop as early the first few months of life (Main, Kaplan, & Cassidy, 1985). When parents are warm, responsive, and caring, children are thought to develop positive internal working models characterized by a positive self-concept and a secure sense of confidence in their parents and the larger world (Cummings & Cicchetti, 1990). On the other hand, emotional insensitivity and unresponsiveness by parents is linked with the children viewing their parents as unreliable and psychologically unavailable and themselves as unworthy and undeserving of love and affection (Bowlby, 1973; Bretherton, 1985; Cummings & Cicchetti, 1990). A consequence may be a general lack of self-efficacy (White, 1959). The negative self-cognitions of children with depressed parents may be precursors of subsequent depression (Hammen, 1988; Jaenicke et al., 1987; Rose & Abramson, this volume). Further, such cognitions are linked with the symptomatology of childhood depression (Asarnow & Bates, 1988; Carlson & Kashani, 1988; Kashani & Carlson, 1987; Stavrakaki & Gaudet, 1989).

The negative internal representations and models that develop from parental behavior in parent-child interactions that are emotionally insensitive may extend to other situations and color the children's perceptions of the social world. Negative parent-child interactions may have particularly strong consequences for young children, whose experience is largely limited to the context of the family and interactions with their depressed parents. Children may respond to what they perceive as a noncontingent social environment by losing interest in the world and ultimately withdrawing into themselves. Alternatively, negative representations of the external world may foster feelings of hostility and anger towards others — a disposition that could contribute to the development of externalizing difficulties.

Impairments in Child Management Techniques

A heterogeneous and diverse array of problems in child management have been linked with parental depression. On the one hand, depressed parents have been reported to be inconsistent, lax, and generally ineffective in child management and discipline activities (Davenport et al., 1984; Gaensbauer et al., 1984; Zahn-Waxler et al., 1984; 1990), and, on the other, they also have been found to be more likely to engage in direct, forceful control strategies (Fendrich et al., 1990). Further, depressed parents are likely to use the least effortful discipline and teaching strategies. Compared to nondepressed parents, depressed parents are more prone to avoid conflict by submitting to child noncompliance, but, when not yielding to the demands of the child, are also least likely to end disagreements in a compromise (Kochanska et al., 1987).

This pattern of child management has been linked with the development of externalizing disorders in children. For example, Patterson and his colleagues have reported relations among inconsistent, power assertive, and lax parental monitoring practices and the development of antisocial and aggressive behaviors in children (Patterson, 1983; Loeber & Dishion, 1984). Based on path analyses of parental and child responses, Olweus (1980; 1984) concluded that parental permissiveness and power assertion contribute to the development of externalizing behaviors in children. Further, Loeber and Dishion (1984) found that lax monitoring and discipline techniques were associated with stable and robust aggressive dispositions. In a subsequent attempt to tease out the direction of effects of parental discipline through the use of structural equation modeling, Dishion (1990) reported that parental inconsistency and ineffectiveness contributed to the development of antisocial behavior and low academic achievement in school age children, which, in turn, were associated with rejection and unpopularity among peers. In the next section we consider several possible mechanisms for how child management practices of depressed parents might contribute to increased risk for the development of psychopathology in their children.

Coercive Process

Patterson and his colleagues have argued that the behavioral contingencies underlying coercive child management practices function as reinforcers for child noncompliance, aggression, and other deviant behaviors. A powerful behavioral contingency involves the parents' inadvertent use of negative reinforcement during an episode of child misbehavior (Patterson, Capaldi, & Bank, 1991). This typically occurs within the context of escalating, negative exchanges between parents and children. Thus, as the child becomes increasingly negative, the parent acts in a positive or neutral manner as a means of escaping the aversive interaction. However, escaping the negative interactions also is reinforcing for the child. The end result is the negative reinforcement of the child's aversive behavior that preceded the parental submission. As a result, in future conflict situations, the parent will be predisposed to submit to the child, and the child will become increasingly inclined to be more aversive and antisocial (Patterson, 1982, 1983; Patterson & Bank, 1989; Patterson et al., 1990).

Due to their lethargy and irritability, depressed parents may, in fact, be particularly inclined to fall into the negative reinforcement trap of maximizing immediate rewards (e.g., submitting to demands of children, using ineffective power assertive techniques) and also minimizing effort and energy expended in managing children (e.g., avoiding compromise with the child). Applying the above scenario to families with depressed parents, when children misbehave, depressed parents may tend to scold or nag children. This, in turn, could result in a negative and escalating conflict in which the parent and child direct aversive behaviors at one another. Eventually, as a means of escaping the aversive and energy draining situation the depressed parent may submit to the child. As a consequence, however, the child's aversive behavior is reinforced. As this process is repeated over and over again, the child is reinforced to engage in increasingly intense, frequent, and persistent aversive behaviors which may ultimately result in the development of a stable disposition towards behavior problems. The inconsistent use of discipline by depressed parents and their lax monitoring of children's behavior may add to the difficulties depressed parents encounter with childrearing, since the former introduces a partial reinforcement schedule likely to lead to the persistence of negative behavioral patterns and the latter communicates to children that they can do almost anything they want because their parents are not watching them.

Affect Regulation

The use of power-assertive techniques by depressed parents may also activate another mechanism, that is, processes of arousal and sensitization, that serve to increase the child's disposition to respond aversively. Zillman (1983) has argued that pairing an arousal-inducing stimulus with a negative provocation increases the individual's disposition to become highly aroused and aggressive in subsequent situations. Thus, over time and with repeated exposure, the negative and emotionally arousing qualities of interactions between depressed parents and their children could also contribute to the development of problems with aggression and difficulties with arousal-regulation. Relatedly, marital couples' history of conflict and hostility has been associated with higher baseline levels of arousal and greater difficulties with regulating negative affect and behavior in the context of interactions (e.g., Levenson & Gottman, 1983).

Interrelations Between Interparent Anger and Child-Rearing Practices

The discussion thus far should not be interpreted to imply that the psychopathology of children with depressed parents originates from parallel and independent disturbances in both the parent-child relationship (e.g., disturbances in childrearing practices) and the marital dyad (e.g., interparent conflict). Rather, interdependencies between these systems surely exist, with disturbances in one family dyad often being transmitted to other family subsystems (Coyne et al., this volume; Minuchin, 1985). Recent theory proposes a powerful pathway for the transmission of disturbance that runs from the marital subsystem to the parent-child subsystem. More specifically, it is thought that the stress, frustration, and hopelessness accompanying marital conflict may be carried over into parental interactions and relationships with their children (Belsky, 1984; Christensen & Margolin, 1988; Downey & Coyne, 1990; Emery, 1982; Emery & O'Leary, 1984; Margolin, 1981).

In support of these speculations, Goldberg and Easterbrooks (1984) found that marital conflict was associated with parental insensitivity and lack of support. Further, a number of correlational studies have identified a constellation of co-occurring factors that includes interparent conflict and violence, lax monitoring practices, poor discipline techniques, parental rejection, and the development of both externalizing and internalizing problems in children (Holden & Ritchie, 1991; Jouriles, Pfiffner, & O'Leary, 1988; Loeber & Dishion, 1984). One possible interpretation is that interparent conflict increases disruptions in parent-child interactions, and that these disturbances, in turn, facilitated the development of child psychopathology (for a review, see Crockenberg & Covey, 1991; Holden & Ritchie, 1991). However, the correlational nature of these prevents certain determination of the directionality of influences between these family subsystems.

More convincing in this regard are findings from sequential analyses performed by Christensen and Margolin (1988) indicating that marital conflict increases subsequent problems in parent-child interaction. Also, Jouriles et al. (1987) found that parent-child aggression largely accounted for the relationship between interparent violence and the development of internalizing and externalizing difficulties in children. Further, a study by Fauber, Forehand, McCombs-Thomas, and Wierson (1990) employing structural equation modelling identified a similar pathway in which marital conflict was associated with disruptions in parenting practices, and these disruptions, in turn, were strongly associated with problems of undercontrol and overcontrol in children.

In addition to its apparent impact on parenting practices, marital conflict also may effect the parent-child relationship by drawing the child into interparent disputes. For example, children may be pressured to side with parents during and following marital conflicts (Emery, 1988; Grych & Fincham, 1990; Johnston, Gonzalez, & Campbell, 1987; Vuchinich, Emery, & Cassidy, 1988). Another possibility is that high levels of marital conflict may cause distressed parents to depend on their children increasingly for comfort and support. Eventually, the role reversals and pressures to ally with parents are likely to place undue psychological burdens on children and may eventually result in withdrawal, anxiety, dysphoria, and other internalizing symptomatology in children (Johnston et al., 1987). As noted earlier in this chapter, there is empirically-based evidence that children may attend to and try to take care of parents during and following conflicts involving parents, particularly when there is a history of marital conflict (e.g., Cummings, Hennessy, Rabideau, & Cicchetti, 1991; J. S. Cummings et al., 1989).

Although most of these studies have utilized nondepressed samples, it is not unreasonable to expect that similar results would apply to families with depressed parents. In fact, interrelations among marital conflict, disrupted parent-child relations, and the development of psychopathology in children may be even more pronounced in families with depressed parents. For example, Hops et al. (1987; 1990) have argued that individuals in families with a depressed parent may be particularly affected in an adverse way by negative interactions with other family members. Consequently, the deleterious impact of negative marital interactions on parent-child subsystems may be even stronger in families with depressed parents. In sum, there is accumulating evidence to suggest that marital and parent-child subsystems are likely to be interrelated, rather than independent, in their influence on children.

Other Dysfunctions in the Family System

Other familial caretaking and interactional processes also may act to increase the risk for the development of psychopathology in children of depressed parents; the treatment above is not intended to be exhaustive. For example, parents with depression may not adequately prepare the child for contexts outside of the immediate family environment. Bipolar depressed parents have been reported both to encourage children to be overly dependent on them and to set unrealistically high standards of achievement and conformity (Davenport et al., 1979; 1984). The former might lead to an increased likelihood of the development of insecure attachments (Bowlby, 1988) and problems with separation/ individuation, that is, problems with the development of autonomy and independence in children. The latter, by making it inevitable that children experience repeated or chronic failure, could lead to a reduction in motivation, emotional dysregulation, and learned helplessness, and thus may be linked with the subsequent development of internalizing difficulties (Brown, 1985; Seligman, 1975).

The pathogenic environment associated with parental depression also may extend beyond the depressed parent-child dyad. Children of depressed parents are more often reared in single parent families (Davenport et al., 1984). When the marital dyad is intact, spouses of depressed parents are more likely to suffer from depression and other forms of psychopathology (Coyne et al., 1990; Downey & Coyne, 1990; Rutter & Quinton, 1984; Zahn-Waxler et al., 1990). Thus, children may have few opportunities to obtain warmth, support, and sensitivity, and all too many avenues to rejection, insensitivity, and conflict (Billings & Moos, 1983; 1985; Fendrich et al., 1990).

Families with a depressed parent are also likely to be characterized by general social maladjustment and alienation (Davenport et al., 1984). For example, Zahn-Waxler et al. (in press) reported that depressed mothers were less willing to encourage and assimilate their young children into social groups and events outside the immediate family. This isolation acts to prevent the child from developing an adequate extrafamilial support network of extended kin, neighbors, peers, and perhaps most importantly, close friends (Davenport et al., 1984; Pellegrini et al., 1986). When familial isolation prevents children's development of close relationships with peers, children are more vulnerable to psychological difficulties (Pellegrini et al., 1986). Moreover, the few contacts children have access to outside of the family are frequently neighbors and friends who are also depressed (Zahn-Waxler et al., 1990). Consequently, children of depressed parents may also be exposed to extrafamilial environments that are deficient and pathogenic.

Towards a Process-Oriented Empirical Model

Research to date thus outlines a variety of issues and areas that may begin to account for relations between parental depression and children's development of psychopathology, but there is clearly a need for process-oriented research that advances understanding of specific relations, particularly with regard to relations among parental depression, marital discord and children's development of psychopathology (Downey & Coyne, 1990). On a more positive note, it is important to recognize that children of depressed parents often, perhaps typically, develop quite well, with no evidence of psychopathology. It also is very important to be able to account for and understand these more positive outcomes. In the following section conceptual and methodological themes are outlined as a possible guide for future research in this area, based upon the process-oriented model outlined by Cummings and colleagues (Cummings & Cummings, 1988; Cummings & El-Sheikh, 1991) and are also generally consistent with principles of the discipline of developmental psychopathology (Cicchetti, 1984; Cicchetti, 1990; Sroufe & Rutter, 1984).

Utilization of Experimental Designs

In the area of research on parental depression the use of experimental or quasi-experimental designs was, until recently, very rare. Instead, most studies have relied upon correlational methods, with the implicit assumption that independent variables cause or at least partially contribute to child outcome measures when effects are found (Dodge, 1990a). As is well known, however, even when high correlations are discovered between variables, little can be known with certainty about the direction of causality or the process(es) involved, the possibility that extraneous and unassessed variables account for relations always exists, and the precise mechanism(s) — whether biological and/ or environmental — behind relations cannot be identified with confidence.

While the most desirable approach is undoubtedly a multi-method one, experimental designs surely have been under-utilized among the methods used to investigate these issues, and have the potential to be instrumental in further advancing understanding of process relations and mechanisms in families with depression. As an example, Cohn and Tronick (1983) set up a procedure in which normal mothers simulate depressive symptoms in interactions with their infants under controlled circumstances. The finding was that infants responded with negative affective expressions and eventually with disengagement to such behaviors by mothers. The fact that these behaviors could be induced based only on the manipulation of the mother's interpersonal interactions with infants adds convincingly to the case that environmental mechanisms, rather than solely biological or genetic mechanisms, are contributors to emotional and behavioral dysregulation in infants.

Researchers would do well to employ similar techniques in order to advance further the understanding of process relations in the link between depressed parents and child pathology.

The parental depression project conducted at NIMH provides another illustration of the use of experimental designs for the purpose of unraveling precursors and behavioral antecedents to later dysfunction in children of depressed parents. Zahn-Waxler, Cummings, McKnew, and Radke-Yarrow (1984), for example, exposed toddlers of depressed and well mothers to a set of social and emotional simulations that were designed to be mildly stressful. Efforts were made to select simulations that reflected everyday stressors that children typically experience in the home and might be particularly pertinent to the home experiences of children of depressed mothers. The specific stressors examined included: (1) an episode of interadult anger and hostility, (2) a simulation of sadness and distress by an unfamiliar adult, (3) an enactment of distress by the mother, and (4) a maternal separation episode followed by a maternal reunion with the toddler. The findings, because they emerged from a controlled experimental context, provided powerful support for the notion that children of bipolar depressed parents have difficulty with affect regulation even in early childhood in a number of ecologically valid, naturally occurring social contexts.

Depression as a Multidimensional Construct

A significant flaw in many investigations in the area of parental depression is the tacit treatment of depression as a homogeneous, unidimensional construct. For instance, parents are often simply dichotomized into depressed and well groups, or, less commonly, the depressed group is divided into categories of bipolar and unipolar depression. Such an approach to the "stimulus" of parental depression does not adequately capture the multi-dimensional complexities of depression and family environments associated with depression.

The manifestation of symptoms alone can take many forms that, in turn, may differ in terms of frequency, duration, time of onset, and the number of recurrences. Yet, only a few investigations (e.g., Radke-Yarrow et al., 1985) have empirically examined how specific dimensions of depression (e.g., type of symptoms, duration and intensity of episode) influence family and child outcomes. The family context within which depression occurs should also be differentiated in a complex characterization of depressionogenic environments, consistent with the fact that a wide variety of parental and family behaviors may play a major role in the intergenerational transmission of psychopathology (e.g., Zahn-Waxler et al. in press). The variety of environmental stressors that commonly co-occur with the onset of depression should also be considered, including intense marital and family conflict, parental hospitalization and physical absence, additional forms of pathology in both parents, adverse socioeconomic conditions, and inadequate social support systems (for a review, see Coyne et al., this volume). A process-oriented approach ideally attempts to tackle these complexities in the pursuit of precisely identifying specific risk factors and mechanisms involved in the intergenerational transmission of maladjustment.

Assessment of Multiple Dimensions of Children's Responses and Higher-Order Patterns of Responding

Problems similar to those found in the empirical conceptualization of depression are also prevalent in the conceptualization of child outcome variables. Most investigations develop or select measures of child outcome that do not fully represent the intricate complexities of child functioning. Two approaches are evident in the literature. A first strategy emphasizes global "diagnostic" outcomes and includes a variety of classifications such as competence, adjustment, internalizing difficulties, and conduct disorders. This perspective has its origins in the discipline of clinical psychology and psychiatry where the primary goal is to identify children who suffer from some form of psychopathology. An emphasis on the global identification of pathology, however, precludes a sophisticated analysis of the mechanisms and processes underlying children's difficulties.

A second assessment approach has its origins in developmental psychology where specialization in areas such as emotion and cognition are typically encouraged. Consequently, an individual comes to be viewed in terms of his or her functioning on separate, independent behavioral domains. This perspective is commonly reflected in the developmental psychologist's focus on the assessment of a single domain of behavior (e.g., emotion) to the exclusion of most, or all, others. Such a microanalytic view, however, works against obtaining a perspective on the complete development and functioning of the organism.

Another approach, and one utilized by the process-oriented model, advocates the integration of macro- and micro-analytic perspectives. Consistent with a major theme of the discipline of developmental psychopathology, a process-oriented approach views behavior and development in terms of an interrelated constellation of response domains that are integrated into and together constitute higher order patterns and forms of functioning (Cicchetti, 1989; Cicchetti, 1990; Cicchetti & Schneider-Rosen, 1986; Izard & Schwartz, 1986). Consequently, a process-oriented approach to assessment is concerned not only with single response domains and global diagnostic measures, but also with coherent patterns that are evident across multiple response domains (Cummings & Cummings, 1988; Cummings & El-Sheikh, 1991). Only a handful of studies in the parental depression literature reflect this approach (e.g. Zahn-Waxler, Chapman, & Cummings, 1984). Only through the simultaneous examination of multiple response domains will it be possible to achieve a full understanding of how and why children of depressed parents are at risk for developing difficulties.

In addition to an emphasis on the measurement and characterization of higher-order patterns in children assessed at precise and multiple levels of analysis, a process-oriented approach focuses on children's responses over time. Of particular interest are children's delayed response patterns and coping styles after exposure to everyday stressors. Assessments of child behavior in an NIMH-based research project provides an excellent illustration of the value of the assessment of multiple micro-analytically measured dimensions of response and of the significance of assessing responses over time (Zahn-Waxler et al., 1984; Zahn-Waxler, Cummings, Iannotti, & Radke-Yarrow, 1984; Zahn-Waxler, McKnew, Cummings, Davenport, & Radke-Yarrow, 1984; Zahn-Waxler et al., 1984). In this research, observations of the children's behavior **after** exposure to various stressful events revealed differences between the responses of children of depressed parents and normal mothers not evident in children's immediate response patterns. For example, it was found that children with normal parents quickly regulated their aggressive tendencies soon after exposure to interparent anger. Children of depressed parents, at first, appeared to suppress their arousal under the same conditions. However, after exposure to parental separation, in addition to interadult anger, these children became quite aggressive and remained emotionally dysregulated for some time thereafter (Zahn-Waxler et al., 1984). Without the assessment of responses to multiple contexts and the measurement of delayed responses, it might have been falsely concluded that children of depressed parents were not behaviorally affected by certain social stressors. This illustrates how more sophisticated assessment strategies can be quite useful in the precise characterization of response processes.

Age-Related Changes and Developmental Course

Another theme of the process-oriented model focuses on the empirical identification of age-related or developmental continuities and changes in child behavior. Such issues, however, have received little attention in the parental depression literature. An exception is the recent cross-sectional study conducted by Zahn-Waxler, Kochanska, Krupnick, & McKnew (1990). Specifically, marked differences in guilt were found between children of depressed and well parents that changed as a function of age. For the normal group, 5- to 6-year-olds exhibited little guilt, responsibility, or involvement in response to hypothetical situations involving another person in distress. On the other hand, 7- to 9-year-old children with well mothers evidenced substantial guilt and involvement. By contrast, 5- to 6-year-old children of depressed parents expressed significantly more guilt, emotional arousal, and involvement than 7- to 9-year-old children of depressed parents.

Another concern of the process-oriented strategy is examining how children of depressed parents approach and resolve salient developmental themes.

The latter, also referred to as "stage-salient issues", recognizes development as a series of developmental tasks which become salient at a given period and remain important throughout an individual's lifetime (for more information, see Cicchetti, 1989, 1990; Cicchetti & Aber, 1986; Cicchetti, Toth, Bush, & Gillespie, 1988). For example, stage salient developmental tasks range from "homeostatic regulation" between birth and three months to emotional regulation at 12 to 30 months of age (Cicchetti, 1989; Cicchetti & Schneider-Rosen, 1986). Successful resolution of these tasks is hypothesized to facilitate normal development whereas unsuccessful resolution places the child at greater risk for maladaptive developmental trajectories.

An examination of how children of depressed parents approached stage salient issues was conducted at NIMH. Findings from this project indicate that toddlers with depressed parents have difficulties achieving the salient developmental task of emotional modulation. Consistent with theoretical proposals, unsuccessful resolution of the emotional regulation theme during toddlerhood predicted subsequent behavioral problems for school age children of depressed parents (Zahn-Waxler et al., 1990).

Despite the recent empirical efforts to examine age-related changes and developmental trajectories, there is still a paucity of explicitly developmental research in the parental depression literature. Research emphasizing this theme, however, is necessary in order to understand fully how the mechanisms and pathways of children with depressed parents are both similar and different from children of normal parents. It is only through the delineation of these developmental trajectories that we can begin to comprehend which pathways and precursors should be considered aberrant and which ought to be considered normative (Cicchetti et al., 1988; Sroufe & Rutter, 1984).

Individual Adaptation and Maladaptation

Consistent with the tenets of developmental psychopathology, a process-oriented approach places emphasis on studying individual adaptation and maladaptation from several different orientations (Cummings & Cummings, 1988; Sroufe & Rutter, 1984). One investigatory orientation involves examining individual behavioral styles or the higher-order patterns that exist across multiple response domains. That is, efforts are made to identify the consistencies in emotional, behavioral, cognitive, and physiological responding to a given social stressor that is indicative of a general style of responding. In the interadult anger literature, for example, as we have noted above, El-Sheikh et al. (1989) reported stable patterns of responding across behavioral, emotional, and physiological systems. Based on these response measures, children were characterized as responding to anger with a hyposensitive, appropriately sensitive, or hypersensitive pattern (Cummings & Cummings, 1988; Cummings & El-Sheikh, 1991). Despite the apparent promise of this approach, however, investigators, to our knowledge, have not examined whether styles of responding to everyday stressors exist at this level of analysis in children of depressed parents.

A related orientation is to study the developmental trajectories of individual differences in adaptation. One project that examined individual differences in the development of children with depressed parents was conducted by Zahn-Waxler et al. (1990). This investigation, which spanned the course of early childhood, suggested that children of depressed parents exhibit continuity in patterns of aggression and other externalizing difficulties indicative of emotional dysregulation. The study of individual adaptation and maladaption is not restricted to the examination of individual children in the course of development. Issues concerning the stability of responding patterns across contexts are equally important. Several investigations have assessed the behavior of children of depressed parents across the contexts of home and school (e.g., Cytryn, McKnew, Bartko, Lamour, & Hamovit, 1982). However, a number of limitations in these studies preclude the examination of individual differences at a process-oriented level, including: (a) child behavior was measured only in terms of global "diagnostic" outcomes; (b) only a single method of assessment was used (typically questionnaires or diagnostic interviews); and (c) children's responses were examined in global contexts (e.g. school and home settings) rather than in specific, tightly defined situations (e.g., interadult verbal conflict or maternal separation episode). In order to identify the specific process relations that underlie individual differences in patterns of adaptation and maladaptation, it is, at the very least, necessary to: (1) employ multi-method techniques, including objective observational assessments; (2) construct child outcome measures that tap specific domains of behavioral responding as well as their interrelated patterns; and (3) assess children's responses to specific, well-defined situations.

Risk and Normal Samples

The field of developmental psychopathology, as one of its core theoretical foci, emphasizes the need to examine both normative and deviant development in order to achieve an understanding of the full continuum of processes and mechanisms involved in children's development (Cicchetti 1984, 1990; Garber, 1984; Sroufe & Rutter, 1984). This theoretical emphasis is most effectively realized through the study of normal and risk populations within the process-oriented framework.

Utilization of heterogeneous and ill-defined samples, characteristic of much of the empirical literature in the area of parental depression, precludes the identification of specific process-relations involved in child development. Recently, however, investigators have developed more sophisticated methodologies that employ precisely defined samples. Moreover, studies are now including a number of different samples that more adequately represent the continuum of risk and normal samples extant in the general population, and also permits for more precise identification of the psychopathological correlates of outcomes. Research designs developed by Hammen and her associates, for example, included four groups of mothers defined as unipolar, bipolar, well, and medically ill (Hammen, this volume; Hammen et al., 1987). Comparison of these groups, in part, facilitated the process of identifying specific risk factors and possible mechanisms contributing to the development of psychopathology in their children. In general, comparing the responses of risk and normal groups to conditions sheds more light upon the coping processes that may mediate the occurrence and development of problematic behaviors.

Buffers and Resilience Factors

Finally, the concern with psychopathological outcomes in children of depressed parents should not cause researchers to overstate the risk associated with being a child of a depressed parent, as children often cope effectively with these conditions, nor cause investigators to neglect the existence and important role of buffers and resilience factors in even very depressionogenic environments. Garmezy (e.g., Garmezy, 1985) has lead the way in articulating this general issue for developmental and clinical research. In fact, Garmezy has argued that the notion of stress and coping focuses too much attention on psychopathology and negative outcomes in childhood, when children are typically successful in overcoming the challenges and stresses with which they are faced. Further, Garmezy contends that the concept of "competence" should be added to the "stress and coping" lexicon to reflect the important role of children's own capacities in overcoming experiential threats and challenges (Garmezy & Masten, 1991). Inclusion of such notions in research programs may both improve the prediction of childhood outcomes as well as provide a more encompassing descriptor of the nature of children's response processes. Unfortunately, relatively little work has been directed towards identifying factors that might buffer or protect children against negative effects associated with growing up in homes in which parents are depressed; this is surely an important domain for future research that merits emphasis.

Summary

In this chapter we present a framework in the context of a review of recent evidence for a process-oriented investigation of relations among parental depression, marital discord, and child adjustment problems. In addition, the process-oriented strategy is expanded to include consideration of broader aspects of family functioning. Finally, the utility and application of the process-oriented approach and the related approach of developmental psychopathology to the specific problem of understanding relations between family functioning and child outcomes in families with parental depression is described. The goal is to provide bases for a "next step" in research on this issue of significant social concern.

REFERENCES

Ablon, S. L., Davenport, Y. B., Gershon, E. S., & Adland, M. L. (1975). The married manic. *American Journal of Orthopsychiatry, 45*, 854–866.

Ainsworth, M. D. S. (1979). Attachment as related to mother-infant interaction. In J. S. Rosenblatt, R. A. Hinde, C. Beer, & M. Busnel (eds.), *Advances in the study of behavior* (Vol. 9, pp. 1–51). New York: Academic Press.

Ainsworth, M. D. S., & Bell, S. M. (1974). Mother-infant interaction and the development of competence. In K. Connolly & J. Bruner (eds.), *The Growth of Competence* (pp. 97–118). London: Academic Press.

Ainsworth, M. D. S., Bell, S. M., Stayton, D. J. (1974). Infant-mother attachment and social development: Socialization as a product of reciprocal responsiveness to signals. In M. P. M. Richards (ed.), *The integration of the child into a social world* (pp. 99–135). London: Cambridge University Press.

Ainsworth, M. D. S., Blehar, M. C., Waters, E., & Wall, S. (1978). *Patterns of attachment: A psychological study of the strange situation.* Hillsdale, NJ: Erlbaum.

Arend, R., Gove, F. L., Sroufe, L. A. (1979). Continuity of individual adaptation from infancy to kindergarten: A predictive study of ego-resiliency and curiosity in preschoolers. *Child Development, 50*, 950–959.

Asarnow, J. R., & Bates, S. (1988). Depression in child psychiatric inpatients: Cognitive and attributional patterns. *Journal of Abnormal Child Psychology, 16*, 601–615.

Ballard, M., & Cummings, E. M. (1990). Response to adults' angry behavior in children of alcoholic and non-alcoholic parents. *Journal of Genetic Psychology, 151*, 195–210.

Ballard, M. E., Cummings, E. M., & Larkin, K. (in press). *Emotional and cardiovascular responses to adults' angry behavior and challenging tasks in children of hypertensive and normotensive parents. Child Development.*

Baumrind, D. (1966). Effects of authoritative parental control on child behavior. *Child Development, 37*, 887–907.

Baumrind, D., & Black, A. (1967). Socialization practices associated with dimensions of competence in preschool boys and girls. *Child Development, 38*, 291–307.

Beardslee, W., Bemporad, J., Keller., M. B., & Klerman, G. L. (1983). Children of parents with a major affective disorder: A review. *American Journal of Psychiatry, 140*, 825–832.

Bell, S. M., & Ainsworth, M. D. S. (1972). Infant crying and maternal responsiveness. *Child Development, 43*, 1171–1190.

Belsky, J. (1984). The determinants of parenting: A process model. *Child Development, 55*, 83–96.

Biglan, A., Hops, H., Sherman, L., Freidman, L., Arthur, J., & Osteen, V. (1985). Problem solving interactions of depressed mothers and their spouses. *Behavior Therapy, 16*, 431–451.

Biglan, A., Rothlind, J., Hops, H., & Sherman, L. (1989). Impact of distressed and aggressive behavior. *Journal of Abnormal Psychology, 98*, 218–228.

Billings, A. G., & Moos, R. H. (1983). Comparison of children of depressed and nondepressed parents: A social environmental perspective. *Journal of Abnormal Child Psychology, 11*, 483–486.

Blehar, M. C., Lieberman, A. F., & Ainsworth, M. D. S. (1977). Early face-to-face interaction and its relation to later infant-mother attachment. *Child Development, 48*, 182–194.

Bowlby, J. (1973). *Attachment and loss: Vol. 1. Separation.* New York: Basic Books.

Bowlby, J. (1988). Developmental psychiatry comes of age. *American Journal of Psychiatry, 145*, 1–10.

Bretherton, I. (1985). Attachment theory: Retrospect and prospect. In I. Bretherton & E. Waters (eds.), Growing points of attachment theory and research. *Monographs of the Society for Research in Child Development, 50* (1–2, Serial No. 209), 167–193.

Brown, D. M. (1985). First-grade boys' responses to a new task following noncontingent feedback. *Journal of Experimental Child Psychology, 39,* 413–420.

Carlson, G. A., & Kashani, J. H. (1988). Phenomonology of major depression from childhood through adulthood: Analysis of three studies. *American Journal of Psychiatry, 145,* 1222–1225.

Christensen, A., & Margolin, G. (1988). Conflict and alliance in distressed and non-distressed families. In R. A. Hinde & J. Stevenson-Hinde (eds.), *Relationships within families* (pp. 263–282). New York: Oxford University Press.

Cicchetti, D. (1984). The emergence of developmental psychopathology. *Child Development, 55,* 1–7.

Cicchetti, D. (1989). How research on child maltreatment has informed the study of child development: Perspectives from developmental psychopathology. In D. Cicchetti & V. Carlson (eds.), *Child maltreatment: Theory and research on the causes and consequences of child abuse and neglect* (pp. 377–431). New York: Cambridge University Press.

Cicchetti, D. (1990). An historical perspective on the discipline of developmental psychopathology. In J. Rolf, A. Masten, D. Cicchetti, K. Nuechterlein, & S. Weintraub (eds.), *Risk and protective factors in the development of psychopathology.* (pp. 2–28). New York: Cambridge University Press.

Cicchetti, D., & Aber, J. L. (1986). Early precursors of later depression: An organizational perspective. In L. Lipsitt & C. Rovee-Collier (eds.), *Advances in infancy* (Vol. 4, pp. 87–137). Norwood, NJ: Ablex.

Cicchetti, D., & Schneider-Rosen, K. (1986). An organizational approach to childhood depression. In M. Rutter, C. E. Izard, & P. B. Read (eds.), *Depression in young people: Developmental and clinical perspectives* (pp. 71–134). New York: Guilford Press.

Cicchetti, D., Toth, S., Bush, M., & Gillespie, J. (1988). Stage-salient issues: A transactional model of intervention. *New Directions for Child Development, 39,* 123–145.

Cicchetti, D., & White, J. (1988). Emotional development and affective disorders. In W. Damon (ed.), *Child development today and tomorrow* (pp. 177–198). San Francisco: Jossey-Bass.

Cohn, J. F., Campbell, S. B., Matias, R., & Hopkins, J. (1990). Face-to-face interactions of postpartum depressed and nondepressed mother-infant pairs at 2 months. *Developmental Psychology, 26,* 15–23.

Cohn, J., & Tronick, E. (1983). Three-month-old infants' reaction to simulated maternal depression. *Child Development, 54,* 185–190.

Cohn, J. F., & Tronick, E. Z. (1989). Specificity of infants' response to mothers' affective behavior. *Journal of the American Academy of Child and Adolescent Psychiatry, 28,* 242–248.

Coyne, J. C., Burchill, S. A. L., & Stiles, W. B. (1991). An interactional perspective on depression. In C. R. Snyder & D. O. Forsyth (eds.), *Handbook of social and clinical psychology: The health perspective* (pp. 327–348). New York: Pergamon.

Crockenberg, S., & Covey, S. L. (1991). Marital conflict and externalizing behavior in children. In D. Cicchetti & S. Toth (eds.), *Research and clinical contributions to a theory of developmental psychopathology: Vol. 3. Rochester symposium on developmental psychopathology.* Rochester: University of Rochester Press.

Cummings, E. M. (1987). Coping with background anger in early childhood. *Child Development, 58,* 976–984.

Cummings, E. M., Ballard, M., & El-Sheikh, M. (1991). Responses of children and adolescents to interadult anger as a function of gender, age, and mode of expression. *Merrill-Palmer Quarterly, 37,* 543–560.

Cummings, E. M., Ballard, M., El-Sheikh, M., & Lake, M. (1991). Resolution and children's responses to interadult anger. *Developmental Psychology, 27*, 462–470.

Cummings, E. M., & Cicchetti, D. (1990). Towards a transactional model of relations between attachment and depression. In M. Greenberg, D. Cicchetti, & E. M. Cummings (eds.), *Attachment in the preschool years: Theory, research, and intervention* (pp. 339–372). Chicago and London: The University of Chicago Press.

Cummings, E. M., & Cummings, J. L. (1988). A process-oriented approach to children's coping with adults' angry behavior. *Developmental Review, 8*, 296–321.

Cummings, E. M., & El-Sheikh, M. (1991). Children's coping with angry environments: A process-oriented approach. In M. Cummings, A. Greene, & K. Karraker (eds.), *Life-span developmental psychology: Perspective on stress and coping* (pp. 131–150). Hillsdale, NJ: Erlbaum.

Cummings, E. M., & Grogg, C. M. (1991). *Adolescent response to nonverbal anger.* Unpublished manuscript, West Virginia University, Morgantown, WV.

Cummings, E. M., Hennessy, K. D., Rabideau, G. J., & Cicchetti, D. (1991). *Maltreatment and children's responses to angry adult behavior.* Manuscript submitted for publication.

Cummings, E. M., Iannotti, R. J., & Zahn-Waxler, C. (1985). The influence of conflict between adults on the emotions and aggression of young children. *Developmental Psychology, 21*, 495–507.

Cummings, E. M., Iannotti, R. J., & Zahn-Waxler, C. (1989). Aggression between peers in early childhood: Individual continuity and developmental change. *Child Development, 60*, 887–895.

Cummings, E. M., & Simpson, K. S. (1991). *Explanation of conflict and children's responses to interadult anger.* Unpublished manuscript, West Virginia University, Morgantown, WV.

Cummings, E. M., Vogel, D., Cummings, J. S., El-Sheikh, M. (1989). Children's responses to different forms of expression of anger between adults. *Child Development, 60*, 1392–1404.

Cummings, E. M., & Wilson, A. (1991). *The effects of covert vs. overt resolution on children's perception of anger.* Unpublished manuscript, West Virginia University, Morgantown, WV.

Cummings, E. M., & Zahn-Waxler, C. (in press). Emotions and the socialization of aggression: Adults' angry behavior and children's arousal and aggression. In A. Fraczek & H. Zumkley (eds.), *Socialization and aggression.* New York and Heidelberg: Springer-Verlag.

Cummings, E. M., Zahn-Waxler, C., & Radke-Yarrow, M. (1981). Young children's responses to expressions of anger and affection by others in the family. *Child Development, 52*, 1274–1282.

Cummings, E. M., Zahn-Waxler, C., & Radke-Yarrow, M. (1984). Developmental changes in children's reactions to anger in the home. *Journal of Child Psychology and Psychiatry, 25*, 63–74.

Cummings, J. S., Pellegrini, D., Notarius, C., & Cummings, E. M. (1989). Children's responses to angry adult behavior as a function of marital distress and history of interparent hostility. *Child Development, 60*, 1035–1043.

Cytryn, L., McKnew, D. H., Bartko, J. J., Lamour, M., & Hamovit, J. (1982). Offspring of patients with affective disorders II. *Journal of the American Academy of Child Psychiatry, 21*, 389–391.

Davenport, Y. B., Adland, M. L., Gold, P. W., & Goodwin, F. K. (1979). Manic-depressive illness: Psychodynamic features of multigenerational families. *American Journal of Orthopsychiatry, 49*, 24–35.

Davenport, Y. B., Ebert, M. H., Adland, M. L., & Goodwin, F. K. (1977). Couples group therapy as an adjunct to lithium maintenance of the manic patient. *American Journal of Orthopsychiatry, 47*, 495–502.

Davenport, Y. B., Zahn-Waxler, C., Adland, M. L., & Mayfield, A. (1984). Early child-rearing practices in families with a manic-depressive parent. *American Journal of Psychiatry, 141*, 230–235.

Dishion, T. J. (1990). The family ecology of boys' peer relations in middle childhood. *Child Development, 61*, 874–892.

Dix, T. (1991). The affective organization of parenting: Adaptive and maladaptive processes. *Psychological Bulletin, 110*, 3–25.

Dodge, K. (1990a). Developmental psychopathology in children of depressed mothers. *Developmental Psychology, 26*, 3–6.

Dodge, K. A. (1990b). Nature versus nurture in childhood conduct disorder: It is time to ask a different question. *Developmental Psychology, 26*, 698–701.

Downey, G., & Coyne, J. C. (1990). Children of depressed parents: An integrative review. *Pychological Bulletin, 108*, 50–76.

El-Sheikh, M., Cummings, E. M., & Goetsch, V. (1989). Coping with adults' angry behavior: Behavioral, physiological, and self-reported responding in preschoolers. *Developmental Psychology, 25*, 490–498.

Emery, R. E. (1982). Interparental conflict and the children of discord and divorce. *Psychological Bulletin, 92*, 310–330.

Emery, R. E. (1988). *Marriage, divorce, and children's adjustment.* Newbury Park, CA: Sage.

Emery, R. E., & O'Leary, K. D. (1984). Marital discord and child behavior problems in a nonclinic sample. *Journal of Abnormal Child Psychology, 12*, 411–420.

Emery, R., Weintraub, S., & Neale, J. M. (1982). Effects of marital discord on the school behavior of children of schizophrenic, affectively disordered, and normal parents. *Journal of Abnormal Child Psychology, 10*, 215–228.

Fauber, R., Forehand, R., McCombs-Thomas, A., & Wierson, M. (1990). A mediational model of the impact of marital conflict on adolescent adjustment in intact and divorced families: The role of disrupted parenting. *Child Development, 61*, 1112–1123.

Fendrich, M., Warner, V., & Weissman, M. M. (1990). Family risk factors, parental depression, and psychopathology in offspring. *Developmental Psychology, 26*, 40–50.

Field, T. M. (1987). Affective and interactive disturbances in infants. In J. D. Osofsky (ed.), *Handbook of infant development* (2nd ed., pp. 972–1005). New York: John Wiley.

Field, T., Healy, B., Goldstein, S., & Guthertz, M. (1990). Behavior-state matching and synchrony in mother-infant interactions of nondepressed vs. depressed dyads. *Developmental Psychology, 26*, 7–14.

Field, T., Healy, B., Goldstein, S., Perry, S., Bendell, D., Schamberg, S., Zimmerman, E., & Kuhn, G. (1988). Infants of depressed mothers show "depressed" behavior even with non-depressed adults. *Child Development, 60*, 1569–1579.

Gaensbauer, J. J., Harmon, R. J., Cytryn, L., & McKnew, D. H. (1984). Social and affective development in infants with a manic-depressive parent. *American Journal of Psychiatry, 141*, 223–229.

Garber, J. (1984). Classification of childhood psychopathology: A developmental perspective. *Child Development, 55*, 30–48.

Garmezy, N. (1985). Stress-resistant children. The search for protective factors. In J. J. E. Stevenson (ed.), *Recent research in developmental psychopathology: Journal of Child Psychology and Psychiatry Book Supplement No. 4* (pp. 213–233). Oxford: Pergamon.

Garmezy, N. & Masten, A. (1991). The protective role of competence indicators in children at risk. In E. M. Cummings, A. L. Greene, and K. K. Karraker (eds.), *Life-span developmental psychology: Perspectives on stress and coping* (pp. 151–176). Hillsdale, NJ: Erlbaum.

Gilbreath, B., & Cicchetti, D. (1991). *Psychopathology in maltreating mothers*. Manuscript submitted for publication.

Goldberg, W. A., & Easterbrooks, M. A. (1984). Role of marital quality in toddler development. *Developmental Psychology, 20*, 504–514.

Goodman, S. H., & Brumley, H. E. (1990). Schizophrenic and depressed mothers: Relational deficits in parenting. *Developmental Psychology, 26*, 31–39.

Gordon, D., Burge, D., Hammen, C., Adrian, C., Jaenicke, C., Hirito, D. (1989). Observations of interactions of depressed women with their children. *American Journal of Psychiatry, 146*, 50–55.

Gottman, J. M., & Fainsliber-Katz, L. (1989). Effects of marital discord on young children's peer interaction and health. *Developmental Psychology, 25*, 373–381.

Grych, J. H., & Fincham, F. D. (1990). Marital conflict and children's adjustment: A cognitive-contextual framework. *Psychological Bulletin, 108*, 267–290.

Grych, J., Seid, M., & Fincham, F. (1991, April). Children's cognitive and affective responses to different forms of interparental conflict. In E. M. Cummings (Chair), *Children's responses to adults' conflicts and emotional expressions across contexts*. Symposium conducted at the meeting of the Society for Research in Child Development, Seattle.

Hammen, C. (1988). Self-cognitions, stressful events, and the prediction of depression in children of depressed mothers. *Journal of Abnormal Child Psychology, 16*, 347–367.

Hammen, C., Gordon, G., Burge, D., Adrian, C., Jaenicke, C., & Hirito, G. (1987). Maternal affective disorders, illness, and stress: Risk for children's psychopathology. *American Journal of Psychiatry, 144*, 736–741.

Hay, D. F., Zahn-Waxler, C., Cummings E. M., & Iannotti, R. J. (in press). Young children's views about conflict with peers: A comparison of the daughters and sons of depressed and well women. *Journal of Child Psychology and Psychiatry*.

Hershorn, M., & Rosenbaum, A. (1985). Children of marital violence: A closer look at the unintended victims. *American Journal of Orthopsychiatry, 55*, 260–266.

Holden, G. W., & Ritchie, K. L. (1991). Linking extreme marital discord, child rearing, and child behavior problems: Evidence from battered women. *Child Development, 62*, 311–327.

Hops, H., Biglan, A., Sherman, L., Arthur, J., Friedman, L., & Osteen, R. (1987). Home observations of family interactions of depressed women. *Journal of Consulting and Clinical Psychology, 55*, 341–346.

Hops, H., Sherman, L., Biglan, A. (1990). Maternal depression, marital discord, and children's behavior: A developmental perspective. In G. R. Patterson (eds.), *Depression and aggression in family interaction* (pp. 185–208). Hillsdale, NJ: Erlbaum.

Izard, C. E., & Schwartz, G. M. (1986). Patterns of emotion in depression. In M. Rutter, C. E. Izard, and P. B. Read (eds.), *Depression in young people: Developmental and clinical perspectives* (pp. 33–70). New York: The Guilford Press.

Jaenicke, C., Hammen, C., Zupan, B., Hirito, D., Gordon, D., Adrian, C., & Burge, D. (1987). Cognitive vulnerability in children at risk for depression. *Journal of Abnormal Child Psychology, 15*, 559–572.

Jenkins, J. M., & Smith, M. A. (in press). Marital disharmony and children's behavioural problems: Aspects of a poor marriage that affect children adversely. *Journal of Child Psychology and Psychiatry*.

Johnston, J. R., Gonzalez, R., & Campbell, L. E. (1987). Ongoing post-divorce conflict and child disturbance. *Journal of Abnormal Child Psychology, 15*, 497–509.

Jouriles, E. N., Barling, J., & O'Leary, K. D. (1987). Predicting child behavior problems in maritally violent families. *Journal of Abnormal Child Psychology, 15*, 165–173.

Jouriles, E. N., Murphy, C. M., & O'Leary, K. D. (1989). Interspousal aggression, marital discord, and child problems. *Journal of Consulting and Clinical Psychology, 57*, 453–455.

Jouriles, E. N., Pfiffner, L. J., & O'Leary, S. G. (1988). Marital conflict, parenting, and toddler conduct problems. *Journal of Abnormal Child Psychology, 16*, 197–206.

Kashani, J. H., & Carlson, G. A. (1987). Seriously depressed preschoolers. *American Journal of Psychiatry, 144*, 348–350.

Klaczynski, P. A., & Cummings, E. M. (1989). Responding to anger in aggressive and nonaggressive boys. *Journal of Child Psychology and Psychiatry, 30*, 309–314.

Kochanska, G., Kuczynski, L. Radke-Yarrow, M., & Welsh, J. D. (1987). Resolution of control episodes between well and affectively ill mothers and their young child. *Journal of Abnormal Child Psychology, 15*, 441–456.

LaRoche, C. (1989). Children of parents with major affective disorders. *The Psychiatric Clinics of North America, 12*, 919–932.

Levenson, R. W., & Gottman, J. M. (1983). Marital interaction: Physiological linkage and affective exchange. *Journal of Personality and Social Psychology, 45*, 587–597.

Lewis, M., Feiring, C., McGuffog, C., & Jaskir, J. (1984). Predicting psychopathology in six-year-olds from early social relations. *Child Development, 55*, 123–136.

Loeber, R., & Dishion, T. J. (1984). Boys who fight at home and school: Family conditions influencing cross-setting consistency. *Journal of Consulting and Clinical Psychology, 52*, 759–768.

Lytton, H. (1990). Child and parent effects in boys' conduct disorder: A reinterpretation. *Developmental Psychology, 26*, 683–697.

Main, M., Kaplan, N., & Cassidy, J. C. (1985). Security in infancy, childhood and adulthood: A move to the level of representation. In I. Bretherton & E. Waters (eds.), Growing points of attachment theory and research. *Monographs of the Society for Research in Child Development, 50* (1–2, Serial No. 209), 66–104.

Main, M., & Weston, D. (1981). The quality of the toddlers' relationship to mother and to father: Related to contact behavior and the readiness to establish new relationships. *Child Development, 52*, 932–940.

Margolin, G. (1981). The reciprocal relationship between maritaland child problems. In J. P. Vincent (eds.), *Advances in family intervention assessment and theory* (vol. 2, pp. 131–182). Greenwich, CT: JAI Press.

Matas, L., Arend, R. A., & Sroufe, L. A. (1978). Continuity and adaptation in the second year: The relationship between quality of attachment and later competence. *Child Development*, 547–556.

Minuchin, P. (1985). Families and individual development: Provocations from the field of family therapy. *Child Development, 56*, 289–302.

Olweus, D. (1980). Familial and temperament determinants of aggressive behavior in adolescent boys: A causal analysis. *Developmental Psychology, 16*, 644–660.

Olweus, D. (1984). Development of stable aggressive reaction patterns in males. In R. J. Blanchard & D. C. Blanchard (eds.), *Advances in the study of aggression* (vol.1, pp. 103–137). New York: Academic.

Orvaschel, H. (1983). Maternal depression and child dysfunction. In B. Lahey & A. Kazdin (eds.), *Advances in clinical child psychology* (Vol. 6, pp. 169–197). New York: Plenum Press.

Panaccione, V., & Wahler, R. (1986). Child behavior, maternal depression, and social coercion as factors in the quality of child care. *Journal of Abnormal Child Psychology, 14*, 273–284.

Parke, R. D., & Slaby, R. G. (1983). The development of aggression. In E. M. Hetherington (ed.), *Socialization, personality, and social development* (Vol. 4, pp. 547–641). New York: John Wiley.

Patterson, G. R. (1982). *Coercive family process*. Eugene, OR: Castalia Press.

Patterson, G. R. (1983). Stress: A change agent for family process. In N. Garmezy & M. Rutter (eds.), *Stress, coping, and development in children* (pp. 235–264). New York: McGraw-Hill.

Patterson, G. R., & Bank, L. (1989). Some amplifying mechanisms for pathologic processes in families. In M. Gunnar (ed.), *Minnesota symposium on child psychology*. Vol. 22. (pp. 167–210). Hillsdale, NJ: Erlbaum.

Patterson, G. R., Capaldi, D., & Bank, L. (1990). An early starter model for predicting delinquency. In D. Pepler, & K. H. Rubin (eds.), *The development and treatment of childhood aggression* (pp. 139–168). Hillsdale, NJ: Erlbaum.

Pellegrini, D., Kosisky, S., Nackman, D., Cytryn, L., McKnew, D., Gershon, E., Hamovit, J., & Cammuso, K. (1986). Personal and social resources in children of patients with bipolar affective disorder and children of normal control subjects. *American Journal of Psychiatry, 143*, 856–861.

Radke-Yarrow, M., Cummings, E. M., Kuczynski, L., & Chapman, M. (1985). Patterns of attachment in two- and three-year-olds in normal families and families with parental depression. *Child Development, 56*, 884–893.

Rutter, M., & Quinton, D. (1984). Parental psychiatric disorder: Effects on children. *Psychological Medicine, 14*, 853–880.

Seligman, M. E. P. (1975). *Helplessness: On depression, development, and death*. San Francisco: Freeman.

Shaw, D. S., & Emery, R. E. (1987). Parental conflict and other correlates of the adjustment of school-age children whose parents have separated. *Journal of Abnormal Child Psychology, 15*, 269–281.

Shred, R., McDonnell, P. M., Church, G., & Rowan, J. (1991, April). *Infants' cognitive and emotional responses to adults' anger behavior*. Paper presented at the biennial meeting of the Society for Research in Child Development, Seattle, WA.

Spieker, S. J., & Booth, C. (1988). Family risk typologies and patterns of insecure attachment. In J. Belsky & T. Nezworski (eds.), *Clinical implications of attachment* (pp. 95–135). Hillsdale, NJ: Erlbaum.

Sroufe, L. A., & Fleeson, J. (1986). Attachment and the construction of relationships. In W. Hartup & Z. Rubin (eds.), *Relationships and development* (pp. 51–71). Hillsdale, NJ: Erlbaum.

Sroufe, L. A., & Rutter, M. (1984). The domain of developmental psychopathology. *Child Development, 55*, 17–29.

Stavrakaki, C., & Gaudet, M. (1989). Epidemiology of affective and anxiety disorders in children and adolescents. *The Psychiatric Clinics of North America, 12*, 791–802.

Tronick, E. Z. (1989). Emotions and emotional communication in infants. *American Psychologist, 44*, 112–119.

Vuchinich, S., Emery, R. E., & Cassidy, J. (1988). Family members as third parties in dyadic family conflict: Strategies, alliances, and outcomes. *Child Development, 59*, 1293–1302.

Wahler, R. G. (1990). Who is driving the interactions? A commentary on "Child and Parent Effects in Boys' Conduct Disorder." *Developmental Psychology, 26*, 702–704.

Watson, J. S. (1977). Depression and the perception of control in early childhood. In J. G. Schulterbrandt & A. Raskin (eds.), *Depression in childhood: Diagnosis, treatment, and conceptual models* (pp. 123–133). New York: Raven Press.

Webster-Stratton, C., & Hammond, M. (1988). Maternal depression and its relationship to life stress, perceptions of child behavior problems, parenting behaviors, and child conduct problems. *Journal of Abnormal Child Psychology, 16*, 299–315.

White, R. W. (1959). Motivation reconsidered: The concept of competence. *Psychological Review, 66*, 297–333.

Zahn-Waxler, C., Chapman, M., & E. M. Cummings (1984). Cognitive and social development in infants and toddlers with a bipolar parent. *Child Psychiatry and Human Development, 15*, 75–85.

Zahn-Waxler, C., Cummings, E. M., Iannotti, R. J., & Radke-Yarrow, M. (1984). Young children of depressed: A population at risk for affective problems. In D. Cicchetti and

K. Schneider-Rosen (eds.), *Childhood Depression*, 26, 81–105. San Francisco: Jossey-Bass.

Zahn-Waxler, C., Cummings, E. M., McKnew, D. H., & Radke-Yarrow, M. (1984). Altruism, aggression, and social interactions in young children of manic-depressive parents. *Child Development*, 55, 112–122.

Zahn-Waxler, C., Denham, S., Iannotti, R., & Cummings, E. M. (in press). Peer relations in children with a depressed caregiver. In R. D. Parke & G. W. Ladd (eds.), *Family-peer relationships: Modes of linkage*. Hillsdale, NJ: Erlbaum.

Zahn-Waxler, C., Iannotti, R. J., Cummings, E. M., & Denham, S. (1990). Antecedents of problem behaviors in children of depressed mothers. *Development and Psychopathology*, 2, 271–291.

Zahn-Waxler, C., Kochanska, G., Krupnick, J., & McKnew, D. (1990). Patterns of guilt in children of depressed and well mothers. *Developmental Psychology*, 26, 51–59.

Zahn-Waxler, C., McKnew, D. H., Cummings, E. M., Davenport, Y. B., & Radke-Yarrow, M. (1984). Problem behaviors and peer interactions of young children with a manic-depressive parent. *American Journal of Psychiatry*, 141, 236–240.

Zekoski, E. M., O'Hara, M. W., & Wils, K. E. (1987). The effects of maternal mood on mother-infant interaction. *Journal of Abnormal Child Psychology*, 15, 361–378.

Zillman, D. (1983). Arousal and aggression. In R. G. Geen & E. I. Donnerstein (eds.), *Aggression: Theoretical and empirical reviews: Vol. 1, Theoretical and methodological issues* (pp. 75–101). New York: Academic.

IX Developmental Predictors cf Depressivc Cognitive Style: Research and Theory

Donna T. Rose & Lyn Y. Abramson

Introduction

Why are some people vulnerable to frequent, severe, or long-lasting depressions while others never seem to become depressed or only develop mild, short-lived depressions? We and others within the cognitive perspective on depression suggest that people's characteristic ways of interpreting events, or their cognitive styles, can make them vulnerable to depression (e.g., Abramson, Metalsky and Alloy, 1989; Beck, 1987). Thus, as a complement to work emphasizing biological risk factors for depression, we suggest that cognitive risk for depression also exists.

The point of departure for this chapter is a well-replicated empirical observation: heterogeneity of cognitive style exists among depressives. Whereas many depressives do exhibit the negative cognitive styles featured in the cognitive theories, other depressives do not. Which depressives exhibit the hypothesized cognitive styles? How did these depressives come to exhibit negative cognitive styles? Do adults with negative cognitive styles have a history of aversive or traumatic developmental events? In this chapter, we provide the theoretical background for these questions, review research on heterogeneity of cognitive styles among depressives, note links among aversive developmental events, cognitive styles and depression, and propose a model of the development of negative cognitive styles.

Background: The Cognitive Theories of Depression

During the past two decades, researchers and clinicians have used the frameworks of the cognitive theories of depression to explore the etiology, course and treatment of depression (Abramson, Metalsky and Alloy, 1989; Beck, 1987). Arguing that these theories propose a subtype of depression, "negative cognition depression," Abramson and Alloy (1990) noted that this subtype is defined in part by cognitive styles that provide vulnerability to depression in the face of negative life events. Thus, within a group of depressed individuals, a subset may be "negative cognition depressives" who would be expected to exhibit more negative cognitive styles than would individuals suffering from "noncognitive" (e.g., biologically-based) depressions.

Although research to date has established an association between the proposed cognitive vulnerability styles and depression (Eaves and Rush, 1984; Hamilton and Abramson, 1983; Hollon, Kendall and Lumry, 1986; McCauley, Mitchell, Burke and Moss, 1988; Norman, Miller and Dow, 1988), and has shown that cognitive styles may interact with stressful events to predict onset of symptoms of depression (Metalsky, Halberstadt and Abramson, 1987), there has been little support for the contention that these theories define a subtype of depression. The problem is that investigators have been unable to identify grouping factors that select depressives who exhibit distinctively negative cognitive styles. Further, there has been almost no investigation of possible developmental antecedents of cognitive vulnerability to depression.

The Hopelessness Theory of Depression

The hopelessness theory (Abramson, Metalsky and Alloy, 1989) postulates the existence of hopelessness depression, defined primarily by the causal sequence hypothesized to culminate in onset of symptoms of hopelessness depression. According to the theory, a proximal sufficient cause of hopelessness depression is an expectation that highly desired outcomes will not occur or that highly aversive outcomes will occur and that there is nothing one can do to change the situation. The common language term "hopelessness" captures the core elements of this proximal sufficient cause: an expectation of a negative outcome coupled with an expectation of helplessness.

How does a person become hopeless and develop the symptoms of hopelessness depression? As can be seen in Figure 1, the hypothesized causal sequence begins with the perceived occurrence of negative life events. According to the theory, people may make certain inferences about the occurrence of negative life events that increase the likelihood that they will become hopeless and, in turn, develop the symptoms of hopelessness depression. Three types of hopelessness-inducing inferences are postulated: (1) Inferences about the cause of the event (specifically, stable and global attributions); (2) Inferences about negative consequences that may result from the occurrence of the event; and (3) Inferences about negative characteristics of the self given that the event occurred. For example, a "pre-med" college student failed an exam in an important science class. The student inferred that his lack of intelligence not only caused him to fail the exam, but also caused him to make an unwise decision about the fraternity he pledged (a stable and global causal attribution). He further inferred that a consequence of the failure on the exam was

THE HOPELESSNESS THEORY OF DEPRESSION

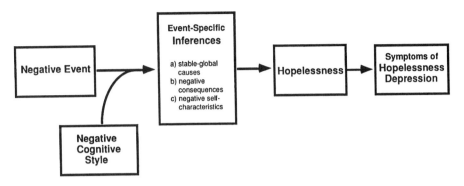

Figure 1. The Hopelessness Theory of Depression. (Abramson, Metalsky and Alloy, 1989).

that he would never be accepted into medical school. He also inferred that his failure on the exam meant that he was a failure as a person due to characteristics including low intelligence and laziness. According to the hopelessness theory, these inferences place the student at risk of becoming hopeless and depressed.

The hopelessness theory further suggests that certain individuals characteristically make such inferences about the occurrence of negative events, and thus are especially vulnerable to hopelessness depression, while other individuals seldom or never make such inferences, and thus are relatively invulnerable to hopelessness depression. This aspect of the theory is conceptualized as a diathesis-stress component (Metalsky, Abramson, Seligman, Semmel and Peterson, 1982). That is, the hypothesized depressogenic inferential styles (the diatheses) are distal contributory causes of the symptoms of hopelessness depression which operate only in the presence of negative life events (the stress). A negative inferential style thus increases the likelihood that a person will make a hopelessness-inducing inference about a particular event, thereby contributing to the development of hopelessness depression.

Beck's Theory of Depression

Abramson, Alloy and Metalsky (1988a) have argued that the diathesis-stress framework of the hopelessness theory may be usefully applied to Beck's theory of depression (1967, 1976). Beck posits that depressive schemas, or dysfunctional attitudes, are activated by negative life events and initiate development of negative views of the self, the environment and the future, the "negative cognitive triad." For example, the pre-med college student who failed the exam might have the schema, "If I make a mistake, I'm a failure as a person." When confronted by a failure, he may conclude that he is a failure as a person (negative view of the self), that the educational system in which he failed is hostile (negative view of the environment), and that he will never be accepted into medical school (negative view of the future). In Abramson et al.'s interpretation of Beck's theory, depressive schemas are the cognitive diatheses, negative events are the stressors, and the negative cognitive triad is the proximal sufficient cause of a subtype of depression, "negative cognitive triad depression."

Even though both the hopelessness theory and Beck's theory postulate traitlike depressogenic cognitive styles, little is known about the origins of these styles. While Beck argues that depressive schemas develop early in life, he does not specify how this process occurs, and the hopelessness theory, while recognizing the need to trace the developmental origins of inferential style, makes no predictions about what these origins may be.

Empirical Evidence of Heterogeneity of Cognitive Style among Depressives

Insofar as both cognitive theories of depression feature specific cognitive patterns as vulnerability factors for negative cognition depression, an inference from these theories is that negative cognition depressives should exhibit the proposed negative cognitive styles to a greater extent than either nondepressed individuals or "noncognitive" depressives. Consistent with this hypothesis, Hamilton and Abramson (1983) reported great heterogeneity of dysfunctional attitudes and attributional styles among a sample of unipolar major depressives, episodic and nonpsychotic type. The cognitive scores of half of the depressed patients fell within the range of nondepressed normal subjects' scores, while the other half of the depressives exhibited more negative cognitions. Although emphasizing the need for research on heterogeneity of cognitive styles in depression, this study was not designed to predict which depressives exhibited the negative cognitive styles. Subsequent studies that divided groups of depressives according to cognitive styles found that more negative cognitive styles predicted differential response to treatment protocols (Miller, Norman and Keitner, 1990), persistence of negative cognitions after clinical improvement (Miller and Norman, 1986), a lower rate of recovery from depression (Williams, Healy, Teasdale, White and Paykel, 1990), and differences in depression history, social support and hopelessness (Norman, Miller and Dow, 1988). While these studies suggest that cognitive style is related to course, treatment and recovery from depression, they do not provide grouping factors to predict which depressives exhibit the worst cognitive styles.

Many studies have attempted to determine which depressives exhibit negative cognitive styles by exploring traditional diagnostic distinctions. Most widely studied has been the melancholic/nonmelancholic distinction, based on the premise that biological or genetic factors may initiate and maintain melancholic depression, while psychological factors may contribute to nonmelancholic depressions. Consistent with this premise, Robins, Block and Peselow (1990) found more dysfunctional attitudes in nonendogenous depressives (see also Zimmerman and Coryell, 1986, and Zimmerman, Coryell and Pfohl, 1986, for similar results when the dexamethasone suppression test was used as the indicator of melancholia). Failing to support the premise of worse cognitive styles among nonendogenous depressives were studies by Eaves and Rush (1984) and Norman, Miller and Dow (1988) which found no cognitive style differences between endogenous and nonendogenous depressives, and the finding of Willner, Wilkes and Orwin (1990) of worse attributional styles in melancholic depressives. Thus, the relationship of melancholia to cognitive style remains unclear. Studies of other diagnostic distinctions have found no cognitive style differences among unipolar, bipolar and substance abusing depressives (Hollon, Kendall and Lumry, 1986) and psychotic and nonpsychotic depressives (Zimmerman, Coryell, Corenthal and Wilson, 1986).

If the cognitive theories of depression are valid, why were these investigators unable to identify a subgroup of depressives whose cognitive styles distinguish them from other depressives? Rose, Leff, Halberstadt, Hodulik and Abramson (1992) argued that these studies did not examine the full range of currently diagnosed depression subtypes. They further suggested that negative cognition depression may cut across traditional depression subtypes rather than map on to any currently diagnosed subtype. Thus, nonnosological factors may be more useful than standard diagnostic systems in identifying depressives with negative cognitive patterns.

With this reasoning, Rose et al. used three approaches with a psychiatric inpatient sample to identify subgroups of depressives whose extremely negative cognitive styles distinguished them from other depressives: (1) They examined the cognitive styles of depressives representing all currently diagnosed depression subtypes; (2) They examined the cognitive styles of depressed patients who spontaneously verbalized cognitions consistent with a negative cognitive style and described characteristics identifying these depressives; and (3) They asked whether nonnosological variables such as sex, developmental events, depression history and severity of depression predicted cognitive styles among depressives.

Rose et al.'s sample consisted of 134 newly-admitted psychiatric inpatients and 54 nondepressed normal control subjects. DSM–III–R diagnoses were determined using information obtained from SADS–Lifetime interviews modified to permit both RDC and DSM–III–R diagnoses. Measures included the Dysfunctional Attitude Scale (DAS, Form A: Weissman and Beck, 1978), the Inferential Styles Questionnaire (ISQ: Rose et al., 1991), the Beck Depression Inventory (BDI: Beck et al., 1961), and the Depressive Milestones Questionnaire (DMQ: Rose et al., 1991). In a follow-up study, a large subset of the original subjects (N=166) also completed the Child's Report of Parent Behavior Inventory (CRPBI: Schaefer, 1965). The DAS is a 40-item scale designed to assess the degree to which individuals endorse the dysfunctional attitudes hypothesized by Beck (1967) to be depressogenic. The ISQ is a modification of the Attributional Styles Questionnaire (Seligman, Abramson, Semmel and von Baeyer, 1979) designed for use with an adult, community sample. The ISQ assesses the inferential styles about cause, consequence and self featured in the hopelessness theory (Abramson et al., 1989). ISQ scores reported by Rose et al. were computed by summing inferences about stable and global causes, consequences and characteristics of the self for negative events. The BDI is a 21-item self-report inventory designed to assess the severity of current depressive symptoms. The DMQ is a 12-item questionnaire that inquires about the occurrence of developmental events hypothesized to be related to adult depression including object loss experiences such as death of a parent, family life characterized by harsh or rigid discipline or perfectionistic parental standards, and sexual assault such as rape or incest. The CRPBI is a 180-item inventory that asks about a wide array of parental behaviors.

Rose et al. identified groups of depressives whose cognitive styles distinguished them from other depressives, and identified nonnosological variables that predicted cognitive style. Using a traditional approach, they found that unipolar depressives with personality disorders (specifically, borderline and schizotypal personality disorders) exhibited more dysfunctional attitudes than did unipolar depressives with chronic or dysthymic patterns. In the analyses of cognitive styles of patients who spontaneously made negative inferences about their lives, Rose et al. found that depressed patients who also earned a diagnosis of borderline personality disorder, reported a history of sexual abuse, had been depressed more than 20% of their lifetimes, and who had early onset of depression exhibited extremely negative cognitive styles when compared with all other depressed patients. Further, this group's Dysfunctional Attitude Scale scores were strikingly worse than any previously reported by other investigators. Finally, examining nonnosological factors, Rose et al. found that depressed patients' reports of having been raised by authoritarian parents who set perfectionistic standards and used harsh, rigid, controlling disciplinary tactics ("family control") predicted negative cognitive styles, as did severity of current depression and patients' reports of having been victims of sexual assault such as rape or incest. Sex, object loss events, age of onset of depression and percent of lifetime spent depressed did not predict cognitive style in this sample (Figure 2). An additional analysis using the Child's Report of Parent Behavior Inventory also found that subjects' reports of emotional abuse by their mothers predicted adult negative cognitive style (Rose and Abramson, 1992).

The approaches employed by Rose et al. (1992) converge on a consistent finding: heterogeneity of cognitive style exists among inpatient depressives and can be predicted. Important predictors of negative cognitive styles include borderline personality disorder, severe depression, and developmental events including sexual abuse, emotional abuse and authoritarian control by parents (see also Crook, Raskin and Eliot, 1981, for a discussion of parent-child relationships and depressive cognitions). These data regarding the adult

Variance in Inferential Style

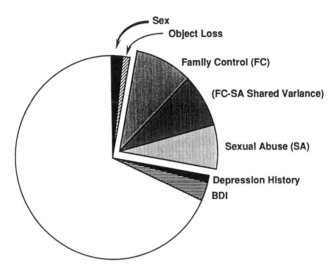

Figure 2. Variance in Inferential Style Questionnaire scores of depressed inpatients. (Rose, Leff, Halberstadt, Hodulik and Abramson, 1991).

negative cognitive styles of individuals who experienced harsh, controlling parenting or sexual or emotional abuse suggest the possibility of a causal pathway to explain the links between these experiences and depression that have been widely noted (e.g., Briere and Runtz, 1988; Bryer, Nelson, Miller and Krol, 1987; Downey and Coyne, 1990; Garnefski, van Egmond, Straatman, 1989).

A Model of Development of Cognitive Vulnerability to Depression

The data described by Rose et al. (1992) indicate a substantial link among aversive or traumatic developmental events, adult cognitive styles and depression. How are these factors related? Rose (1987) proposed that the logic of the hopelessness theory of depression supports a causal model to account for these associations. According to the hopelessness theory, negative life events elicit cognitive activity as the affected individual strives for understanding of the cause and meaning of the event. This interplay between negative events and cognitive activity is the foundation of this model, which traces a progression from the occurrence of negative events, to generation of specific cognitions about the events, to development of cognitive styles (Figure 3). This model thus adds two new links to the causal chain proposed by the hopelessness theory by explaining the origins of the cognitive styles featured as contributory causes of hopelessness depression. It is important to note that while this model focuses on childhood events that may lead to the development of negative cognitive styles, there may be analogous adult experiences with the power to induce negative cognitive styles in an individual who reached adulthood with a normal cognitive style (e.g., chronic, inescapable violent abuse by a spouse). Thus, while development of negative cognitive styles is probably most likely during childhood and adolescence, this model is intended to apply across the life span.

I. The Expanded Causal Chain: Link #1: Negative Developmental Events Elicit Specific Cognitions.

An individual who is confronted with a negative event is motivated to begin an epistemic search for probable causes, consequences and meanings of the event (Kelley, 1967, Kruglanski and Klar, 1987, Ulman and Brothers, 1988, Weiner, 1985, Wortman and Dintzer, 1978). In this process, the individual acts as a "lay scientist," generating and testing hypotheses (Kelley, 1967). An adaptive goal of this epistemic process is to develop hypotheses about the occurrence of the event that can be used to guide future behaviors in an attempt to prevent recurrence of the event, thus inspiring hopefulness.

Situational factors and motivation for epistemic activity

Several situational factors may increase the motivation to engage in epistemic activity:

(1) *Degree of threat or unpleasantness of the negative event* (Wong and Weiner, 1981). The more threatening or unpleasant the event, the greater the motivation to understand its causes, consequences and meaning. Thus, a severely-beaten child who feared that the abuser might eventually kill him may have greater motivation to engage in epistemic activity than would a child who expected only bruises from the beating.

(2) *Repetition of the event.* As long as a negative event has occurred only once, the individual has the option of coding it as a rare occurrence that is unlikely to recur. However, once a negative event is repeated, the rare event hypothesis is disconfirmed and may be abandoned, causing the individual to search for alternative hypotheses which lack the security of the rare event hypothesis because they must account for the likelihood of repeated occurrences.

(3) *In abuse situations, the physical proximity of the abuser to the abused individual.* Because physical proximity may increase the likelihood of repetition of an abuse event, epistemic activity may be particularly desirable when

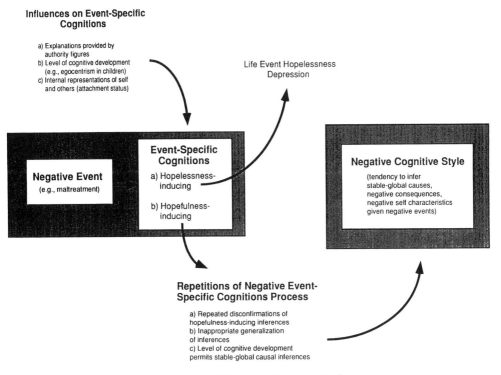

Figure 3. A model of Development of Negative Cognitive Style.

an individual's abuser cannot be easily avoided, such as when the abuser is a family member or other person who has frequent access to the abused individual.

(4) *In maltreatment situations, the nature and quality of the relationship between the abuser and the abused individual.* If the negative event occurs within the context of an important relationship (i.e., parent-child), the security of the relationship might be threatened, leading to high motivation to understand the event and take action to restore the relationship (Berscheid, Graziano, Monson and Dermer, 1976; Erber and Fiske, 1984, Kruglanski and Klar, 1987). For example, when a mother tells her child that she wishes the child had never been born, the child's security in the relationship is compromised. Because the relationship may be vital to the child's physical and emotional well-being, the motivation to understand the mother's dissatisfaction and try to remediate it is great. By comparison, if an acquaintance or stranger maltreated the child there would be less threat to the child and less need to engage in epistemic activity. Maltreated children's struggles to reconcile need of their caregivers with fear of abuse are evident in their behavior when they are briefly separated from their caregivers. Maltreated children show a disorganized/disoriented pattern of attachment behaviors characterized by

concurrent proximity seeking and avoidance. For example, the child approaches the caregiver with head averted, or backs towards the caregiver (Carlson, Cicchetti, Barnett and Braunwald, 1989, Crittenden and Ainsworth, 1989).

(5) *The extent to which the event challenges the individual's positive self-image.* A number of investigators have posited a basic need to maintain a positive view of the self (Arkin and Baumgardner, 1985, Berglass and Jones, 1978, Kruglanski and Ajzen, 1983, Kruglanski and Klar, 1987). When this positive view of the self is threatened, epistemic activity is required to ameliorate the resulting discrepancy between self-image and situational information about the self (Kruglanski and Ajzen, 1983). For example, when a teacher tells a child in front of her classmates, "You are a worthless person who will never succeed at anything," the child's view of herself as a good student and worthwhile person is challenged. The child may then initiate an epistemic process to understand why the teacher made the statement with the goal of explaining it in a way that is consistent with the child's positive self-image (e.g., the teacher is an angry person who often attacks students). While most children develop predominantly positive self-images which they would need to defend when confronted with negative events, it is important to note that children who are maltreated during infancy and early childhood may develop predominantly negative self-representations (Cicchetti, Beeghly, Carlson and Toth, 1990; Cicchetti and Schneider-Rosen, 1986), and thus may passively accept maltreatment as a deserved outcome. Children who are not actively maltreated, but are emotionally neglected (e.g., due to their caregiver's depression), may also develop negative self-representations such as "I am unlovable" (Downey and Coyne, 1990), which may also make them vulnerable to passive acceptance of maltreatment. Once they have developed negative views of themselves and relationships, these children may not attempt to make hopefulness-inducing inferences for negative events.

In addition to situational factors that may motivate epistemic activity, organismic factors such as intelligence, tendencies to use dissociation or repression in response to traumatic events (Fine, 1990; Fish-Murray, Koby and van der Kolk, 1987), and level of cognitive development may modulate the extent to which an individual is able to engage in such activity.

Social cognitive development and the inferential process

Studies in social cognition have indicated that even toddlers engage in social causal reasoning (see Miller and Aloise, 1989, for a review of this literature). However, the content of children's inferences may vary according to age. For example, children's views of the intentionality of behaviors may affect the likelihood of making an internal rather than an external attribution. Before about age 5, children tend to believe that all behaviors are intended, even if they are not (Smith, 1978). Heider (1958) noted that preschoolers' overattributions of intentionality are consistent with an egocentric perspective that the self is responsible for all outcomes connected with it. Egocentrism is a characteristic of children during the preoperational stage of cognitive development, from about ages 2–6 as described by Piaget (Ginsburg and Opper, 1988). Thus, very young children may be more likely to attribute negative events such as abuse to internal causes (e.g., their own behaviors) rather than to other people (Orzek, 1985).

Young children may also be more likely to attribute outcomes to unstable and specific causes, such as specific behaviors, rather than to stable and global causes, such as personality traits. Rholes and Ruble (1986) note that the concept of stability requires the ability to integrate information acquired over time, which is not well developed in young children. Likewise, inferences of globality require integration of information across situations, a process beyond the capabilities of most young children.

Even when young children do understand stable traits (e.g., nice, mean), they may not comprehend the relationship between traits and behavior (Miller and Aloise, 1989). Rather, young children may infer from situational information that transient states such as emotions and motives cause outcomes (e.g., "Mommy spanked me to make me pick up my toys.") Searching situational information for causal relationships is consistent with Shultz's (1982) view that children prefer causes that include an obvious, temporally proximal mechanism that produces outcomes (e.g., "Mommy got mad because my room was messy"), rather than a more subtle, temporally distal mechanism (e.g., "Mommy is mad about everything these days because she's worried about money"). Inferring temporally distal causes is difficult for children in the preoperational stage of cognitive development due to lack of reversibility (Ginsburg and Opper, 1988), the ability to trace a sequence of information back several steps. Thus, explanations focusing on the most recent possible causes of an event are likely to be most available to younger children.

Work in adult social cognition has revealed an "attributional bias" to view one's own behaviors as situationally determined but to view others' behaviors as dispositionally caused (Jones and Nisbett, 1972). Abramovitch and Freedman (1981) found that this bias can be observed even in 4 year olds. When outcomes are negative, children are especially likely to make behavioral rather than characterological inferences about their own behavior (King, Hegland and Galejs, 1986; Mischel, Zeiss and Zeiss, 1974). In summary, young children should be most likely to make internal, unstable and specific attributions for negative events.

As children move into the concrete operational period at about age 7, they begin to acquire the ability to conserve information over time and across situations. With conservation, therefore, children become able to make stable and global causal inferences. In summary, since even very young children make causal inferences about personally meaningful events, the level of a child's cognitive development is therefore likely to affect not whether an inference is made, but the type or content of the inference.

Several investigators have found that some children do make negative causal attributions, and that these attributions are associated with hopelessness and depression (McCauley, Mitchell, Burke and Moss, 1988; Nolen-Hoecksema, Girgus and Seligman, 1986; Seligman et al., 1984).

Adaptiveness of the epistemic process

Certain hypotheses about the occurrence of negative events can serve as frameworks for developing protective strategies to prevent further negative events (Fine, 1990; see also Cicchetti and Schneider-Rosen, 1986, for an analogous treatment of insecure attachment patterns as adaptive responses). To the extent that these strategies seem promising, they may inspire hopefulness: the expectation that one has the ability to prevent entirely the occurrence of an anticipated negative outcome, or to reduce the anticipated negative impact if the outcome cannot be prevented. This model assumes that most individuals exposed to maltreatment respond — at least initially — by interpreting the maltreatment as preventable in the future. Since the alternative — believing that one is helpless to prevent further trauma — may threaten emotional and physical survival (Summit, 1983), a defensive bias towards making hopefulness-inducing inferences psychologically favors survival. These hopefulness-inducing hypotheses about negative events may thus be viewed as provisionally "adaptive" insofar as they (1) suggest protective strategies for preventing additional negative outcomes and (2) increase hopefulness. Note that in our definition, the provisional "adaptiveness" of a hypothesis does not require that protective strategies ultimately be effective. Consistent with the assumption of a bias to make hopefulness-inducing inferences is evidence that young maltreated children may defend against their frightening, unpredictable environments by making inflated self-assessments of their competence to control their environments (Vondra, Barnett and Cicchetti, 1990). Categories of adaptive hypotheses include:

(1) *Causal inferences*. Identification of possible causes may suggest ways that the individual can prevent repetition of the event by avoiding the cause. For example, a boy who was attacked by the neighborhood bully when walking home from school may decide that the cause of the attack was the bully's desire to beat up any boys smaller than himself. The boy may therefore decide to take a different route home to avoid walking by the bully's house. As a consequence, the boy may feel hopeful about avoiding further confrontations.

(2) *Inferences about consequences of negative events*. Identification of possible consequences of events may suggest ways to minimize damage by taking preventive action. For example, a child who has been embarrassed by the behavior of an alcoholic parent and fears the ridicule of her peers may decide never again to bring friends to the family home. This decision may increase the child's hope of keeping a secret about which she is ashamed.

(3) *Inferences about characteristics of the self.* In addition to seeking to understand the causes and consequences of negative events, individuals may wonder whether the occurrence of such an event means that they are flawed in some way. Such an inference would be especially likely for individuals who lack consensus information (Kelley, 1967) suggesting that the negative event happened to many people with a wide spectrum of characteristics. Children's limited experience of the world, and the secrecy that often surrounds abuse, would limit most children's access to such information.

Particularly relevant to developing a tendency to infer negative characteristics of the self are findings from the attachment theory literature that maltreatment of infants and toddlers may contribute to negative internal working models of themselves and of their relationships with caregivers. When caregivers are abusive and/or unavailable, their children may learn to view themselves as unlovable or flawed, and to view other people as rejecting, critical or dangerous (Carlson, Cicchetti, Barnett and Braunwald, 1989; Cicchetti, 1991; Cummings and Cicchetti, 1990). The presence of negative self-representations is suggested by data showing that some maltreated toddlers even display negative affect in response to their own reflections in visual self-recognition experiments (Cicchetti, Beeghly, Carlson and Toth, 1990). When early maltreatment causes negative attributes to be incorporated into the earliest organization of the self system, the later tendency to make negative inferences about the self should be especially strong and resistant to change (Cummings and Cicchetti, 1990). In addition, when a child's basic working model of relationships with others includes images and beliefs that maltreatment is part of interpersonal interactions, the child may more readily believe that people in many areas of life will continue to treat him/her badly (i.e., make stable and global causal inferences for negative interpersonal events).

Identification of flaws in the self may suggest ways that the individual can change (e.g., appearance, behavior) in order to protect against further negative events. For example, some sexually abused individuals infer from the abuse that their appearance or behavior is seductive and is likely to provoke further abuse. An individual who makes this inference about herself may seek to protect herself from further abuse by changing her appearance (e.g., by becoming obese or by wearing voluminous clothing) or by modifying her behavior (e.g., by behaving in a hostile manner towards men).

Inferences that are most likely to be hopefulness-inducing

Hopefulness-inducing inferences admit the possibility of preventing anticipated negative outcomes. Thus, an expectation of change is an important feature of these inferences about causes, consequences and characteristics of the self in response to negative events. Unstable and specific causal inferences suggest that the cause of a negative event may not recur and is limited to a circumscribed aspect of life. For example, attributing a grade of "F" on a spelling test to failure to study the list of words, while noting that studying produced a "B" on a math test suggests that studying the next spelling list will prevent a recurrence of a failing grade. By comparison, a stable and global inference ("I am stupid and will fail tests in all my classes") suggests no possibility of preventing negative outcomes. In the same manner, inferring positive consequences or negative but remediable consequences from a negative event may produce hopefulness, as may inferring negative but modifiable characteristics of the self from a negative event. By comparison, inferring unchangeable negative consequences or characteristics of the self is likely to produce hopelessness.

Situational factors influencing the content of hopefulness-inducing cognitions

An important precursor to generating hopefulness-inducing hypotheses is to determine whether something about the self or something about the environment can be changed to avert further negative outcomes. Thus, a hopefulness-inducing cognition should state or imply an expectation that the individual could change in some way, or that other people or circumstances could change, or both. When a student attributes a failing exam grade to her failure to study due to excessive socializing (an internal-unstable-specific attribution), she could avert further bad grades by changing her own behavior (i.e., reducing her social activities and increasing her study time). If another student attributes a low calculus grade to poor instruction by the professor, he could switch to a different professor, thus changing his circumstances.

To the extent that other people or circumstances seem to be unchangeable, individuals must generate hypotheses that focus on their own capacities to change. Examples of situations in which other people or circumstances may seem unlikely to change are situations in which children are emotionally, physically or sexually abused by their parents or other adults in authority, and situations in which adults are abused by people who have physical or economic power over them (e.g., harassment at work, battered women, "elder abuse"). In such situations, the abused individual may lack the legal, physical, psychological or economic resources to escape from an abuser or to demand that the abuse cease. Individuals may also be especially likely to generate hopefulness-inducing hypotheses that include plans to change their own behavior when they have been victims of unpredictable environmental circumstances, such as violence by strangers. For example, Janoff-Bulman and Lang-Gunn (1988) found that women raped by strangers tended to attribute the rapes to their own behaviors, such as walking alone at night. By invoking behavioral self-blame, the women were able to plan actions to prevent future rapes. An alternative explanation of the rapes — that the world is a dangerous place in which women are defenseless — provides no hope for the future. Thus, at least initially, individuals are likely to feel hopeful when they believe they can change themselves to avoid maltreatment when they are confronted with aversive circumstances they view as unchangeable.

Of course, a pitfall may arise when the individual incorrectly assesses the likelihood of changing the circumstances. A hopefulness-inducing cognition based on the assumption that circumstances cannot be changed, and therefore the self needs to be changed, may actually prevent the individual from escaping from the situation or taking actions that could ameliorate the situation. For example, a woman who is constantly belittled by her domineering husband may infer that she is a failure and vow to improve herself to gain her husband's approval. This inference and plan may be her most hopefulness-inducing response if she assesses her husband's behavior as unchangeable and believes that her marriage must be " 'til death do us part." Paradoxically, her attempts to gain her husband's approval in response to his critical comments may actually reinforce and thus increase his negative behavior and appear to validate her assessment that his negative behavior is unchangeable and that her own behavior is flawed. If the woman had instead demanded that her husband participate in marital therapy or had threatened to leave the marriage if his behavior did not change, she might have improved her circumstances.

Selection among competing hypotheses based upon a hierarchy of needs

It is often possible to generate several mutually exclusive hypotheses about the occurrence of a negative event. When hypotheses contradict, one hypothesis may be adopted over the others in accordance with a hierarchy of needs (Kruglanski and Ajzen, 1983, Kruglanski and Klar, 1987), such as the need to believe that the world is a just place (Lerner, 1980), the need to maintain a positive self-image (Berglass and Jones, 1978), the need to control one's environment (Kelley, 1971, Harvey and Weary, 1984), the need to avoid physical harm (Kruglanski and Ajzen, 1983) or the need to conform to social rules, such as obedience to authority.

An illustration of this process is provided by a child who generated the following two hypotheses to explain a severe beating by his father: (1) I am a good boy and I did not do anything wrong, but my father is a bad man who likes to beat people even when they do not do anything wrong; and (2) I must have done something bad that made my father beat me, because adults know what is right and since I was punished I must have done something wrong. If the boy adopted the first hypothesis, he could maintain his positive self-image, but he would have to live in fear that his father might beat him at any moment, regardless of his own attempts to be good. If the child adopted the second hypothesis, he could believe that his father is a just person who only wants his son to behave properly, and he could hope that by attempting to be good all the time he could avoid future beatings. The second hypothesis may well be more hopefulness-inducing given the child's situation. Since he must live with his father, he can feel safer if he believes he can prevent beatings by modifying his own behaviors. To believe that he must live in constant fear of unpredictable violence would be intolerable (Forward and Buck, 1988, Janoff-Bulman and Lang-Gunn, 1988, Summit, 1983). Thus, in this example, the need to expect physical safety may take precedence over the need to maintain a positive self-image.

The adaptiveness of hopefulness-inducing cognitions: A matter of perspective

A benefit of generating hypotheses about negative events lies in the induction of hopefulness. However, it is important to note that hopefulness-inducing cognitions may be selected regardless of their objective validity. For example, a woman who has been battered by her husband may decide that she can prevent future beatings by keeping the house spotless based upon her external-unstable-specific causal inference that her husband was angered by the untidiness of the house. While an informed observer may expect that the husband is very likely to continue the beatings unless he receives treatment (viewing the husband's temper as a stable-global cause of violence), the wife may embark on her housecleaning with hope of a good outcome and be surprised when the violence recurs in spite of her efforts. Thus, many cognitions that appear maladaptive to others may be selected by an individual because of their power to inspire hopefulness in that individual.

When hopefulness-inducing cognitions cannot be made: Life-event hopelessness depression

While an important goal of generating hypotheses to explain negative events is to inspire hopefulness, some situations are so aversive or traumatic that hopefulness is an extremely unlikely outcome. For example, a girl who has been repeatedly sexually abused by her father under threat of serious physical harm may be unable to generate a hypothesis that would allow her to believe that she has the ability to prevent the repetition of the abuse. In such a case, the girl is likely to become hopeless and develop symptoms of hopelessness depression. Note that according to the hopelessness theory, it is not necessary to have a negative cognitive style in order to experience hopelessness. Instead, cognitions about specific events may initiate hopelessness and the onset of "life event hopelessness depression" (Abramson, Metalsky and Alloy, 1988).

Origins of inferences: internally generated vs. externally supplied

Both internal and external sources of information may be used in making inferences. The individual may make inferences about an event based entirely on his/her own knowledge about the world and human behavior. The objective quality of such internally-generated inferences would depend on the maturity and sophistication of the individual. Children, lacking broad knowledge about the world and human interactions, may be especially prone to make inferences that would seem irrational to better-informed adults. For example, many children of divorced parents blame themselves for the breakup of their parents' marriage (Wallerstein and Blakeslee, 1989). Because abuse experiences are not widely discussed, children may have no knowledge about prevalence and usual causes of abuse, and thus may make inferences that would surprise adults. Cultural information may also contribute to the inference a child makes. For example, frequently viewing scenes of violence on television could lead a child to infer that violence is a normative response to conflict in many areas of life (a stable-global explanation).

Inferences may also be based on information about the event supplied by other people. Bloom and Capatides (1987) suggested that most of what their child subjects knew about subjective causality was based on beliefs, reasons and justifications supplied by adults. In a common instance of such externally-supplied explanations, adults who physically or sexually abuse a child tell the child that the abuse was caused by a characteristic or behavior of the child (e.g., the child was "seductive" or the child misbehaved and deserved punishment; see Berliner and Conte,1990; Crittenden and Ainsworth, 1989). Lacking knowledge that would contradict these externally-supplied explanations, children may adopt the explanations without question, particularly if the adult who supplies the explanation is perceived by the child as an important authority (i.e., a parent or teacher). Emotional abuse often consists of the abuser supplying negative information to the victim. For example, when a parent says to a child, "You're worthless and will never amount to anything," the child has been supplied with an internal, stable, global causal inference for failure events. Because emotional abuse so explicitly provides negative information, this may be a particularly powerful form of abuse leading to development of negative cognitions and depression. By comparison, when an abuser beats a child but does not supply causal information, the child has the option of making a more benign causal inference. In addition to supplying specific negative inferences directly to children, adults may indirectly transmit negative cognitions to children through their own verbal modeling of negative cognitive style (Cummings and Cicchetti, 1990). Depressed parents may be especially likely to model negative cognitions.

II. The Expanded Causal Chain: Link #2: Specific Cognitions about Developmental Events are Elaborated into Traitlike Cognitive Styles

If a goal of generating hypotheses about negative events is to increase hopefulness, how then does a person develop cognitive vulnerability to hopelessness depression? The hopelessness theory posits that characteristic tendencies to infer stable and global causes, negative consequences and negative characteristics of the self given negative events increases the likelihood of becoming hopeless. How do people come to generate these inferences more readily than hopefulness-inducing hypotheses?

Repeated disconfirmations of hopefulness-inducing cognitions contribute to negative cognitive styles

When individuals generate hopefulness-inducing hypotheses, they are in effect designing experiments to test their hypotheses. If these experiments repeatedly fail, they may have to abandon the original hopefulness-inducing hypotheses. For example, when a boy adopts the hypothesis, "My mother beat me because I misbehaved; therefore, if I am very good all the time I will not be beaten again," he has defined an experiment in which good behavior should predict cessation of beatings. The boy is likely to monitor his behavior closely in his mother's presence to be sure that the conditions of the experiment — good behavior — are being met. If beatings ensue in spite of the boy's good behavior, the hypothesis will be disconfirmed and must eventually be abandoned. Given a limited domain of hypotheses to explain the beatings, the boy may ultimately have to adopt a hopelessness-inducing hypothesis such as, "My mother is crazy and will continue to beat me no matter how I behave," or "I'm a bad kid and can't do anything right no matter how hard I try."

Over time, repeated abandonment of hopefulness-inducing hypotheses may result in diminished availability of these hypotheses with concomitant increased availability of hopelessness-inducing cognitions. Since availability refers to the individual's general repertory of knowledge stored in long-term memory (Kruglanski and Klar, 1987), this shift over time from hopefulness- to hopelessness-inducing cognitions eventually yields a negative cognitive style, defined as the tendency to generate hopelessness-inducing cognitions when confronted with negative events. Another factor which may increase the relative availability of hopelessness-inducing cognitions is failure to develop a basic repertory of hopefulness-inducing cognitions due to frequent exposure to negative events early in life coupled with lack of hopefulness validating experiences. In the most extreme cases, in which traumatic negative events occur frequently from early ages and positive experiences are rare, individuals may learn to be chronically hopeless. This "learned hopelessness" may be the source of the chronic patterning of depression frequently seen in individuals with such histories, and may be expressed in statements such as, "I always knew I was doomed."

Inappropriate generalization of cognitions over time and across situations

Another way individuals may develop tendencies to infer stable-global causes, negative consequences and negative characteristics of the self in response to negative events is inappropriate generalization of initially hopefulness-inducing cognitions. As noted above, an individual's hierarchy of needs may lead to adoption of certain objectively negative cognitions as most likely to inspire hopefulness. Thus, when a girl blames her own behavior for her father's violent outbursts, she may be choosing the most hopefulness-inducing cognition for that specific situation. However, if she generalizes that specific cognition to many relationships, she is likely to conclude that something about her will always cause her to be abused. Thus, while certain cognitions may be adaptive (hopefulness-inducing) in specific situations, they are likely to become maladaptive (hopelessness-inducing) if generalized over time and across situations.

Examples of repeated disconfirmation and inappropriate generalization of cognitions: Self-blame in abuse situations

When individuals blame themselves for the occurrence of a negative event (internal causal inference) or infer from the negative event that there must be something wrong with them, they may focus on either stable or unstable factors. Stable factors include relatively enduring characteristics such as intelligence, physical attractiveness or certain aspects of personality. Unstable factors are typically voluntary behaviors. Characterological self-blame refers to inferred stable characteristics while behavioral self-blame refers to inferred unstable factors (Janoff-Bulman and Lang-Gunn, 1988). Because behavioral self-blame allows the possibility of change through modification of behavior, it is likely to be hopefulness-inducing, while characterological self-blame is likely to encourage hopelessness.

Several situations may suggest characterological rather than behavioral self-blame. (1) If a victim of abuse initially made a behavioral self-blame inference for the abuse and modified the suspect behavior without preventing further abuse, she may conclude based on repeated disconfirmation of behavioral self-blame that characterological rather than behavioral factors are involved. (2) Negative experiences that contribute particularly to the development of characterological self-blame are those that suggest an internal cause or trait that is stable over time and across a variety of situations. For example, chronic sexual abuse by several perpetrators may provide the situational information that the abuse is unique to the victim (i.e., something about her must be causing it), that it keeps happening (stable cause) and that it is not specific to one perpetrator. (3) Another experience that may result in characterological self-blame is emotional abuse in which the abuser supplies characterological hypotheses such as "You are stupid" or "You are unlovable."

In summary, negative cognitive styles may develop when hopefulness-inducing cognitions are repeatedly disconfirmed or when hopefulness-inducing but negative cognitions (e.g., "I misbehaved") are inappropriately generalized over time and across situations. According to the hopelessness theory of depression (Abramson, Metalsky and Alloy, 1989), individuals who develop such styles are at risk of becoming hopeless and depressed when confronted by negative events.

Implications of social cognitive development in children for vulnerability to hopelessness depression

While this model of development of negative cognitive style is not intended to apply exclusively to children, it is interesting to speculate on interfaces among levels of children's social cognitive development, inferences about negative events, and vulnerability to hopelessness depression. Because this model describes a process in which repeated disconfirmations of hopefulness-inducing inferences and inappropriate generalizations of inferences over time and across situations produce negative cognitive styles, frequency and ages of onset and cessation of maltreatment experiences should contribute to development of negative cognitive style. Maltreatment which begins early in childhood and persists into the late concrete operations or formal operations periods should be most likely to produce a pattern of initial egocentric internal, unstable and specific causal inferences gradually giving way to stable and global causal inferences. It is important to note that this model predicts that onset of hopelessness and depression would typically not be expected as an initial consequence of a maltreatment event, but would more likely appear some time — perhaps years — after onset of maltreatment. Of course, as noted above, some abuse experiences are so traumatic that life event hopelessness depression may develop immediately. Early childhood onset of maltreatment which ceases prior to development of cognitive conservation, or which is of very limited frequency and duration, should engender a primarily internal, unstable and specific causal inferential style. In some children, cessation of maltreatment in this period may paradoxically instill a positive cognitive style if the child infers that her/his own actions taken in response to behavioral self-blame were instrumental in ending the maltreatment. Unfortunately, early cessation of maltreatment is probably the exception rather than the norm, since maltreatment often occurs in contexts highly conducive to its continuation (e.g., substance-abusing families, highly-stressed, low SES single mothers, and families in which one adult is domineering and violent; Crittenden and Ainsworth, 1989; Pianta, Egeland and Erickson, 1989).

Depression and hopelessness in maltreated children

Many investigators have found increased levels of depression in maltreated children. In studies of physically abused children, Allen and Tarnowski (1989) found that abused children were more depressed and hopeless than nonabused children, and Kaufman (1991) noted that physically and emotionally abused children showed disproportionately high rates of diagnosable depression as compared with prevalence rates in general populations of children. Kazdin, Moser, Colbus and Bell (1985) found that physically abused child psychiatric inpatients were more depressed and hopeless than nonabused child patients. Interestingly, Kazdin et al. also found that children with both past and current abuse were more depressed and hopeless than were children with either past or current abuse only. In fact, children with only past abuse did not differ from nonabused children in depression and hopelessness. Kashani, Shekim, Burk and Beck (1987), studying children of hospitalized mothers with affective disorders, found that those children who had been physically abused had greater psychopathology than did nonabused children. When Kashani et al. analyzed factors that predicted depression in abused children, they found that fear of being abused in the future was the most powerful predictor of depression.

Several studies of sexually abused children and adolescents have noted increased rates of depression. Gidycz and Koss (1989) found that sexually victimized adolescent girls were more depressed than were nonvictimized girls, and that greater extent of victimization predicted more severe depression. Lipovsky, Saunders and Murphy (1989) compared victims of father-child sexual assault with their nonabused siblings, finding that the abuse victims reported higher levels of depression than did their nonabused siblings. Sansonnet-Hayden, Haley, Marriage and Fine (1987) reported greater severity of depression and more suicide attempts among sexually-abused adolescent inpatients than among nonabused patients. Kaufman, Peck and Tagiuri (1954) and Browning and Boatman (1977), in clinical studies of small samples of young female incest victims, noted depression as a predominant feature of their subjects.

While the literature currently available on child maltreatment and depression does not yet include information on cognitive styles and thus does not permit a test of this model of development of cognitive style, many research findings are consistent with predictions of the model. Most of these studies of maltreated children do find a strong association between maltreatment and depression. The prediction that chronic abuse beginning early in childhood and continuing into late childhood or adolescence should be associated with worse cognitive styles and more depression is supported by the Kazdin et al. (1985) finding that children with current and past abuse are more hopeless and depressed than are children with current or past abuse only. The similarities between the past-abused and never-abused groups support the prediction that cessation of abuse prior to late childhood may be associated with better cognitive outcomes. The finding of Kashani et al. (1987) that fear of future abuse strongly predicted depression in physically abused children supports a link between cognitions about abuse, hopelessness and depression.

Conclusion

In this chapter, we have described research data showing links among child maltreatment, cognitive styles and depression, and we have proposed a model to account for these links. Ironically, this work brings us back full circle to the origins of the hopelessness theory: the work of Seligman (1975) on learned helplessness in animals exposed to uncontrollable shock. The helplessness-inducing animal experiments now seem analogous to the maltreatment experienced by many humans. As the learned helplessness concept evolved into the hopelessness theory (Abramson, Seligman and Teasdale, 1978; Abramson, Metalsky and Alloy, 1989), the role of trauma was for a time forgotten. We suggest the importance of reintroducing the concept of trauma to the hopelessness theory.

The model of development of negative cognitive style and vulnerability to hopelessness and depression expands the causal chain featured in the hopelessness theory of depression (Abramson, Metalsky and Alloy, 1989). Expanding the hopelessness theory to include developmental precursors of negative cognitive style has implications for prevention, diagnosis and treatment of hopelessness depression. The model suggests that interventions with maltreated children may reduce their risk of becoming vulnerable to hopelessness depression. Specifically, interventions should encourage children to make unstable, specific causal inferences about abuse experiences, and reframe abuse experiences in ways that permit more positive inferences about consequences and characteristics of the self. However, harm to the child may result if interventions ignore the hopefulness-inducing adaptiveness of inferences that may seem irrational to adults. For example, urging a child to replace the inference, "My dad beats me because I do naughty things" with "My dad is a violent man," may trigger hopelessness and depression. Early detection and cessation of abuse should also protect against development of negative cognitive styles. This model also proposes that emotional abuse may be a particularly noxious contributor to negative cognitive style, suggesting that programs that educate parents about emotional abuse and its effects may be especially beneficial.

This model has implications for diagnosis and treatment of depression. As Rose et al. (1992) showed, developmental experiences such as sexual abuse and growing up in rigidly authoritarian families identify adult depressives with distinctively negative cognitive styles, suggesting that these individuals may be the "negative cognition depressives" described in the hopelessness theory of depression. While the concept of hopelessness depression as a distinct subtype has yet to be fully validated, clinicians should consider cognitive approaches for treating depressives with histories of maltreatment.

We conclude with a statement by one of our research subjects whose theory about the relationships among maltreatment, cognitive style and depression presaged our own:

> We grew up traumatically. We've seen stuff that you've probably never seen your mom and dad do to each other but we're not crazy. And we've been hurt by it. We're very hurt. And that's what causes all these depressionary stages that I've been going through, because I can't cope. If I grew up from a child as a stronger kid, I don't think I'd be having these problems.

REFERENCES

Abramovitch, R. and Freedman, J.L. (1981). Actor-observer differences in children's attributions. *Merrill-Palmer Quarterly, 27*, 53–59.

Abramson, L.Y. and Alloy, L.B. (1990). Search for the "negative cognition" subtype of depression. In C.D. McCann and N.S. Endler (eds.), *Depression: New directions in theory, research and practice* (pp. 77–109). Toronto: Wall Editions.

Abramson, L.Y., Alloy, L.B. and Metalsky, G.I. (1988). The cognitive diathesis-stress theories of depression: Toward an adequate evaluation of the theories' validities. In Alloy, L.B. (ed.), *Cognitive processes in depression* (pp. 31–73). New York: Guilford Press.

Abramson. L.Y., Metalsky, G.I. and Alloy, L.B. (1988). The hoplessness theory of depression: Does the research test the theory? in L.Y. Abramson (ed.), *Social cognition and clinical psychology: A synthesis* (pp. 33–65). New York: Guilford Press.

Abramson, L.Y., Metalsky, G.I. and Alloy, L.B. (1989). Hopelessness depression: A theory-based subtype of depression. *Psychological Review, 96*, 358–372.

Abramson, L.Y., Seligman, M.E.P. and Teasdale, J. (1978). Learned helplessness in humans: Critique and reformulation. *Journal of Abnormal Psychology, 87*, 49–74.

Allen, D.M. and Tarnowski, K.J. (1989). Depressive characteristics of physically abused children. *Journal of Abnormal Child Psychology, 17*, 1–11.

Arkin, R.M. and Baumgardner, A.H. (1985). Self-handicapping. In J.H. Harvey and G. Weary (eds.), *Attribution: Basic issues and applications* (pp. 169–202). New York: Academic Press.

Beck, A.T. (1967). *Depression: Clinical, experimental, and theoretical aspects.* New York: Harper & Row.

Beck, A.T. (1976). *Cognitive therapy and the emotional disorders.* New York: Harper & Row.

Beck, A.T. (1987). Cognitive models of depression. *Journal of Cognitive Psychotherapy, An International Quarterly, 1*, 5–37.

Beck, A.T., Ward, C.H., Mendelson, M, Mock, J.E., and Erbaugh, J.K. (1961). An inventory for measuring depression. *Archives of General Psychiatry, 4*, 561–571.

Berglass, S. and Jones, E.E. (1978). Drug choice as a self-handicapping strategy in response to noncontingent success. *Journal of Personality and Social Psychology, 36*, 405–417.

Berliner, L. and Conte, J.R. (1990). The process of victimization: The victim's perspective. *Child Abuse and Neglect, 14*, 29–40.

Berscheid, E., Graziano, W., Monson, T. and Dermer, M. (1976). Outcome dependency: Attention, attribution and attraction. *Journal of Personality and Social Psychology, 34*, 987–989.

Bloom, L. and Capatides, J.B. (1987). Sources of meaning in the acquisition of complex syntax: The sample case of causality. *Journal of Experimental Child Psychology, 43*, 112–128.

Briere, J. and Runtz, M.A. (1988). Symptomatology associated with childhood sexual victimization in a nonclinical adult sample. *Child Abuse and Neglect, 12*, 51–59.

Browning, D.H. and Boatman, B. (1977). Incest: Children at risk. *American Journal of Psychiatry, 134*, 69–72.

Bryer, J.B., Nelson, B.A., Miller, J.B. and Krol, P.A. (1987). Childhood sexual and physical abuse as factors in adult psychiatric illness. *American Journal of Psychiatry, 144*, 1426–1430.

Carlson, V., Cicchetti, D., Barnett, D. and Braunwald, K.G. (1989). Finding order in disorganization: Lessons from research on maltreated infants' attachments to their caregivers. In D. Cicchetti and V. Carlson (eds.) *Child maltreatment: Theory and research on the causes and consequences of maltreatment* (pp. 494–528). NY: Cambridge University Press.

Cicchetti, D. (1991). Fractures in the Crystal: Developmental psychopathology and the emergence of self. *Developmental Review, 11*, 271–287.

Cicchetti, D., Beeghly, M., Carlson, V. and Toth, S. (1990). The emergence of the self in atypical populations. In D. Cicchetti and M. Beeghly (eds.), *The self in transition: Infancy to childhood* (pp. 309–344). Chicago: University of Chicago Press.

Cicchetti, D. and Schneider-Rosen, K. (1986). An organizational approach to childhood depression. In M. Rutter, C. Izard and P. Read (eds.), *Emotions, cognition and behavior* (pp. 71–134). New York: Cambridge University Press.

Crittenden, P.M. and Ainsworth, M. (1989). Attachment and child abuse. In D. Cicchetti and V. Carlson (eds.), *Child maltreatment: Theory and research on the causes and consequences of child abuse and neglect* (pp. 432–463). New York: Cambridge University Press.

Crook, T., Raskin, A. and Eliot, J. (1987). Parent-child relationships and adult depression. *Child Development, 52*, 950–957.

Cummings, E.M. and Cicchetti, D. (1990). Toward a transactional model of relations between attachment and depression. In M.T. Greenberg, D. Cicchetti and E.M. Cummings (eds.), *Attachment in the preschool years: Theory, research and intervention* (pp. 339–372). Chicago: University of Chicago Press.

Downey, G. and Coyne, J.C. (1990). Children of depressed parents: An integrative review. *Psychological Bulletin, 108*, 50–76.

Eaves, G. and Rush, A.J. (1984). Cognitive patterns in symptomatic and remitted unipolar major depression. *Journal of Abnormal Psychology, 93*, 31–40.

Erber, R. and Fiske, S.T. (1984). Outcome dependency and attention to inconsistent information. *Journal of Personality and Social Psychology, 47*, 709–726.

Fine, C.G. (1990). The cognitive sequelae of incest. In R.P. Kluft (ed.), *Incest-related syndromes of adult psychopathology* (pp. 161–182). Washington, D.C.: American Psychiatric Press.

Fish-Murray, C.C., Koby, E.V. and van der Kolk, B.A. (1987). Evolving ideas: The effect of abuse on children's thought. In B.A. van der Kolk (ed.), *Psychological Trauma* (pp. 90–110). Washington, D.C.: American Psychiatric Press.

Forward, L. and Buck, C. (1988). *Betrayal of innocence: Incest and its devastation*. New York: Penguin Books.

Garnefski, N., van Egmond, M. and Straatman, A. (1989). The influence of early and recent life stress on severity of depression. *Acta Psychiatrica Scandinavica, 81*, 295–301.

Gidycz, C.A. and Koss, M.P. (1989). The impact of adolescent sexual victimization: Standardized measures of anxiety, depression, and behavioral deviancy. *Violence and Victims, 4*, 139–149.

Ginsberg, H.P. and Opper, S. (1988). *Piaget's theory of intellectual development*, 3rd Edition. Englewood Cliffs, N.J.: Prentice Hall.

Hamilton, E.W. and Abramson, L.Y. (1983). Cognitive patterns in major depressive disorder: A longitudinal study in a hospital setting. *Journal of Abnormal Psychology, 92*, 173–184.

Harvey, J.H. and Weary, G. (1984). Current issues in attribution theory and research. *Annual Review of Psychology, 35*, 427–459.

Heider, F. (1958). *The psychology of interpersonal relationships*. New York: Wiley.

Hollon, S.D., Kendall, P.C. and Lumry, A. (1986). Specificity of depressotypic cognitions in clinical depression. *Journal of Abnormal Psychology, 95*, 52–59.

Janoff-Bulman, R. and Lang-Gunn, L. (1988). Coping with disease, crime and accidents: The role of self-blame attributions. In L.Y. Abramson (ed.), *Social cognition and clinical psychology: A synthesis* (pp. 116–147). New York: Guilford Press.

Jones, E.E. and Nisbett, R.E. (1972). The actor and observer: Divergent perceptions of the causes of behavior. In E.E. Jones et al. (eds.), *Attribution: Perceiving the causes of behavior* (pp. 79–94). Morristown, N.J.: General Learning Press.

Kashani, J.H., Shekim, W.O., Burk, J.P. and Beck, N.C. (1987). Abuse as a predictor of psychopathology in children and adolescents. *Journal of Clinical Child Psychology, 16*, 43–50.

Kaufman, J. (1991). Depressive disorders in maltreated children. *Journal of the American Academy of Child and Adolescent Psychiatry, 30*, 257–265.

Kaufman, I. Peck, A.L., and Tagiuri, C.K. (1954). The family constellation and overt incestuous relations between father and daughter. *American Journal of Orthopsychiatry, 24*, 266–279.

Kazdin, A.E., Moser, J., Colbus, D. and Bell, R. (1985). Depressive symptoms among physically abused and psychiatrically disturbed children. *Journal of Abnormal Psychology, 94*, 298–307.

Kelley, H.H. (1967). Attribution theory in social psychology. In D. Levine (ed.), *Nebraska Symposium on Motivation* (Vol. 15, pp. 192–238). Lincoln: University of Nebraska Press.

Kelly, H.H. (1971). Attribution in social interaction. In E.E. Jones, D.E. Kanause, H.H. Kelley, R.E. Nisbett, S. Valins and B. Weiner (eds.), *Attribution: Perceiving the causes of behavior* (pp. 1–27). Morristown, N.J.: General Learning Press.

King, A., Hegland, S. and Galejs, I. (1986). Locus-of-control dimensions in preschool children. *Journal of Psychology, 120*, 37–44.

Kruglanski, A. and Ajzen, I. (1983). Bias and error in human judgment. *European Journal of Social Psychology, 13*, 1–44.

Kruglanski, A.W. and Klar, Y. (1987). A view from a bridge: Synthesizing the consistency and attribution paradigms from a lay epistemic perspective. *European Journal of Social Psychology, 17*, 211–241.

Lerner, M.J. (1980). *The belief in a just world: A fundamental delusion.* New York: Plenum Press.

Lipovsky, J.A., Saunders, B.E. and Murphy, S.M. (1989). Depression, anxiety, and behavior problems among victims of father-child sexual assault and nonabused siblings. *Journal of Interpersonal Violence, 4*, 452–468.

McCauley, E., Mitchell, J.R., Burke, P. and Moss, S. (1988). Cognitive attributes of depression in children and adolescents. *Journal of Consulting and Clinical Psychology, 56*, 903–908.

Metalsky, G.I., Abramson, L.Y., Seligman, M.E.P., Semmel, A. and Peterson, C.R. (1982). Attributional style and life events in the classroom: Vulnerability and invulnerability to depressive mood reactions. *Journal of Personality and Social Psychology, 43*, 612–617.

Metalsky, G.I., Halberstadt, L.J. and Abramson, L.Y. (1987). Vulnerability of depressive mood reactions: Toward a more powerful test of the diathesis-stress and causal mediation components of the reformulated theory of depression. *Journal of Personality and Social Psychology, 52*, 386–393.

Miller, P.H. and Aloise, P.A. (1989). Young Children's understanding of the psychological causes of behavior: A review. *Child Development, 60*, 257–285.

Miller, I.W. and Norman, W.H. (1986). Persistence of depressive cognitions within a subgroup of depressed inpatients. *Cognitive Therapy and Research, 10*, 211–224.

Miller, I.W., Norman, W.H. and Keitner, G.I. (1990). Treatment response of high cognitive dysfunction depressed inpatients. *Comprehensive Psychiatry, 30*, 62–71.

Mischel, W., Zeiss, R. and Zeiss, A. (1974). Internal-external control and persistence: Validation and implication of the Stanford Preschool Internal-External Scale. *Journal of Personality and Social Psychology, 29*, 265–278.

Nolen-Hoeksema, S., Girgus, J.S. and Seligman, M.E.P. (1986). Learned helplessness in children: A longitudinal study of depression, achievement, and explanatory style. *Journal of Personality and Social Psychology, 51*, 435–442.

Norman, W.H., Miller, I.W. and Dow, N.G. (1988). Characteristics of depressed patients with elevated levels of dysfunctional cognitions. *Cognitive Therapy and Research, 12*, 39–52.

Orzek, A. (1985). The child's cognitive processing of sexual abuse. *Child and Adolescent Psychotherapy, 2*, 110–114.

Pianta, R., Egeland, B, and Erickson, M.F. (1989). The antecedents of maltreatment: Results of the Mother-Child Interaction Research Project. In D. Cicchetti and V. Carlson (eds.), *Child maltreatment: Theory and research on the causes and consequences of child abuse and neglect* (pp. 203–253). Cambridge: Cambridge University Press.

Rholes, W.S. and Ruble, D.N. (1986). Children's impressions of other people: The effects of temporal separation of behavioral information. *Child Development, 57*, 872–878.

Robins, C.J., Block, P. and Peselow, E.D. (1990). Endogenous and non-endogenous depression: Relations to life events, dysfunctional attitudes and event perceptions. *British Journal of Clinical Psychology, 29*, 201–207.

Rose, D.T. (1987). Childhood sexual abuse and child and adolescent depression. Unpublished manuscript. University of Wisconsin-Madison.

Rose, D.T. and Abramson, L.Y. (1992). Childhood maltreatment, cognitive style and psychopathology. Manuscript in preparation.

Rose, D.T., Leff, G., Halberstadt, L.J., Hodulik, C.J. and Abramson, L.Y. (1992). Heterogeneity of cognitive style in depressed inpatients. Under editorial review.

Sansonnet-Hayden, H., Haley, G., Marriage, K. and Fine, S. (1987). Sexual abuse and psychopathology in hospitalized adolescents. *Journal of the American Academy of Child and Adolescent Psychiatry, 26*, 753–757.

Schaefer, E.S. (1965). A configurational analysis of children's reports of parent behavior. *Journal of Consulting Psychology, 29*, 552–557.

Seligman, M.E.P. (1975). *Helplessness: On depression, development, and death.* San Francisco: Freeman.

Seligman, M.E.P., Abramson, L.Y., Semmel, A. and von Baeyer, C. (1979). Depressive attributional style. *Journal of Abnormal Psychology, 88*, 242–247.

Seligman, M.E.P., Peterson, C.R., Kaslow, N.J., Tananbaum, R.L., Alloy, L.B. and Abramson, L.Y. (1984). Attributional style and depressive symptoms among children. *Journal of Abnormal Psychology, 93*, 235–238.

Shultz, T.R. (1982). Causal reasoning in the social and nonsocial realms. *Canadian Journal of Behavioral Sciences, 14*, 307–322.

Smith, M.C. (1978). Cognizing the behavior stream: The recognition of intentional action. *Child Development, 49*, 736–743.

Summit, R.C. (1983). The child sexual abuse accommodation syndrome. *Child Abuse and Neglect, 7*, 177–193.

Ullman, R.B. and Brothers, D. (1988). *The shattered self: A psychoanalytic study of trauma.* Hillsdale, N.J.: The Analytic Press.

Vondra, J.I., Barnett, D. and Cicchetti, D. (1990). Self-concept, motivation and competence among preschoolers from maltreating and comparison families. *Child Abuse and Neglect, 14*, 525–540.

Wallerstein, J. and Blakeslee, S. (1989). *Second chances: Men, women and children a decade after divorce.* New York: Ticknor and Fields.

Weiner, B. (1985). An attributional theory of achievement motivation and emotion. *Psychological Review, 92,* 548–573.

Weissman, A.N. and Beck, A.T. (1978, November). Development and validation of the Dysfunctional Attitudes Scale: A preliminary investigation. Paper presented at the meeting of the American Educational Research Association, Toronto, Canada.

Williams, J.M.G., Healy, D., Teasdale, J.D., White, W. and Paykel, E.S. (1990). Dysfunctional attitudes and vulnerability to persistent depression. *Psychological Medicine, 20,* 375–381.

Wilner, P., Wilkes, M. and Orwin, A. (1990). Attributional style and perceived stress in endogenous and reactive depression. *Journal of Affective Disorders, 18,* 281–287.

Wong, P.T.P. and Weiner, B. (1981). When people ask "why" questions, and the heuristics of attributional search. *Journal of Personality and Social Psychology, 40,* 650–663.

Wortman, C.B. and Dintzer, L. (1978). Is an attributional analysis of the learned helplessness phenomenon viable?: A critique of the Abramson-Seligman-Teasdale reformulation. *Journal of Abnormal Psychology, 87,* 75–90.

Zimmerman, M. and Coryell, W. (1986). Dysfunctional attitudes in endogenous and nonendogenous depressed inpatients. *Cognitive Therapy and Research, 10,* 339–346.

Zimmerman, M., Coryell, W., Corenthal, C. and Wilson, S. (1986). Dysfunctional attitudes and attribution style in healthy controls and patients with schizophrenia, psychotic depression and nonpsychotic depression. *Journal of Abnormal Psychology, 95,* 403–405.

Zimmerman, M., Coryell, W. and Pfohl, B. (1986). Melancholic subtyping: A qualitative or quantitative distinction? *American Journal of Psychiatry, 143,* 98–100.

X Childhood Maltreatment and Adult Depression: A Review of Research

JULES R. BEMPORAD, M.D. & STEVEN J. ROMANO, M.D.

Current conceptualizations of depression consider this disorder the final outcome of a variety of predisposing factors. A genetic predisposition (Dunner, 1982), current stressful circumstances (Paykel, 1979), learned methods of processing experience (Beck, 1976), as well as specific childhood events, have been proposed as predisposing to the vulnerability to depressive disorders. In this chapter we focus on the last parameter, first documenting the evidence for the occurrence of specific childhood events in the life history of adult depressives and later attempting to relate early experiences to adult disorder through a perspective that is cognizant of the complexities of the myriad pathways that link temporal events throughout development. A major reason for concentrating on the role of childhood events as predisposing to adult depression is the relative neglect that has been accorded these potentially significant factors, as depression has been viewed increasingly as a medical disorder whose fundamental pathology resides in a genetic vulnerability to stress.

This neglect of possible childhood antecedents to adult depression represents a very recent shift in the conceptualization of most psychopathological conditions, including mood disorders. In prior decades childhood experiences were considered pertinent etiological factors, particularly as described in the psychoanalytic and early psychiatric literature on depression. Freud (1917) proposed a pathological solution to an early loss of love or love object as predisposing to adult depression. Abraham (1924) postulated the occurrence of a childhood depressive episode (primal parathymia) due to early maternal rejection which is reexperienced in adult melancholia. These two pioneer contributions anticipated a large literature by others who, in the following decades, reported their findings on the childhood conditions of depressed adults engaged in psychotherapeutic treatment. The major themes stressed in these single case reports or small patient series were: (1) the occurrence of a significant childhood loss; (2) an adverse childhood environment which did not adequately reward or acknowledge the individual; and (3) parental or familial needs that interfered with the attainment of expected psychological individuation (see Arieti & Bemporad, 1978, and Mendelson, 1979, for reviews). In recent decades, these reports have been largely ignored by American psychiatry, partially on the basis that the data presented were not objectively collected and suffered from the particular author's personal theoretical bias, or from the depressed patient's own distortion of his or her distant past.

This prevailing attitude of contemporary American psychiatry may have obscured the findings of researchers, mostly in other countries, who in the past two decades have conducted large scale, systematic studies on the relationship of childhood experience and adult depression. While cognizant of potential genetic or acquired biological vulnerabilities, these studies have tended to consider these as only some of a greater number of variables which might culminate in a depressive disorder in adult life, thereby constructing complex models of illness which approximate realistic life conditions such as those seen in clinical practice. The purpose of this chapter is to present a review of these studies together with a consideration of the vulnerability to depression according to newer conceptions of causality in psychopathology. The identification of specific childhood events or modes of childhood experience as occurring significantly more frequently in the life history of adult depressives than in adults without depression would have obvious ramifications for an etiological theory of this disorder. It might be possible to demonstrate how these vulnerabilities, together with other risk factors, may culminate in the clinical disorder. The ultimate aim would be to tease apart psychological, social and biological factors that vary from the norm so as to gauge the participation of each in the pathogenic process at specific points in development. For example, some studies have implicated childhood bereavement as a powerful predictor of adult depression while other studies have not (Finkelstein, 1988). One possible explanation for this discrepancy in research results might be that childhood loss expresses its effect only in the presence of other factors, which synergistically either magnify or express the pathogenicity of early abandonment. In keeping with the principles of developmental psychopathology, any vulnerability factors should be considered in the context of other influences on the maturational process at that particular moment in time. On a larger scale, such information could help in identifying aberrations in developmental processes adding to our knowledge of pathogenesis and suggesting successful interventions at appropriate phases of the life cycle.

Reconstruction of Childhood Events

Although the psychoanalytic effort to reconstruct allegedly significant events of childhood through the recall of memories, the interpretation of dreams and the analysis of transferential behavior is well known, an equally valid line of inquiry which also was initiated at the end of the nineteenth century has received less attention. This latter investigation concerns the construction of instruments to assess objectively the child's attitude towards his/her parents. In a comprehensive review of studies on the child's perception of his/her relationship to parents, covering the years 1894–1936, Stodgill (1937) reported that toward the end of the last century, the pioneering questionnaire studies of G. Stanley Hall led to a large number of objective investigations of parent-child interactions. For example, Barnes, Schallenberger and others (cited in Stodgill) analyzed the type of punishment and attitudes toward punishment in over 7,000 school children in 1894, finding decreasing amounts of corporeal punishment with increasing age of the child and that children resented unjust punishment rather than punishment in itself. These pioneer studies were followed by investigations into idealization of parents, child gender discrepancies in relationship to the male and female parent, differences in familial relationships between delinquent and nondelinquent children, and the effect of parental religious beliefs on the later religious life of their children. Other studies examined the influence of external factors on child-parent relationships, such as frequency of attending movies (in a pre-television era), rural versus urban environments, and familial church membership. In the 1950s and 1960s Schaefer (1965) and Roe and Siegelman (1963) built on the work of prior investigators to produce questionnaires that attempted to assess systematically and to derive major themes of the child's conceptualization of his/her parent's behavior. Utilizing a variety of discrete components of possible parental behaviors, Schaefer found that three replicated factors emerged from repeated questionnaire or interview trials: Acceptance versus Rejection, Psychological Autonomy versus Psychological Control, and Firm Control versus Lax Control. These dimensions were found to differentiate children with disparate levels of adjustment and who came from contrasting socioeconomic levels. Roe and Siegelman (7) independently derived dimensional factors that were remarkably similar from their questionnaire studies of children, as did Becker (1964) from psychologists' ratings of parental behavior. The prevailing themes could be summarized as Acceptance — Rejection, Involvement-Detachment, and Strict versus Permissive Control, which appeared to capture the essential elements of child-parent relationships, and showed high validity and reliability upon later testing (Renson, Schaefer, & Levy, 1968). The most frequently utilized measure to emerge from these studies was the Children's Report of Parental Behavior Inventory (CRPBI), which is still in use, particularly in studies of childhood abuse, neglect or other forms of maltreatment. This highly reliable instrument primarily analyzes boys' and girls' perceptions of their mothers' and fathers' behaviors on the dimensions of love versus hostility and autonomy versus control.

Based on these early studies, as well as comparable work of others, Parker, Tupling and Brown (1979) in Australia and Perris, Jacobson, Lindstrom et al. (1980) in Sweden extended the questionnaire methodology to assess child-parent relationships as recalled by adults. Parker, partially influenced by Levy's (1943) classic study on maternal overprotection, constructed the Parent Bonding Instrument (PBI) to investigate the long term effects of parental overprotection. He administered a series of multi-item questionnaires to a non-clinical sample, subsequently examining the data for resultant factor loading. Two major dimensional factors emerged: a "care" component ranging from affectionate warmth to cold rejection and an "overprotection" component ranging from excessive intrusion to promotion of autonomy. Subsequently, the PBI was examined repeatedly for validity (utilizing independent witnesses such as sibs and others to verify subject's recall of childhood and subjects to verify sib's recall) and reliability (utilizing test-retest methodologies) (See Parker (1983) for a detailed review). General conclusions from multiple trials with the PBI are that there is a high correlation between reports of subjects, siblings, parents and others concerning prior parent-child interactions. There was also a high correlation of scores between testing occasions (9 weeks apart) when subjects were depressed and non-depressed. Comparable results were found for subjects tested in Sydney, Australia and Oxford, England, with higher maternal scores for care in higher socio- economic groups, but neither age nor sex of respondent, influencing the PBI scores. Since these initial tests for validity and reliability, the PBI has been used extensively as a measure of the adult subject's perception of the degree of warmth — rejection and overprotection — autonomy allowed by each parent.

Perris, Jacobsson, Lindstrom, et al. (1980) independently developed a similar inventory named the EMBU (an acronym for "own memories of child-rearing experiences") based on factor analysis of items given initially to non clinical populations. This structured instrument was also based on items from prior inventories and reformulated to capture adult recollections of childhood experiences. Perris' group found the following factors emerging from their data: one relating to parental control and performance-orientation, one to parental acceptance versus rejection, and one to parental overprotection which applied to questions regarding the mother only. Since its development, the EMBU has been used with a variety of populations.

Other researchers have used structured amnestic interviews rather than questionnaires in assessing memories or perception of childhood rearing experiences. Still others have relied on objective events that can be measured with certainty, such as death of a parent, or separation. The literature on loss or separation while extensive, has yielded contradictory finding. (Finkelstein, 1988). This literature will not be considered here except in those instances where both childhood loss and childhood maltreatment were simultaneously investigated.

Review of Studies

The relevant studies are presented in Table I, in chronological order of date of publication, specifying investigator, method of assessment, index subjects and controls, and findings. The number of subjects pooled from all studies totals close to four thousand with roughly equal numbers of index cases and controls. The most common type of experimental method was to divide subjects into depressed and non-depressed cohorts according to established research interviews and diagnostic criteria and subsequently to examine differences in remembered childhood experiences between the two groups.

Findings

The following literature review focuses on research illuminating the relationship between early childhood experiences and the development of adult depression. The purpose of this review is to evaluate the impact of maltreatment in childhood on the eventual evolution of affective psychopathology in adulthood.

First, some mention of research in associated areas of child development is in order. There is a body of research which assesses experiential variables linked to childhood depression. Included in this category are those studies addressing the effects of maltreatment and parental psychopathology on child behavior, more specifically on the development of depression in children exposed to negative environmental situations. Much of this literature focuses on the presence and influence of abuse and neglect. A recent study by Kaufman (1991) highlights a number of issues germane to this field. Kaufman examined the prevalence of depressive disorders in fifty-six 7- to 12-year-old maltreated children. Maltreatment in this work included physical abuse, "emotional maltreatment" (exposure to parental drug use, spousal violence, verbal abuse and rejection), neglect and sexual abuse. The reported prevalence of depressive disorders in this study was 18% for major depression and 25% for dysthymia, a figure similar to the incidence of depressive disorders in children at-risk secondary to familial history of affective pathology. In addition, the majority of those meeting criteria for major depression also met criteria for dysthymia. In this study, children with major depression and/or dysthymia were more likely to have experienced severe injuries over an extended period of time, and to have had psychologically unavailable or drug dependent parents. These children were also more apt to have had frequent out-of-home placements. Significantly, those maltreated children with fewer conflictual relationships and a greater number of positive supports were less likely to be depressed, underscoring the influence and potentially buffering effects of social support on the development of affective disturbance. With

Table 1. Summary of Studies Addressing Childhood Experiences and Adult Depression

		SAMPLE		ASSESSMENT		Childhood Experience/Report of Parental Characteristics Associated with Adult Depression
Year	Investigator	Subjects	Controls	Depression	Relations	
1969	Abrahams and Whitlock	152 (Depressed)	152	Hamilton	Bene-Anthony Family Relations Clinical Interview	Yes
1971	Raskin, et al.	371 (Hospitalized-Depressed) 174 (Hospitalized-Depressed)	254	Not Specified	Abbreviated CRPBI	Yes
1975	Jacobsen, Fasman and DiMascio	347 (Depressed Women Inpatients) 114 (Depressed and Outpatients)	198 (Normal Women)	Not Specified	Author's Assessment Depriving Events and Child-rearing Practices	Yes

Year	Author		Sample	Measure	Author's Rating Procedure – Osgood Semantic Differential	
1979	Blatt, et al.	—	83 Women 38 Men (Non-clinical College Students)		The Zung DEQ Semantic Differential	Yes
1979	Parker	52	52 (Neurotic-Depressive)	Clinical Interview and History	PBI	Yes
		70	70 (Manic-Depressives)	Clinical Interview and History	PBI	No
			236 (Non-clinical Students)	Interview & History Costello-Comrey Scales	PBI	Yes
1980	Parker		124 Women (Non-clinical) 112 Men (Non-clinical)	Costello-Comrey Trait Depression Measure	PBI	No (for assessment of parental characteristics as vulnerability factors for depression)
1981	Parker Study 1	none	36 (Depressives)	Beck Depressive Inventory	PBI	Yes
	Study 2	none	100 (Mothers of Post-graduate Students)	Costello-Comrey Wilson-Laubond	PBI	Yes

		SAMPLE		ASSESSMENT		Childhood Experience/Report of Parental Characteristics Associated with Adult Depression
Year	Investigator	Subjects	Controls	Depression	Relations	
1981	Crook, Raskin, and Eliot	714 (Hospitalized, Depressed)	347 (Normal Adults)	Not Specified	CRPBI (Modified) Clinical Interviews	Yes
1982	Parker	109 (Non-clinical Adoptees)	109 (General Practice Patients)	Costello-Comrey Rating Scale	PBI	Yes
1985	Cadoret, et al.	443 (Adoptees)	—	SADS, DIS or Structured Interview Based On Feighner Criteria	Environmental Factors Established Through Adoptive Parent Interview and Adoption Records	Yes
1985	Perris, et al.	54 (Bipolars) 52 (Unipolars)	200 (Normals)	Not Specified	EMBU	Yes

Year	Author						
1986	Perris	47 (Unipolars) 21 (Bipolars) 34 (Neurotic-reactive) 39 (Unspecified)	205 (Normals)	Not Specified	EMBU	Yes
1987	Hallstrom	60	400	Interview	Interview	Yes
1987	Parker, Kiloh and Hayward	26 (Endogenous Depressives) 40 (Neurotic Depressives)	26 (General Practice) 40 (General Practice)	SADS	PBI	Yes (Neurotic Depressives)
1988	Gaszner	50	259 (Normals)	Not Specified	EMBU	Yes
1988	Gorayeb	10	121	BDI	EMBU	Yes (Preliminary Results)
1989	Torgersen	298	—	SCID-I CPRS-D	Interview	Yes

regard to parental psychopathology, depressed children were more apt to have parents with higher depression scores.

A study by Walker, Downey and Bergman (1989) addressed the effects of parental psychopathology and maltreatment on child behavior. These authors reviewed the interactive effects of multiple risk factors on childhood maladjustment, primarily identifying parent psychiatric disorder and maltreatment. Their findings supported a diathesis-stress model of psychopathology, noting a significant relation between risk factors and child behavior, the latter including aggression, withdrawal and delinquency. Though their sample did not lend itself to the evaluation of parental affective disorder on child behavior, nor specifically explore the incidence of depressive reactions in their subjects, their findings did underscore the need to explore risk factors simultaneously.

An earlier study by Kazdin, Moser, Colbus, and Bell (1985) reported on depressive symptoms among physically abused and psychiatrically disturbed children. Seventy-nine child psychiatric inpatients, ages 6 to 13, were examined to elucidate associations between physical abuse and depression. Compared to non-abused subjects in the patient control group, abused children evidenced higher levels of depression and hopelessness, in conjunction with lower levels of self-esteem. The authors stated that for a psychiatric patient sample, physical abuse was associated with depressive symptomatology, which arose in close temporal proximity to the perpetrated abuse. In their discussion, Kazdin, et al. suggested that physically abused, depressed children might be at risk for long-term consequences, such as suicide or maladaptive child-rearing practices.

Such conjecture leads one to consider more thoughtfully the possibility of identifying those children at risk for later depressive episodes, and the potential for prevention or early intervention. To explore and elucidate further the impact of childhood experience and its subsequent influence on the development of depression in *adulthood*, we will now turn to a review of the growing body of literature addressing this issue.

Greater than half the studies reviewed utilized carefully developed instruments for the identification of parental characteristics, the significance of which were established through factor analysis. These inventories included Parker's PBI and the EMBU, developed by Perris and colleagues. Though the studies reviewed differed with regard to design and psychometric assessment, some summarizing comments can be proposed. Sixteen of the seventeen studies abbreviated in Table 1 were suggestive of childhood experience and perceived parental attitudes and rearing practices influencing the development of adult depression.

Parker observed an association of parental characteristics to depressive disorders in a number of studies conducted (Parker, 1979, 1981, 1982, 1987), a finding more prominent in those subjects classified as neurotic depressives (Parker, 1979, 1987). This group reported less parental care and greater maternal overprotection. A similar trend was noted in a non-clinical group of students (Parker, 1979). Parker offers three broad explanations to account for these findings in both neurotic depressives and his non-clinical group of students (Parker, 1979). First, judgement of parental and subsequent relationships by those with a depressive or neurotic temperament might tend to be more negatively expressed. Parker sites previous studies implicating neurotics and depressives selectively monitoring negative events, being more sensitive to negative interpersonal interactions, and attributing responsibility inaccurately (Beck, 1976). This, he suggested, may lead to the scoring of parents on the PBI as lower on care and higher on overprotection. After conducting further analysis of the influence of neuroticism and depression on the scoring of this measure, Parker concluded that neuroticism may exert influence on the PBI's overprotection scale, but not depression. A second explanation offered was that depressives may elicit less parental care or greater overprotection. There is considerable evidence that infants and children do influence the behavior of adult caregivers. Lastly, he proffers that antecedent causes of depressive experience may be low parental care and/or parental overprotection, affecting a child's self-esteem and modulation of affective states. Parker also stressed the significance of "affectionless" control as a risk factor for depression. In his discussion of these results, Parker suggested that object loss or threatened object loss may be the most likely situation to precipitate depression in a non-clinical group, within the context of an interpersonal relationship. Interestingly, bipolar patients did not differ from controls, and there was no evidence that a patient's manic depressive illness negatively influenced recall of parental attitudes and behaviors (Parker, 1979). Parker (1987) summarized his cumulative findings utilizing the PBI with depressed individuals as indicating a considerable degree of specificity with regard to type of depression most influenced by parental attitudes and behavior, with relevancy to neurotic depression (currently classified as dysthymic disorder), but not to endogenously depressed individuals.

Other researchers also have identified significant associations between childhood experience and depressive disorders. Perris (1985, 1986), Gaszner (1988), and Gorayeb (1988, preliminary results), assessed parental rearing practices through use of the EMBU. In Perris' study, four groups of depressives were examined, including unipolar, bipolar, neurotic-reactive, and a group with unspecified depressive disorder. The findings were described as a general trend of depressed patients to report earlier parental deprivation, and did not provide evidence to support a clear specificity with regard to type of depressive syndrome more significantly affected. They did note, though, that neurotic reactive patients rated both parents as more rejecting, reporting father as globally less severe and less consistent in child-rearing practices, and mothers as more severe and less consistent than the groups of both unipolar and bipolar individuals. Perris cited the variables of low emotional warmth and overprotection as important, recognizing that these variables corresponded roughly to Parker's construct of "affectionless control". Concluding, Perris purports that the aforementioned results supported the hypothesis that deprivation of love represents a risk factor for depressive disorders. Gazner approximated and confirmed Perris' findings in a series of fifty depressed Hungarian individuals, illustrating that depressives experienced parents as less emotionally warm and more rejecting and overprotecting as compared to normals. The preliminary results reported by Gorayeb concurred with these findings. In his review of childrearing practices in Brazil, Gorayeb found that depressed patients experienced their parents as more guilt engendering, more depriving and less affectionate.

Earlier studies employing abbreviated or modified versions of the Reports of Parental Behavior Inventory CRPBI, developed by Schaefer (1965), also yielded results in support of childhood experiences affecting adult depression (Crook et al., 1981; Raskin, 1971). Raskin reported that depressives rated parents more negatively than normals and Crook and colleagues commented that depression in adult life may be related to parental rejection and control. Method of assessment for depression in these investigations was not specified.

The studies of Abraham and Whitlock (1969), Blatt, Wein, Chevron, and Quinlan (1979) and Jacobsen, Fasman and DiMascio (1978) suggest a link between early childhood experiences and adult depression, though most did not utilize a more structured and established method to assess these experiences. In their study of 152 depressed patients with controls matched for age, sex, and socio-economic status, Abraham and Whitlock examined the relationship between childhood bereavement and negative childhood experiences to the development of affective illness. The depressed patients described more unhappy experiences in childhood than did controls, and those with mixed and neurotic depressions had a significantly higher incidence of such experiences as compared with controls and those with manic-depressive or endogenous affective illness. Interestingly, though not statistically significant, was the fact that more of the controls had experienced childhood loss of one or both parents. The authors concluded that qualitative differences in the child-parent relationship contribute to the formation of affective disorder in adults, adding that physical loss of a parent does not necessarily influence development of adult depression. Jacobson et al., examined childrearing processes and assessed depriving events in a group of 461 depressed women, both inpatient and outpatient, and a normal reference population of 198 females. Childhood deprivation in this study was defined as "the lack, loss, or absence of an emotionally sustaining relationship prior to adolescence". They, too, found no association with overt childhood loss, such as parental death or separation, but did discover evidence supporting an association between depriving childrearing processes and adult depression. This finding was more prominent in the backgrounds of depressed inpatients, possibly in association with greater severity of affective illness. Data obtained from Blatt et al.'s investigation of parental representations and depression in normal young adults supported their contention that cognitive levels of parental representation, obtained through both open-ended description and a more structured rating method, may be a central dimension in depression. Negative ratings of parents and qualities attributed to parents were significantly correlated with measures of depression and the intensity and type of depressive experience. Significant were descriptions of parents as lacking in nurturance, support and affection.

The more recent investigations of Alnaes and Torgersen (1989) and Hallstrom (1987) further address the increasing evidence in support of the association of early childhood relationships and parental rearing practices to depression. In Hallstrom's retrospective study of 60 middle-aged women suffering a major depressive episode, subjects more frequently reported an unhappy childhood with a higher incidence of corporal punishment, feeling misunderstood by parents and a poor relationship with mother. These differences were significant in comparison to a control group of 400 females without a history of major depression. Hallstrom also found that parents of subjects were in contact with psychiatric services twice as often as nondepressed study participants. Alnaes and Torgersen studied the characteristics of patients with major depression in combination with dysthymic or cyclothymic disorders in their investigation of childhood experience and precipitating events. Two hundred and ninety-eight (298) non-psychotic outpatients were included, categorized into four groups utilizing DSM–III criteria. These included major depression only, major depression with dysthymic or cyclothymic disorders, dysthymic or cyclothymic disorder without major depression, and one group of other psychiatric disorders. Summarizing their findings, they found that patients in the mixed group reported a greater incidence of traumatic experiences in childhood than did subjects in either "pure" group. This finding was augmented in comparison to those patients with other psychiatric disorders. In addition, patients with major depression in combination with pure dysthymic-cyclothymic disorder remembered their childhood as generally more traumatic and with a less satisfying relationship to parents. There was no significant difference in the severity of depression between the mixed group and those with pure major depression, nor significant age and sex differences in comparison to the other groups. Based on this, the authors concluded that their results supported a difference with regard to early traumata between those with mixed chronic and major depression and both pure affective groups.

Two of the studies employed adoptees as subjects (Cadoret et al., 1985, and Parker, 1982). Cadoret summarized that environmental factors, including for males, an adoptive home with an alcoholic individual, and for females, death of an adoptive parent prior to adoptee age 19 and adoptive family with a behaviorally disturbed individual, predisposed adoptees to depression. Parker described parental characteristics of low care and overprotection linked with depression and anxiety in adoptees.

With regard to overt childhood loss, two studies revealed no association between adult depression and loss (Abraham & Whitlock, 1969; Jacobsen, Fasman, and DiMascio, 1975), but evidenced support for the association of depriving and unsatisfactory child-parent relations with depression in adulthood. Parker (1980), though, attempting to isolate vulnerability factors to

normal depression, commented that object loss or threatened loss may precipitate depression within an interpersonal relationship in a non-clinical
sample. Blatt et al. (1979) purported that the quality of a depressive's internalized object representations may contribute to a vulnerability to depression
associated with object loss. Brown, Harris, and Bifulco (1986), in their discussion of the long-term effects of early parental loss, underscored the complexity of the experiences linking loss to adult depression. These authors
stressed a psychosocial model, whereby vulnerability factors, in conjunction
with provoking events, determine depressive reactions. Early loss of a mother,
via its role as a vulnerability factor, influences onset of depression only in the
presence of a provoking agent. After conducting research aimed at evaluating
a number of variables and potential psychosocial markers of increased vulnerability, these researchers concluded that there is greater evidence to suggest
familial environment than the impact of loss in the genesis of later depression.
They recognized that, in certain populations, loss of a mother led to the
development or exacerbation of negative circumstances which set the stage
for the emergence of depression when combined with an inciting event. Lack
of care in childhood was cited as the most crucial and influential experiential
measure, often following object loss in the history of adult depressives. With
the exception of the aforementioned, the cumulative data de-emphasizes
overt loss *per se* in the genesis of adult depression.

In summary, the majority of studies reviewed support the hypothesis that
early childhood experiences, perceived parental characteristics, and child-rearing practices are associated with the development of depressive disorders in
adulthood. Further, it appears that overt loss in childhood is often of a more-
limited significance as compared with the perceived nature of the object
relationship.

Discussion

Sixteen of seventeen studies reviewed showed a significantly greater history
of childhood maltreatment in unipolar depressives, than in healthy controls
or in patients with other diagnoses, including schizophrenia and bipolar disorder. The finding that these severely ill individuals, who could be expected to
be as demoralized or negativistic as unipolar depressives, recalled childhoods
indistinguishable from normal controls supports a lack of retrospective distortion as a result of adult functioning. The presence of childhood maltreatment
was more strongly correlated with adult depression than was childhood separation or loss, suggesting that the vulnerability to depression from a childhood
loss may be expressed through post-loss negative events and may be buffered
by post-loss favorable experiences. Therefore, later lack of care may be the
variable through which loss becomes a vulnerability factor for depression. A
follow up study conducted by Brown, Harris, and Bifulco (1986), which is
discussed below, examines just this question, since a loss may result in variable
amounts of aberrant care which may be the critical variable. The form of

childhood maltreatment also appears somewhat specific. Parker and colleagues consistently report a combined childhood experience of high over protection and low emotional warmth as particularly relevant to adult depression. Perris and colleagues have also found a pattern of affectionless control. Others have focussed on lack of care experiences, including repeated rupture of affectionate relationships through multiple placements and late adoption following losses.

Implications for Developmental Psychopathology

(A) Theoretical Framework

These findings have immediate relevance for the burgeoning field of developmental psychopathology. This recent area of study (Cicchetti, 1984) attempts to consider psychiatric disorders from a longitudinal, developmental framework, conceptualizing most clinical syndromes as the culmination of multiple causes which may make their appearance throughout the life cycle and are the result of a balance between predisposing and sparing factors. The field of developmental psychopathology is therefore concerned: (1) with the processes or mechanisms which result in relative health or illness; (2) with both developmental continuity and discontinuity of behaviors from one maturational stage to another; (3) with the effects of sensitizing and/or "steeling" effects; (4) with the degree of adaptation at each developmental level; and (5) with the particular susceptibility to possible precipitating events. As such, early childhood experiences are but one of a multitude of factors that may determine adult functioning. Genetic factors, post childhood experiences and presence of adult stressors, to name only a few, are additional variables that can strongly influence the eventual psychological fate of the individual.

Therefore the presence or absence of particular childhood experiences should not, by itself, account for the later occurrence of a particular disorder. At the same time, such experiences are not to be discounted and may strongly predispose to later illness in the presence of other vulnerability factors. Rutter (1986) has enumerated seven major ways by which early experience may be linked to psychiatric disorders occurring some years later:

(1) Childhood experience may lead to an immediate disorder (i.e., depression) which persists into adult life for reasons that are independent of the initial causation or provocation.

(2) Childhood experiences may induce physiological changes which in turn influence later functioning.

(3) Childhood experiences may lead directly to altered patterns of behavior which only some years later take the overt form of a clinical disorder.

(4) Childhood experiences may lead to changed family circumstances, which in turn predispose to later disorder.

(5) Childhood experiences may alter sensitivities to stress or modify styles of coping which may predispose to disorders in later life only in the presence of later stressors.

(6) Childhood experiences may alter the individual's self concept, attitudes or cognitive set, which in turn influence later responses.

(7) Childhood experiences may impact on later functioning by opening up or closing down opportunities.

These seven paths through which childhood experiences may affect later life demonstrate that it is usually difficult, if not impossible, to demarcate a clear one-to-one, linear causal relationship between early experience and later disorder. Consideration must be given to the possibility that not all disorders have their origins in childhood and the content of these early years may not be particularly relevant. Furthermore, even if one grants possible etiological significance to certain experiences, development does not come to a halt with the cessation of these experiences and later influences may modify, even negate, the impact of these early events. For example, individuals who abuse their children are often found to have been childhood victims of abuse themselves. Yet, if the question is reversed and one asks how many abused children become adult abusers, the answer varies to as low as 30% (Erickson, 1991). Therefore, the majority of abused children manage to compensate for their prior traumatization and to break the intergenerational pattern of abuse.

(B) The Nature of Vulnerability

When examined in the light of this overall theoretical framework of developmental psychopathology, the exact significance of the finding of childhood maltreatment in the history of depressed adults must be scrutinized carefully. No obvious conceptual linking bridging the childhood maltreatment and adult disorder becomes immediately apparent. As stated above, earlier psychoanalytic theories attempted to related childhood experience and adult pathology in a linear causal manner. According to this formulation the memory of a childhood "trauma" was re-evoked by some familiar situation in adult experience causing a breaking down of repression and the emergence of painful ideation or affects which, in concert with pathological defenses, were thought to comprise the major clinical syndrome. Therefore, a direct relationship between the early trauma and later illness was thought to exist.

More recent considerations of illness utilize a multi-causal concept of psychopathology with vulnerability conceived of as the accumulation of predisposing factors and/or experiences which still requires a particular precipitant to become transformed into clinical illness (Sroufe & Rutter, 1989). Prior vulnerabilities may decrease the threshold to illness, just as prior sparing factors may raise this threshold. For example, Perris (1988) reports that patients with rejecting mothers as children became ill after experiencing fewer negative life events than patients with responsive mothers. Therefore, maternal stimulation versus rejection does not insure lack of psychopathology, but seems to increase relative resistance to later provoking agents. Often the finding of a variety of vulnerability factors leads to their exerting their effect through a common result. For example, Perris (1988) found that depressed individuals with an affected family member experienced the onset of depression at an earlier age than depressed patients with no family history of illness, suggesting a genetic vulnerability. However, the data also revealed that having an affected family member was closely correlated with dysfunctional parenting so it is unclear if the resultant adult syndrome is due to a genetic predisposition, aberrant childhood experience or, possibly, both factors in combination.

A similar compounding of effects has been supported by investigations of childhood loss and later depression. Some studies have shown a correlation while others have not. Possibly, the best explanation for these contradictory results comes from a study of Brown, Harris, and Bifulco (1986), whose impetus was the unexpected finding that childhood mother loss strongly correlated with depression in an epidemiological study of depressed women (Brown and Harris, 1978). These researchers attempted to assess the relationship of childhood bereavement to adult depression by examining a group of women all of whom had suffered loss of the mother (through death or prolonged separation) but of whom only some exhibited depression as adults. On the basis of 225 appropriate female subjects, Brown, Harris, and Bifulco found that those who progressed toward depression as adults had experienced a markedly different life situation following maternal loss than did those who presented without psychopathology as adults. Briefly, those women who became depressed came from lower socio-economic backgrounds so that after maternal loss they could not be cared for by the remaining parent and had to be sent to institutions or to relatives who generally did not welcome an additional burden. These post loss situations were recalled as so unfavorable that the subjects never felt accepted, secure or acknowledged. The researchers describe the post separation experience as typified by "lack of care". As the subjects passed puberty they attempted to escape their situations by an early marriage, often to an unsuitable mate and as the result of a premarital pregnancy. This precocious acceptance of an adult role at a very early age also prevented the subjects from finishing school (and thus obtaining an important avenue for independence and self-esteem). Other significant resultants were a poor marriage and an early burden of motherhood. These external characteristics: lack of outside employment, lack of a confiding relationship with a spouse, and numerous young children at home, which typified the adult lives of these subjects were just those vulnerability factors for depression that had been identified in the earlier epidemiological study of adult depression. Therefore, maternal separation in less affluent girls sets in motion a life path that appears to lead to a situation in adults that is vulnerable to depression.

In contrast, those subjects who experienced maternal loss but were better off economically described a different set of circumstances following separation. Their fathers were able to keep them at home, and to supply maternal substitutes in the form of nannies, housekeepers or step mothers. Their quality of life was sufficiently positive so they did not marry early or become pregnant as adolescents so as to escape from home. They were able to complete their educations, select more appropriate spouses and become mothers at a more judicious age. As a result, their adult lives were more rewarding and satisfying. A few of the economically disadvantaged girls were also kept at home or fell into favorable circumstances following separation and did well as adults. The converse was also found. A few affluent girls met with adverse circumstances following separation and set out on a life path that resulted in an adult situation that was typical of vulnerability to depression.

This study strongly suggests that maternal separation is a powerful vulnerability factor for adult depression if it leads to adverse circumstances which then progress to poor life choices culminating in external factors that predispose to depression. However, it is the experience of lack of care rather than the preceding separation that appears to be the key childhood experience. Furthermore, as Brown, Harris and Bifulco clearly indicate, the progression to adverse external circumstance is but one aspect of the vulnerability to depression. A more powerful factor may be the internal psychological development of their subjects who were exposed to a series of negative experiences over which they had no control. It is easily understandable how such a series of events and the continued negative reflected appraisals of significant others can form a self concept typified by helplessness and hopelessness in the face of later difficulties. For example, in a related study, Bifulco, Brown, and Harris (1987) found that women who had experienced lack of care as children were twice as likely to develop a negative self image than those who had experienced adequate care. Furthermore, in later detailed analyses of their data, these researchers found a considerable degree of continuity of helplessness between childhood and adulthood (Harris, Brown, & Bifulco, 1990). They conclude that lack of care in childhood combines with childhood helplessness, which in conjunction with other environmental circumstances leads to a high probability in adulthood of continued helplessness and a variety of adverse environmental experiences, such as poor emotional support, predisposing to clinical depression. Therefore, depression appears to result from an interplay of internal cognitive sets or attitudes, such as hopelessness or poor self-regard, which appear continuous between childhood and adult life, and of external circumstances, such as premarital pregnancy or poor current emotional support, which result from unfortunate choices or factors outside the control of the individual. Depression is ultimately considered as a pathological state resulting from a complex career path of which the first step, but by no means the last, may be lack of care subsequent to parental loss.

The studies of Brown, Harris and Bifulco implicate both external circumstances and internal attitudes in the etiology of depression. Other investigators have focussed on the psychological sequelae of early maltreatment, allotting a pivotal role to the formation of cognitive sets which perpetuate vulnerability by the idiosyncratic processing of every day events resulting in depressogenic conclusions. On the basis of clinical experience with depressed adults, Bowlby (1980) has delineated three chronic experiential modes that he has found in therapeutic work to typify the childhood recollections of depressed adults. These experiential modes can be summarized as follows: (1) never having attained a stable or secure relationship with the parent despite repeated efforts; (2) having been told repeatedly that one is incompetent or inadequate; and (3) having experienced an actual loss of a parent with disagreeable consequences which could not be altered. Each of these experiences, or their combination, results in the formation of depression-prone cognitive schemas, according to Bowlby, so that later experience is processed in an idiosyncratic manner, eventually leading to clinical depression in the presence of a provoking event. The principal issue over which the depression prone individual feels helpless is the ability to maintain affectional relationships. This vulnerability, together with the life circumstances that such a belief creates, is carried on into adult life and predisposes to clinical illness. Abramson, Seligman, and Teasdale (1978; see also Rose & Abramson, this volume) have speculated that maltreatment creates a persistent cognitive set of low self-esteem and of helplessness, predisposing to adult psychopathology. These authors maintain that depressive symptoms are associated with a learned attributional style that utilizes internal, stable and global causes for negative events that befall the self. These often erroneous assumptions and generalizations are said to produce depression following life stressors.

Perris (1988) has singled out the development of a pathological childhood self concept as particularly germane to adult depression. He conceives of adult depression as being the result of multiple possible vulnerabilities of which a dysfunctional self-schema is most influential. This self-schema consists of pathognomonic systematic cognitive distortions which are the result of dysfunctional parental rearing practices and can be characterized as the individual's assumption that he/she has no control over significant events which can greatly affect him/her.

The formation of a self schema as the result of parent-child interactions and the stability of such self schemata into adult life have been reported upon in the literature on normal development. Some developmental theorists, such as Sroufe and Fleeson (1986), or ethologists, such as Hinde (1979), believe that relationships should be used as the unit of scientific analysis of behavior. Sroufe and Fleeson (1986), conceive of the individual's relationships as coherent wholes that may not be reduced to the characteristics of interacting members in isolation. They contend that relationships exhibit continuity and stability across time and contexts, with relational behavior in one time context predicting relational behavior years later. For example, a mother's care giving behavior with a 6-month-old infant can predict her care giving behavior with a subsequent child three years later. In addition, Sroufe and Fleeson maintain that relationships can be internalized by individuals and form inner representations that guide subsequent behaviors. Therefore, an individual not only learns his or her own expected behaviors, but also anticipates the behaviors of others in the relational system. These automatic expectations of the self and others which approximated closely Perris' concept of self schema, are carried forward in time through the developmental process and greatly influence the selection and response to later social experiences. Sroufe and Fleeson propose that through the internal perpetuation of relationships, others are selected, responded to and influenced in a manner congruent with previous relationship learning. The expectation of self and others in a relational system can generate the myriad behavior reactions seen in everyday life. These expectations may result in both the construction of external circumstances and the internal coping reactions of the individual.

The links between childhood maltreatment, as well as other factors, and adult depression could be conceptualized as a multistrand continuum, as represented in Figure 1, adapted from Richman and Flaherty's (1985) paradigm of social causation of illness in a life cycle perspective. From this model, it can be seen that a variety of aberrant childhood experiences can result in an equally dysfunctional self schema and an external limitation of choices in the normal pursuit of a more satisfactory adult life. As these limitations consolidate during the progression out of childhood, the vulnerability to depression is manifested as a marginal psychological adjustment which may continue, as such, or evolve into a clinical episode if provoked by a stressor. Neither the establishment of dysfunctional self schemata nor the limitation in external social supports need ultimately doom the individual. According to this view of vulnerability, compensatory experiences (such as marriage to a caring spouse, the development of a rewarding interest or career) may offset the vulnerability and result in greater resilience to stress.[1] These circumstances probably account for some of the non-depressed subjects who reported childhood maltreatment.

(C) Specificity of Childhood Experience

The types of childhood experiences recalled by depressed individuals suggest the shaping of a specific and chronic personality type that is repeatedly vulnerable to depressive episodes. The consideration of premorbid personality variables as important in depression is supported by research indicating that this illness involves more than a single episode in the life of an affected individual. Akiskal (1982) and Clayton (1985) found that depression is most commonly an episodic disorder with residual as well as pre-episode pathology. Keller and Shapiro (1982) report that 40% of those who suffer a major

---

[1] In this regard, it is of interest that Hooley, Orley and Teasdale(1986) found a 59% relapse rate within one year for depressives who lived with a critical spouse and a zero relapse rate for depressives with an emotionally supportive non-critical spouse.

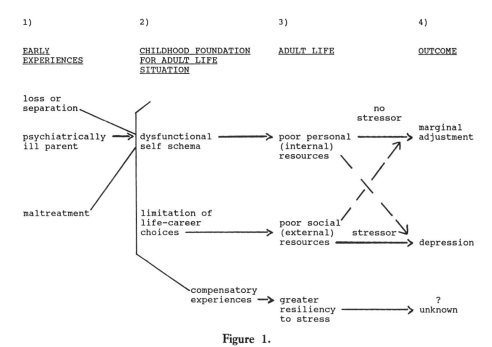

Figure 1.

depressive episode suffer from a more enduring chronic dysthymia. In addition, personality malfunctioning is so common in depressed individuals that there is some impetus to create a diagnostic category of Depressive Personality Disorder (Phillips, Gunderson, & Hirschfeld, 1990). The vulnerability to depression may reside in pre-morbid personality patterns that render the individual helpless and hopeless in the face of some significant deprivation or frustration. This adult characteristic may be derived from the *specific* types of childhood experience reported in retrospective studies which emphasize childhood overprotection and lack of care. Overprotection could produce the perpetuation of atavistic dependency needs and a lack of autonomy necessary to overcome adverse experiences. Lack of care could produce a low sense of personal self worth and the belief that others or the environment have little to offer. Such experiences would lead naturally to distorted perceptions of oneself and of others as well as to a paucity of adaptive mechanisms which would allow for the substitution of narcissistic supplies following a major loss or disappointment. The difficulties of depressives in believing they can continue satisfactory relationships as described by Bowlby and the findings of "affectionless control" in retrospective studies may be linked conceptually to empirical investigations on the vicissitudes of parent-child attachment. Cummings and Cicchetti (1990) propose that insecure attachment found in children of psychologically unavailable parents may result in a vulnerability to later depression. The lack of security in attachment to parental figures is perpetuated as an internalized and autonomous insecurity regarding all future intimate relationships, affecting expectations from others and crystalizing in depressogenic modes of processing everyday experience. The observable mode of attachment which can be measured in the young child is assumed to correspond to internal psychological schemas regarding expectations of others and of oneself. Insecure or anxious attachment behavior in the young child may be the forerunner of other means of expressing low self-regard or negative expectations that are more developmentally appropriate to adults. This observable and measurable behavior could be further investigated as to its correlation with later negative expectation of self and others and therefore as a precursor of adult depression.

Overprotection and lack of care have been identified as important childhood experiences in increasing the vulnerability to later affective disorders. The correlation of particular childhood experience with adult disorders has been found in regard to other psychiatric entities, indicating the specificity of certain childhood experience for certain adult disorders. Adults with multiple personality or borderline disorder have been found to have a history of repeated sexual abuse (Herman, Perry, & VanderKolk, 1989) Severe adolescent delinquents seem to have never experienced a long lasting emotional bond with an adult (Rutter, 1979). Therefore, not only do aberrant childhood experiences appear to predict later disorders, but also specific experiences may predict specific disorders.

Conclusion

The seventeen studies reviewed largely support the role of childhood maltreatment as a precursor of adult depression. While subject to all the difficulties implicit in retrospective investigations, the relative uniformity of results strongly suggests that there is validity in these findings. Therefore, childhood experience appear to comprise one aspect of the vulnerability to later affective disorders.

These studies are also of interest in defining further aspects of depression from the framework of developmental psychopathology. For example, childhood bereavement which has been correlated inconsistently with adult depression may become a vulnerability factor when it leads to post loss maltreatment. Furthermore, these studies indicate that specific forms of childhood maltreatment, such as affectionless control, are predictive of depression just as other particular dysfunctional childhoods seem to lead to discrete adult disorders, suggesting a specificity in the development of psychopathology. The developmental link between the aforementioned childhood maltreatment and later depression has been described as the creation of a certain self schema, which includes expectations from one self and from significant others. This self schema may persist in the form of helplessness and hopelessness in reaction to negative life events or may contribute to constraining external circumstances, such as premature parenthood, which contribute to the vulnerability to depression. Such self schemas are formed in the context of early relationships and are believed to shape the nature of future relationships. The early introduction of healthier relationships might do much to alter the formation of dysfunctional attitudes toward the self and others and thus eliminate one precursor to adult depression. It is speculated that the observable behavior of anxious attachment parallels and predicts the creation of depressogenic self schemas and thus could serve as a means of identifying children in need of intervention.

REFERENCES

Abraham, K. (1927). A Short Study of the Development of the Libido. In *Selected Papers on Psychoanalysis*, London: Hogarth Press, 418–502.

Abrahams, M.J. & Whitlock, F.A. (1969). Childhood experience and depression. *Brit. J. Psychiat.*, Vol. 115, 883–888.

Abramson, L.Y., Seligman, M., & Teasdale, J. (1978). Learned helplessness in humans: critique and reformulation. *J. of Abnormal Psychology*, Vol. 87, 32–48.

Akiskal, M.S. (1982) Factors associated with incomplete recovery in primary depressive illness. *J. of Clinical Psychiatry*, Vol. 43, 266–271.

Alnaes, R. & Torgersen, S. (1989). Characteristics of patients with major depression in combination with dysthymic or cyclothymic disorders. *Acta Psychiatr. Scand.*, Vol. 79, 11–18.

Arieti, S. & Bemporad, J.R. (1978). *Severe and Mild Depression*. New York: Basic Books.

Beck, A.T. (1976). *Cognitive therapy and the emotional disorders*. New York: International Universities Press.

Becker, W.C. (1964). Consequences of different kinds of parental discipline. In M.L. Hoffman & L.W. Hoffman (eds.) *Review of Child Development Research*. New York: Russell Sage, 169–208..

Bifulco, A., Brown, G., & Harris, T. (1987). Childhood loss of parent, lack of adequate parental care and adult depression: a replication. *J. of Affective Disorders*, Vol. 12, 115–128.

Blatt, S.J., Wein, S.J., Chevron, E., & Quinlan, D.M. (1979). Parental representations and depression in normal young adults. *J. of Abnormal Psychology*, Vol. 88 (4), 388–397.

Bowlby, J. (1980). *Loss*. New York: Basic Books.

Brown, G.W., & Harris, T. (1978). *Social Origins of Depression: A study of psychiatric disorder in women*. London: Tavistock.

Brown, G.W., Harris, T.O., & Bifulco, A. (1986). "Long-Term effects of early loss of parent". In M. Rutter, C. E.Izard & P.B. Read (eds.) *Depression in Young People*, New York: The Guilford Press, 251–296.

Cadoret, R.J., O'Gorman, T.W., Heywood, E., & Troughton, E. (1985). Genetic and environmental factors in major depression. *J. of Affective Disorders*, Vol. 9, 155–164.

Cicchetti, D. (1984). The Emergence of developmental Psychopathology. *Child Development*, 55:1–7.

Clayton, P.J. (1983). The prevelance and course of the affective disorders. In J.M. Davis & J.W. Maas (eds.) *The Affective Disorders*. Washington: American Psychiatric Press, 193–201.

Crook, T., & Raskin, A. (1981). Parent-child relationships and adult depression. *Child Development*, Vol. 52, 950–957.

Cummings, E.M. & Cicchetti, D. (1990). Toward a transactional model of relations between attachment and depression. In M. Greenberg, D. Cicchetti, & E.M. Cummings (eds.) *Attachment in the Preschool Years: Theory, Research and Intervention*, Chicago: University of Chicago Press, 339–372.

Dunner, D.L. (1982). High risk studies in affective disorders. In E. Usdin & I. Hanin (eds.) *Biological markers in psychiatry and neurology*. Oxford: Pergamon Press, 3–11.

Erickson, M.F. (1991). How often do abused children become child abusers? *Harvard Medical School Mental Health Letter*. Vol. 8, 8.

Finkelstein, H. (1988). The Long term effects of early parent death: a review. *J. of Clinical Psychology*, 44:3–9.

Freud, S. (1957). Mourning and melancholia. Standard Edition. London: Hogarth Press, 14: 293–358.

Gaszner, P., Perris, C., Eisemann, M., & Perris, H. (1988). The early family situation of Hungarian depressed patients. *Acta Psychiatr. Scand.*, Vol. 78: (343), 111–114.

Gorayeb, R. (1987) Child rearing patterns in Brazil. *Acta Psychiatr. Scand.*, Vol. 78 (344), 147–149.

Hallstrom, T. (1987). Major depression, parental mental disorder and early family relationships. *Acta Psychiatr. Scand.*, Vol. 75, 259–263.

Harris, T., Brown, G., & Bifulco, A. (1991). Loss of parent in childhood and adult psychiatric disorder: a tentative overall model. *Development and Psychopathology*, 2: 311–327.

Herman, J.L., Perry, J.C., & Van der Kolk, B. (1989). Childhood trauma in borderline personality disorder. *American J. of Psychiatry*, 146: 490–495.

Hinde, R.A. (1979). *Toward understanding relationships*. London: Academic Press.

Hooley, J., Orley, J., & Teasdale, J. (1986). Levels of expressed emotion and relapse in depressed patients. *British J. of Psychiatry*, 148: 642–647.

Jacobson, S., Fasman, J., & DiMascio, A. (1975). Deprivation in the childhood of depressed women. *J. of Nervous Mental Disease*, Vol. 160 (1), 5–14.

Kaufman, J. (1991). Depressive disorders in maltreated children. *J. Am. Acad. Child Adolesc. Psychiatry*, 30: 2, 257–265.

Kazdin, A.E., Moser, J., Colbus, D., & Bell, R. (1985). Depressive symptoms among physically abused and psychiatrically depressed children. *J. Abnormal Psychology* 94, No. 3, 298–307.

Keller, M.D., & Shapiro, R.W. (1982). "Double depression": Superimposition of acute depressive episodes on chronic depressive disorders. *American J. of Psychiatry*, 139: 438–442.

Levy, D. (1943). *Maternal Overprotection*. New York: Columbia University Press.

Mendelson, M. (1979). *Psychoanalytic concepts of depression* (2nd ed.), New York: Spectrum.

Parker, G. (1979). Parental characteristics in relation to depressive disorders. *Brit. J. Psychiat.*, Vol. 134, 138–147.

Parker, G. (1980). Vulnerability factors to normal depression. *J. of Psychosomatic Res.*, Vol. 24, 67–74.

Parker, G. (1981). Parental reports of depressives: An investigation of several explanations. *J. of Affective Disorders*, Vol. 3, 131–140.

Parker, G. (1982). Parental representations and affective symptoms: Examination for an hereditary link. *British J. of Med. Psychology*, Vol. 55, 57–61.

Parker, G. (1983). *Parental Overprotection*. New York: Grune & Stratton.

Parker, G., Kiloh, L., & Hayward, L. (1987). Parental representations of neurotic and endogenous depressives. *J. of Affective Disorders*, Vol. 13, 75–82.

Parker, G., & Lipscombe, P. (1981). Influences on maternal overprotection. *Brit. J. Psychiat.*, Vol. 138, 303–311.

Parker, G., Tupling, H., & Brown, L.B. (1979). A parental bonding instrument. *Brit. J. of Med. Psychology*, 52: 1–10.

Paykel, E.S. (1979). Recent life events in the development of the depressive disorders. In R.A. Depue (ed.) *The Psychobiology of the depressive disorders*. New York: Academic Press, 245–262.

Perris, C. (1988). A theoretical framework for linking the experience of sysfunctional parental rearing attitudes with manifest psychopatholgy. *Acta Psychiatr. Scand.*, 78 (supp): 93–109.

Perris, C., Arrindell, W.A., & Perris, H. et al. (1986). Perceived depriving parental rearing and depression. *Brit. J. of Psychiatry*, Vol. 148, 170–175.

Perris, C., Jacobson, L., Lindstrom, H., VonKnorring, L., & Perris, H. (1980). Development of a new inventory for assessing memories of parental rearing behavior. *Acta Psychiatr. Scand.*, 61: 265–274.

Perris, C., Maj, M., Perris, H., & Eisemann, M. (1985). Perceived parental rearing behavior in unipolar and bipolar depressed patients: A verification study in an Italian sample. *Acta Psychiatr. Scand.*, Vol. 72, 172–175.

Phillips, K.A., Gunderson, J.G., & Hirschfeld, R.M.A. (1990). A review of the depressive personality. *Amer. J. of Psychiatry*, 147: 830–837.

Raskin, A., Boothe, H.H., Reatig, N.A., & Schulterbrandt, J.G. (1971). Factor analyses of normal and depressed patients' memories of parental behavior. *Psychological* Vol. 29, 871–879.

Renson, G.J., Schaeffer, E.S., & Levy, B.I. (1968). Cross-national validity of a spherical conceptual model for parent behavior. *Child Development*, 39: 1229–1235.

Richman, J.A., & Flaherty, J.A. (1985). Stress, coping resources and psychiatric disorders: alternate paradigms from a life cycle perspective. *Comprehensive Psychiatry*, 26: 456–465.

Rutter, M. (1979). Maternal deprivation, 1972–1978: new findings, new concepts, new approaches. *Child Development*, 50: 283–305.

Rutter, M. (1986). The Developmental psychopathology of depression: Issues and perspectives. In M. Rutter, C.E. Izard, and P.F. Read (eds.) *Depression in young people*. New York: Guilford Press, 3–30.

Schaefer, E.S. (1965). Children's reports of parental behavior: An inventory. *Child Development*, Vol. 36, 413–424.

Schaefer, E.S. (1965). A Configurational analysis of Children's reports of parent behavior. *J. of Consulting Psychology*, Vol. 29 (6), 552–557.

Sroufe, L.A., & Fleeson, J.C. (1986). Attachment and the construction of relationships. In W. Hartup & Z. Rubin (eds.). *Relationships and Development*. Hillsdale, New Jersey: Erlbaum, 51–71.

Sroufe, L.A., & Rutter, M. (1984). The Domain of developmental psychopathology. *Child Development*, 55: 17–29.

Stodgill, R.M. (1937). Survey of experiments of children's attitudes toward parents: 1894–1936. *J. of Genetic Psychology*, 51: 293–303.

Walker, E., Downey, G., & Bergman, A. (1989). The effects of parental psychopathology and maltreatment on child behavior: a test of the Diathesis-Stress model. *Child Development* 60: 15–24.

Index of Authors

Index of Subjects